Nancy Clark's
SPORTS NUTRITION
Guidebook

SIXTH EDITION

Nancy Clark, MS, RD, CSSD
Sports Nutrition Services, LLC
Newton, MA

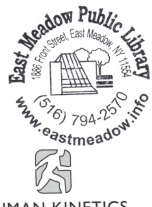

HUMAN KINETICS

Library of Congress Cataloging-in-Publication Data

Names: Clark, Nancy, 1951- author.
Title: Nancy Clark's sports nutrition guidebook / Nancy Clark, MS, RD, CSSD.
Description: Sixth edition. | Newton, MA : Sports Nutrition Services, LLC,
  2020. | Includes bibliographical references and index.
Identifiers: LCCN 2019009410 (print) | LCCN 2019013919 (ebook) | ISBN
  9781492591580 (epub) | ISBN 9781492591597 (PDF) | ISBN 9781492591573
  (print)
Subjects: LCSH: Athletes--Nutrition. | Cooking. | LCGFT: Cookbooks.
Classification: LCC TX361.A8 (ebook) | LCC TX361.A8 C54 2020 (print) | DDC
  613.7/11--dc23
LC record available at https://lccn.loc.gov/2019009410

ISBN: 978-1-4925-9157-3 (print)

Managing Editors: Dominique J. Moore, Miranda Baur, Anne E. Mrozek; **Copyeditor:** Annette Pierce; **Indexer:** Nancy Ball; **Permissions Manager:** Dalene Reeder; **Senior Graphic Designer:** Joe Buck; **Graphic Designer:** Dawn Sills; **Cover Designer:** Keri Evans; **Cover Design Associate:** Susan Rothermel Allen; **Senior Art Manager:** Kelly Hendren; **Illustrations:** © Human Kinetics, unless otherwise noted; **Printer:** Kingery Printing – United Graphics Division

Human Kinetics books are available at special discounts for bulk purchase. Special editions or book excerpts can also be created to specification. For details, contact the Special Sales Manager at Human Kinetics.

Printed in the United States of America   10 9 8 7 6 5 4 3 2

The paper in this book is certified under a sustainable forestry program.

Human Kinetics
1607 N. Market Street
Champaign, IL 61820
USA

United States and International
Website: **US.HumanKinetics.com**
Email: info@hkusa.com
Phone: 1-800-747-4457

Canada
Website: **Canada.HumanKinetics.com**
Email: info@hkcanada.com

Tell us what you think!
Human Kinetics would love to hear what we can do to improve the customer experience. Use this QR code to take our brief survey.

With appreciation for their love and support,
I dedicate this sixth edition to my husband, John,
and to our children, Mary and John Michael. They
warm my heart, nourish my soul, and balance my life.

CONTENTS

Preface   vii

Acknowledgments   ix

PART I   Everyday Eating for Active People

1 Building a High-Energy Eating Plan   3

2 Eating to Stay Healthy for the Long Run   35

3 Breakfast: The Key to a Successful Sports Diet   61

4 Lunch and Dinner: At Home, on the Run,
      and on the Road   79

5 Between Meals: Snacking for Health
      and Sustained Energy   99

6 Carbohydrate: Simplifying a Complex Topic   111

7 Protein: Building and Repairing Muscles   139

8 Fluids: Replacing Sweat Losses
      to Maintain Performance   161

PART II   The Science of Eating and Exercise

9 Fueling Before Exercise   183

10 Fueling During and After Exercise   201

11 Supplements, Performance Enhancers,
      and Engineered Sports Foods   219

12 Nutrition and Active Women   239

13 Athlete-Specific Nutrition Advice   253

PART III   Balancing Weight and Activity

14 Assessing Your Body: Fat, Fit, or Fine?   275
15 Gaining Weight the Healthy Way   295
16 Losing Weight Without Starving   311
17 Dieting Gone Awry: Eating Disorders
        and Food Obsessions   335

PART IV   Winning Recipes for Peak Performance

18 Breads and Breakfasts   359
19 Pasta, Rice, and Potatoes   375
20 Vegetables and Salads   393
21 Chicken and Turkey   403
22 Fish and Seafood   419
23 Beef and Pork   429
24 Beans and Tofu   437
25 Beverages and Smoothies   453
26 Snacks and Desserts   463

Appendix A: For More Information   479
Appendix B: Selected References   497
Index   515
About the Author   525

PREFACE

We all want to be healthy and enjoy high energy; it's much more fun than the alternative. According to this Instagram post, eating well for health, energy and weight management is simple:

> *Just eat five small meals a day. But eat only lunch and dinner. Eat lots of protein and lift weights. But don't eat too much protein; it might hurt your kidneys. Don't do any cardio; it's bad for your joints. Make sure you are sleeping a lot, but don't be sedentary. And don't be too active. Make sure you replace all of your lost salt. But never eat too much sodium. Just eat vegetables. Don't eat potatoes, though, or corn. Fruit is good for you but it's all sugar. Sugar is bad for you. Oh, I forgot to mention, sugar is a vital source of quick-burning carbohydrate that your brain needs to survive. But you should avoid it at all costs.*

Huh??? Eating well is not so simple, is it?

This commentary highlights the confusion that abounds, largely due to today's abundance of nutrition information. I repeatedly hear from Internet-surfing casual exercisers and competitive athletes they feel more confused than ever about what and when to eat; how to fuel before, during, and after exercise; and how to choose the best sports foods.

Whether you are a Millennial or a Baby Boomer, you don't want nutrition to be your missing link. Yet, if you get caught up in trendiness, you can fail to eat well, fail to get the most out of your workouts, and fail to feel good about your bodies and your eating patterns. My hope is the sensible information in *Nancy Clark's Sports Nutrition Guidebook, Sixth Edition,* clarifies your confusion about how much carbohydrate, protein, and fat you should consume and teaches you how to enjoy a variety of tasty, nutrient-rich foods that can give you the winning edge. You'll learn the latest information about the topics that confuse active people:

- How to schedule preexercise eating so you don't run out of gas during workouts (or the workday, for that matter!)
- How to lose undesired body fat and have energy to exercise
- How to choose the right balance of carbohydrate to fuel your muscles and protein to build your muscles including sample menus and suggestions

- How to consume enough protein at meals, even if you are a vegetarian
- How to choose health-protective foods
- How to assemble meals with minimal effort and clean-up
- How to tame the cookie monster
- How to eat greener

If your goal is to move to the next level of performance and health, the science-based, up-to-date information in this book can help you get there. You'll find answers to your questions about the Paleo Diet, Keto Diet, gluten-free foods, energy drinks, commercial sports foods, muscle cramps, organic foods, hyponatremia, amenorrhea, and recovery foods as well as tips on how to apply this information to your busy lifestyle.

As you navigate your way through today's confusing web of nutrition advice, I invite you to enjoy this sixth edition as a resource that offers a sustainable approach to finding success with food and weight. I use the word *sustainable* because too many trendy diets are not easily sustainable for the long term. They commonly end up creating "diet backlash," including sub-optimal athletic performance, binge eating, guilt, weight gain, and depression. This *Sports Nutrition Guidebook* will help you embrace a healthy eating pattern that fits your lifestyle, fuels your muscles and your brain, and also nourishes your soul. Your job is to be responsible, use the information in this book to show up for winning meals and sports snacks, and enjoy the success that comes with having high energy. Why be just a good athlete when you can be great?

With best wishes for a yummy journey,
Nancy Clark, MS, RD, CSSD
Sports Nutrition Services, LLC
P.O. Box 650124
Newton, MA 02465
www.nancyclarkrd.com

ACKNOWLEDGMENTS

With sincere thanks to my husband, John, and our (now adult) children Mary and John Michael. Without their love and support, I would lack the purpose, meaning, and balance that energizes my life. I'm grateful that Mary and JM now teach me the food ways of Millennials, as well as offer valuable technical support.

With gratitude to my clients, who educate me as much as I try to educate them. I feel honored they entrust me with their food, weight, and nutrition concerns. Throughout this book, I have shared their stories but have changed their names and occupations to protect their privacy.

I am very appreciative of the dietitians who contributed so many yummy recipes. I am also honored by and grateful for all the dietitians who have supported my work throughout the years. So many of them have recommended the first five editions of this book, and they have helped it to thrive. Thank you one and all.

I acknowledge the recipe testers, primarily my husband and our neighbors, Joan and Rex Hawley. My kids managed to escape most of the testing this time around, given the nest is now empty, but they have paid their dues in past editions. Instead, our English Setter, Charlie Brown, earns recognition for his "help" with recipe testing, and constant companionship, both when I was cooking and writing. A faithful buddy, for certain!

I'm grateful for my soul-mates in this marathon called life, Jean Smith and Catherine Farrell. They are forever supportive, adding friendship to life's menu.

And last but not least, a big thank you to the staff at Human Kinetics for their support of this book since 1990. This includes Jason Muzinic, Dominique Moore, Susan Outlaw, Joe Buck, and Keri Evans.

PART I

EVERYDAY EATING FOR ACTIVE PEOPLE

CHAPTER 1

BUILDING A HIGH-ENERGY EATING PLAN

I'm so confused by the overwhelming amount of nutrition information that is available on the Internet, in the news, and from my friends. I want to eat well so I have energy to exercise well, but I don't know what to eat anymore. Help!

—*Joshua*

If you are like Joshua (and the majority of my clients), you know that food is important for fueling the body and investing in overall health, but you feel confused about what's best to eat—and when to eat it. Student athletes, sports parents, casual exercisers, fitness fanatics, and competitive athletes alike repeatedly express their frustrations about trying to choose high-quality diets. Long work hours, attempts to lose weight, and time spent exercising can all contribute even more to food becoming a source of stress rather than one of life's pleasures. Given today's good food–bad food culture, eating well has become more confusing than ever.

In this chapter, you'll learn how to eat well and fuel your body appropriately all day long, even if you have a busy lifestyle. Whether you work out at the health club, compete with a varsity team, aspire to be an Olympian, or simply actively play with your kids, you can nourish yourself with a nutrient-dense diet that supports good health and high energy, even if you are grabbing food to eat on the run.

In the upcoming chapters, I offer information on how to manage meals—breakfasts, lunches, dinners, and snacks—but in this chapter, I cover the day-to-day basics of how to build a winning, well-balanced sports diet. You'll learn how to eat more of the best foods, eat less of the rest, and create a food plan that results in high energy, good health, top performance, and weight management.

CREATE A WINNING FOOD PLAN

A fundamental key to eating well is to prevent yourself from getting too hungry. When people get too hungry, they tend to care less about the nutritional quality of the food they eat and more about grabbing whatever food is in sight. By evenly distributing your calories throughout the day, you can prevent hunger, curb your physiological desire to eat excessively, and tame your psychological desire to treat yourself with goodies. This is contrary to the standard pattern of skimping by day only to overindulge at night.

As you start to create your winning food plan, keep in mind these two key concepts:

1. Eat at least three, preferably four, and ideally five, different kinds of nutrient-dense food at meals. The government's food plate (www.ChooseMyPlate.gov) suggests five kinds of foods per meal: protein, grain, fruit, vegetable, and dairy/calcium-rich food (figure 1.1). The more types of foods you eat, the more vitamins, minerals, and other nutrients you consume.

Many of my clients eat a limited diet: oatmeal, oatmeal, oatmeal; apples, apples, apples; protein bars, protein bars, protein bars. Repetitive eating keeps life simple, minimizes decisions, and simplifies shopping, but it can result in an inadequate diet and chronic fatigue. Instead of repeatedly eating the same 10 to 15 foods each week, target 35 different types of foods

Go With Your Gut

When you eat, you are actually feeding your microbiome, the 100 trillion bacteria that live in your gut. This microbiome sends signals to your brain and affects your mood, immune system, and weight. Gut microbes thrive on fruits, vegetables, legumes, beans, and whole grains and are bolstered by fermented foods such as yogurt and kefir. Luckily, the same nutrient-dense diet that supports your gut health also enhances sports performance.

In contrast, nutrient-poor processed foods contribute to a less diverse microbiome, inflammation, and reduced health. Hence, as often as possible, choose minimally processed whole foods. For instance, choose bananas rather than commercial energy bars, and microwaved sweet potato rather than ramen noodles. These wholesome foods can sway your microbiome in a positive direction—away from chronic disease and toward lifelong health.

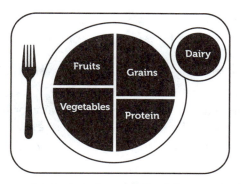

FIGURE 1.1 Does your plate look similar to MyPlate? If not, make the effort to include *at least three or four*—if not all five—of the food groups in each meal so that you will consume a healthy balance of vitamins, minerals, proteins, and carbohydrates.

USDA's Center for Nutrition Policy and Promotion.

per week. You can do this by eating not just bran flakes with milk and a banana for breakfast, but many different cereals topped with a variety of fruits and nuts; not just a plain turkey sandwich for lunch, but different types of breads with additional fillings, such as turkey on rye bread with low-fat cheese, avocado, and a side of baby carrots. Start counting!

2. Think moderation. Enjoy a foundation of healthy foods, but don't deprive yourself of enjoyable foods. Rather than categorize a food as being good or bad for your health, think about moderation, assess the entire day's menu, and aim for a diet that offers at least 85 to 90 percent nutrient-dense foods and, if desired, 10 to 15 percent fun foods with fewer nutritional merits. This way, even a cookie and some chocolate can fit into a nourishing diet; you just need to balance them with healthier choices during the majority of the day.

DON'T JUST EAT, EAT WELL

The fundamental key to building a healthy sports diet is to consume a variety of nutrient-dense foods from the five basic food groups (fruits, vegetables, grains, lean protein, and low-fat dairy (or calcium-rich) foods. To guide your food choices, the U.S. government offers updated nutrition recommendations every five years. The overarching concepts in the *2015-2020 Dietary Guidelines for Americans* are to develop healthy eating patterns that include a variety of nutrient-dense foods and maintain a healthy body weight. Although I will address these guidelines in more detail throughout this book, here is a summary of the foods you should emphasize in your daily diet:

- Eat more vegetables and fruits.
- Enjoy a variety of colorful vegetables, especially dark green, red, and orange vegetables.
- Replace refined grains with whole grains until at least half of all the grains you eat are whole.
- Increase your intake of fat-free or low-fat dairy (or soy) milk and milk products such as milk, yogurt, kefir, and cheese.
- Choose a variety of protein foods, which include beans, legumes, nuts, seeds, soy products, eggs, seafood, poultry, and lean meat.
- Include seafood twice a week by choosing fish in place of other animal protein.
- Replace protein foods that are higher in solid fat (such as greasy burgers and spareribs) with choices that are lower in solid fat and calories (such as chicken and eggs) or are sources of healthful oils (such as fish and nuts).
- Use oils (such as olive and canola) to replace solid fat (such as butter and stick margarine) where possible.
- Choose foods that provide more potassium, dietary fiber, calcium, and vitamin D, which are nutrients of concern in American diets. These foods include vegetables, fruits, whole grains, beans, legumes, and milk and milk products or alternatives.

The following information can help you not just eat, but also eat well— even if you are eating on the run and rarely cook meals at home.

Whole Grains and Starches

If you eat well, there is a "whole" in your diet—whole grains! Wholesome breads, cereals, and other grain foods are the foundation of a high-performance sports diet, as well as any diet, for that matter. Grains that are unrefined or only lightly processed are excellent sources of carbohydrate, fiber, and B vitamins. They fuel your muscles, protect against needless muscular fatigue, and reduce problems with constipation if they're fiber rich. And despite popular belief, the carbohydrate in grains is not fattening; excess calories are fattening. Excess calories often come from the various forms of fat (butter, mayonnaise, gravy) that accompany rolls, sandwich bread, potatoes, and other types of carbohydrate. If weight is an issue, I recommend that you limit the fat but enjoy fiber-rich breads, cereals, and other whole grains. These foods help curb hunger and assist with weight management. Wholesome forms of carbohydrate should be the foundation

Put a "Whole" in Your Diet

Whole grains offer hundreds of phytochemicals that play key roles in reducing the risk of heart disease, diabetes, and cancer. For a food to be called a whole grain, one of the following should be first in the ingredient list on the food label:

Amaranth	Sorghum
Brown rice	Triticale
Buckwheat	Whole-grain barley
Bulgur (cracked wheat)	Whole-grain corn
Farro	Whole oats or oatmeal
Millet	Whole rye
Popcorn	Whole wheat
Quinoa	Wild rice

Look for the word *whole* at or near the top of the ingredient list on the food label. Note that the word *wheat* on a label may not mean whole wheat, and a dark color might be from food coloring, so be sure to look for the word *whole*. Ideally, choose foods with at least 8 grams (a half serving) of whole grain per serving. Your daily goal is at least 48 grams of whole grain—three servings.

Note: The term *high fiber* does not equate to *whole grain*; high-fiber foods may contain just the bran layer of the grain, not the germ and endosperm that comprise the whole grain.

of both a weight-management program and a sports diet. (See chapters 6 and 16 for more information on carbohydrate and weight.)

Grains account for about 25 percent of the calories consumed in the United States. Most Americans still consume more than half their grains in highly processed, refined foods (white bread, white rice, products made with white flour), and that does not support a healthy eating pattern. The refining process strips grains of their bran and germ, thereby removing fiber, antioxidants, minerals, and other health-protective compounds. People who habitually eat diets based on refined grains tend to have a higher incidence of chronic diseases, such as adult-onset diabetes and heart disease. That said, the *2015-2020 Dietary Guidelines for Americans* state that *at least half of grains should be whole*. The Dietary Guidelines Committee's choice of "at least half" rather than 100 percent does not represent a compromised position, because enriched and fortified grains also play an important role in providing nutrients of concern, including folic acid (to prevent birth defects) and iron (to prevent anemia). Refined grains can certainly be included in a balanced diet.

How Much Is Enough?

To get adequate carbohydrate to fully fuel your muscles, you need to consume carbohydrate as the foundation of each meal. You can do this by eating at least 200 calories of grain foods per meal—such as one bowl of cereal, two slices of bread, or one cup of rice. This is not much for hungry exercisers who require 600 to 900 calories per meal. Most active people commonly need to eat (and should eat) double or even triple the standard servings listed on the labels of cereal and pasta boxes.

Top Choices

If refined white grains (white flour, bread, rice, pasta) dominate your grain choices, here are tips to boost your intake of whole grains. And whatever you do, don't try to stay away from grains, thinking they are fattening. That is not the case.

• **Whole-grain cereals.** Wheaties, Cheerios, Total, Kashi, and Shredded Wheat are examples of cereals with the words *whole grain* on the cereal box or in the list of ingredients.

• **Oatmeal.** When cooked into a tasty hot cereal, soaked overnight in milk, or eaten raw as in muesli, oatmeal makes a wonderful breakfast that helps lower cholesterol and protect against heart disease. Some people even keep microwavable packets of instant oatmeal in their desk drawers for cozy afternoon snacks. Oatmeal (instant and regular) is a whole-grain food with slow-to-digest carbohydrate that offers sustained energy and is perfect for a preexercise snack.

• **Whole-grain breads.** Select the hearty brands that have whole wheat, rye, or oatmeal listed as the first ingredient. Keep sliced bread in the freezer so that you have a fresh supply on hand for toast, sandwiches, or snacks. When at the sandwich shop, request the turkey with tomato on dark rye.

• **Whole-grain and graham crackers.** These low-fat munchies are a perfect high-carbohydrate snack for your sports diet. Be sure to choose wholesome brands of crackers with low fat content, not the ones that leave you with greasy fingers. Look for brown rice cakes, Ak-Mak, Dr. Kracker,

---

FACT OR FICTION

Quinoa is a superior whole grain.

The facts: Quinoa (which is actually a seed, although we eat it as a grain) is touted as being a superior grain because it offers more protein than other grains. But 200 calories (1/3 cup when uncooked) of quinoa provides only 8 grams of protein; pasta offers 7 grams, and rice offers 4. None are what I call protein powerhouses. Be sure to balance the meal by combining quinoa with tofu, beans, or yogurt to reach the target of 20 to 30 grams of protein per meal. Quinoa is also expensive: $8 per pound ($18/kg), as compared to brown rice at $1.50 per pound ($3.30/kg). But it is quick cooking (less than 15 minutes), versatile, and a wholesome addition to any meal.

Finn Crisp, RyKrisp, Triscuit Thin Crisps, Wasa, and Mary's Gone Crackers (among others). Enjoy graham crackers topped with peanut butter for a yummy snack.

- **Popcorn.** Whether popped in air or in a little canola oil, popcorn is a fun way to boost your whole-grain intake. The trick is to avoid smothering it in butter or salt. How about sprinkling it with Mexican or Italian seasonings or a seasoned popcorn spray?

Against the Grain?

You may need to stay away from wheat because you have celiac disease, are gluten intolerant, or simply choose to limit your intake of wheat for personal reasons. With careful planning, you can still consume an excellent sports diet. Please refer to chapter 6 for more information about how to plan a wheat-free, gluten-free sports diet.

Vegetables

Vegetables, like fruits, contribute important carbohydrate to the foundation of your sports diet. Vegetables (and fruits) are what I call nature's vitamin pills because they are excellent sources of vitamin C, beta-carotene (the plant form of vitamin A), potassium, magnesium, and many other vitamins, minerals, and health-protective substances. In general, vegetables offer slightly more nutritional value than fruits. Hence, if you don't eat much fruit, you can compensate by eating more veggies. You'll get similar vitamins and minerals, if not more.

How Much Is Enough?

The recommended intake is at least 2 1/2 cups of vegetables (about 400 g) per day (preferably more). Many busy people rarely eat that much in a week. If you are a vegetable minimalist, the trick is to eat large portions when you do eat vegetables—a big pile rather than a standard serving—and that can equate to 2 1/2 cups in one sitting. Then, to really invest in your health, try to do that twice a day, such as eating a big colorful salad with lunch and a bunch of broccoli with dinner. The food industry is working hard to make eating vegetables as easy as opening a bag of leafy greens, baby carrots, peeled and cubed butternut squash—or frozen bags of broccoli that you can simply toss into the microwave oven.

Top Choices

Any vegetable is good for you. Of course, vegetables fresh from the garden are best, but they are often difficult to obtain. Frozen vegetables are a good second choice; freezing retains the nutritional value. Canned vegetables are also a good choice; rinsing them with plain water can reduce their higher sodium levels. Because canned vegetables are processed quickly, they retain many of their nutrients. Overcooking is a prime nutrient destroyer, so cook fresh or frozen vegetables only until they are tender-crisp, preferably in a microwave oven, steamer, or wok. Heat canned vegetables just until warm; there's no need to boil them.

Dark, colorful vegetables usually have more nutritional value than paler ones. If you are struggling to improve your diet, boost your intake of colorful broccoli, spinach, peppers, tomatoes, carrots, and winter squash. They are more nutrient dense than pale lettuces, cucumbers, zucchini, onions, and celery. (In no way are these pale vegetables bad for you; the colorful ones are just more nutrient dense, giving you more vitamins and minerals per calorie.) Here's the scoop on a few of the top vegetable choices.

FACT OR FICTION

White foods are nutritionally worthless.

The facts: Some white foods are fantastic sources of nutrients—including bananas, cauliflower, onions, and parsnips. Egg whites are protein rich, as are white beans and white yogurt. White bread and other foods made from refined white flour are less nutrient dense, but they can also be balanced into an overall healthy sports diet, particularly if they are enriched with B vitamins and iron.

• **Broccoli, spinach, and peppers (green, red, or yellow).** These low-fat, potassium-rich vegetables are loaded with vitamin C and the health-protective carotenes that are the precursors of vitamin A. One medium stalk (1 cup) of steamed broccoli offers a full day's worth of vitamin C, as does half a large pepper. I enjoy munching on a pepper instead of an apple for a snack; it offers more vitamins and potassium and fewer calories. What a nutrition bargain!

• **Tomatoes and tomato sauce.** In salads or on pasta or pizza, tomato products are another easy way to boost your veggie intake. They are good sources of potassium, fiber, and vitamin C (one medium-size tomato provides half the vitamin C you need each day); carotenes; and lycopene, a phytochemical that might protect against certain cancers. Tomato juice and other vegetable juices are additional suggestions for fast-laners who lack the time to cook or an interest in cooking. They can enjoyably drink their veggies! Commercial tomato products tend to be high in sodium, so people with high blood pressure should limit their intake or choose the low-sodium brands. Some "salty sweaters," however, welcome tomato or V8 juice after a hard workout; the sodium helps replace the sodium lost in sweat (see chapter 8).

What If I Don't Like Kale?

Although kale is nutrient dense, it is not the only nourishing green vegetable. Table 1.1 shows how other vegetables compare (based on a 50-calorie cooked portion).

TABLE 1.1   Kale Versus Other Green Vegetables*

Green vegetable	Vitamin A (IU**)	Vitamin C (mg)	Calcium (mg)	Magnesium (mg)	Folate (mcg)
Kale 1 1/2 cup	1,318 (188%)	80 (106%)	140 (14%)	35 (11%)	25 (6%)
Spinach 1 1/4 cup	1,170 (167%)	22 (30%)	300 (30%)	195 (63%)	325 (82%)
Broccoli 1 1/2 cup	112 (16%)	95 (125%)	60 (6%)	30 (10%)	155 (40%)
Asparagus 1 1/4 cup	113 (16%)	17 (23%)	50 (5%)	32 (10%)	335 (83%)

*The number in parentheses refers to the percent of the recommended dietary allowance (RDA) provided by the vegetable.

**International units.

• **Cruciferous vegetables (members of the cabbage family).** Cabbage, broccoli, cauliflower, brussels sprouts, collards, kale, kohlrabi, turnips, and mustard greens may protect against cancer. Do your health a favor by regularly enjoying these choices. You can't go wrong eating piles of these.

If you are eating too few vegetables, be sure the ones you eat are among the best. The information in table 1.2 can guide your choices, as can the information in the salad section in chapter 4.

Fruits

Fruits add to the strong foundation of carbohydrate needed for your sports diet. Fruits are also rich in fiber, potassium, and many vitamins, especially vitamin C. The nutrients in fruits improve healing; aid in recovery after exercise; and reduce the risk of cancer, high blood pressure, and constipation.

How Much Is Enough?

The *Dietary Guidelines for Americans* recommend at least 2 cups of fruit or juice per day—this translates into only two standard pieces of fruit. The U.S. Centers for Disease Control and Prevention (CDC) encourages consuming even more to help prevent many of the diseases of aging. If you are a fruit minimalist, I recommend that you schedule it into your breakfast routine. Whip up a smoothie with pineapple juice, frozen berries, banana, and Greek yogurt, and then pour it into a travel mug. Enjoy a medium banana on your cereal plus a glass of orange juice. Either option will cover your baseline fruit requirement for the entire day, but do strive to consume more fruit throughout the day by eating raisins instead of an energy bar for a preexercise snack, snacking on apple slices with peanut butter, or tossing dried cranberries into your salad.

Top Choices

If daily fruit is not readily available—or if it spoils before you get around to eating it, the following tips will help you better balance your intake. Make the following fruit choices a top priority in your good nutrition game plan.

• **Citrus fruits and juices.** Whether as whole fruit or as fresh, frozen, or bottled juice, citrus fruits such as oranges, grapefruits, clementines, and tangerines surpass many other fruits or juices in vitamin C and potassium content.

If the hassle of peeling an orange or a grapefruit is a deterrent for you, just drink its juice. Any fruit is better than no fruit! Yes, the whole fruit has slightly more nutritional value, but given the option of a quick glass of

TABLE 1.2   Comparing Vegetables

Vegetable	Amount	Calories	Vitamin A (IU*)	Vitamin C (mg)	Potassium (mg)
Asparagus	8 spears cooked	25	1,200	9	270
Beets	1/2 cup boiled	35	30	3	260
Broccoli	1 cup cooked	55	2,415	100	455
Brussels sprouts	8 medium cooked	60	1,300	105	535
Cabbage, green	1 cup cooked	35	120	55	300
Carrot	1 medium raw	30	12,030	5	230
Cauliflower	1 cup cooked	30	15	55	175
Celery	One 7-inch (18 cm) stalk	5	180	2	105
Corn	1/2 cup frozen	60	130	5	145
Cucumber	1/3 medium	15	105	3	145
Green beans	1 cup cooked	45	875	10	180
Kale	1 cup cooked	35	17,700	55	300
Lettuce, iceberg	7 leaves	15	525	3	150
Lettuce, romaine	2 cups shredded	15	8,200	5	230
Mushrooms	1 cup raw pieces	20	0	0	315
Onion	1/2 cup chopped	30	2	5	115
Peas, green	1/2 cup cooked	65	640	10	215
Pepper, green	1 cup diced	30	550	120	260
Pepper, red	1 cup diced	45	4,665	190	315
Potato, baked	1 large with skin	260	30	30	1,500
Spinach	1 cup cooked	40	18,865	15	840
Squash, summer	1 cup cooked	35	380	10	345
Squash, winter	1 cup baked	75	10,700	20	500
Sweet potato	1 medium baked	100	21,900	25	540
Tomato	1 small raw	15	760	15	215
RECOMMENDED INTAKE					
Men:			>3,000	>90	>4,700
Women:			>2,310	>75	>4,700

*International units.

Data from USDA National Nutrient Database for Standard Reference.

juice or nothing, juice does the job. Just 8 ounces (240 ml) of orange juice provides carbohydrate to fuel your muscles, more than the daily reference intake of 75 milligrams of vitamin C; all the potassium you may have lost in an hour-long workout; and folic acid, a B vitamin needed for building protein and red blood cells. Choose the OJ with added calcium to give your bone health a boost.

• **Bananas.** This low-fat, high-potassium fruit is perfect for busy people, and it even comes in a biodegradable wrapper! Bananas are excellent for replacing sweat losses of potassium, an electrolyte (mineral) that also protects against high blood pressure. To boost your banana intake, add sliced banana to cereal, blend it into a smoothie, pack a banana in your lunch bag for a satisfying dessert (buy a banana saver to prevent it from getting squished), and keep bananas on hand for a quick and easy preexercise snack. My all-time favorite combination is banana with peanut butter, graham crackers, and a glass of low-fat milk—a well-balanced meal or snack that includes four kinds of foods (fruit, nuts, grain, dairy), with a nice foundation of carbohydrate (banana, crackers) plus protein (peanut butter, milk) for the accompaniment.

To prevent bananas from becoming overripe, store them in the refrigerator. The skin may turn black from the cold, but the fruit itself will be fine. Another trick is to keep (peeled) banana chunks in the freezer. They blend nicely with milk to make creamy smoothies. (See the recipes for fruit smoothies in chapter 25.)

Without a doubt, bananas are among the most popular sports snacks. I once saw a cyclist with two bananas safely taped to his helmet, ready to grab when he needed an energy boost.

• **Cantaloupe, kiwi, strawberries, and all other berries.** These nutrient-dense fruits are also good sources of vitamin C and potassium. Many of my clients keep berries and chunks of melon in the freezer, ready to be made into a smoothie for breakfast or a pre- or postworkout refresher.

• **Dried fruits.** Convenient and portable, dried fruits are rich in potassium and carbohydrate. They travel well; keep baggies of dried fruit and nuts (as in a trail mix) in your gym bag or car instead of yet another energy bar.

If you are eating too little fruit, be sure that the fruit you eat is nutritionally the best. The information in table 1.3 can guide your choices.

TABLE 1.3 Comparing Fruits

Fruit	Amount	Calories	Vitamin A (IU*)	Vitamin C (mg)	Potassium (mg)
Apple	1 medium	80	80	5	160
Apple juice	1 cup	115	2	2	250
Apricots	10 halved dried	85	1,260	1	400
Avocado	1 medium	240	215	15	710
Banana	1 medium	105	75	10	425
Blueberries	1 cup raw	85	80	15	115
Cantaloupe	1 cup pieces	60	6,000	65	475
Cherries	10 sweet	50	50	5	180
Cranberry juice	1 cup	140	20	110	35
Dates	5 dried	120	5	0	240
Figs	1 medium raw	35	70	1	115
Grapefruit	1/2 medium pink	50	1,415	40	165
Grapefruit juice	1 cup white	95	20	70	380
Grapes	1 cup	60	90	5	175
Honeydew melon	1 cup cubes	60	85	30	390
Kiwi	1 medium	45	60	65	215
Orange, navel	1 medium	70	350	83	230
Orange juice	1 cup fresh	110	500	125	500
Peach	1 medium	60	570	10	285
Pineapple	1 cup raw	80	95	80	180
Pineapple juice	1 cup	130	10	25	325
Prunes	5 dried	115	370	0	350
Raisins	1/3 cup	145	0	1	360
Strawberries	1 cup raw	50	20	90	235
Watermelon	1 cup	45	875	10	170
RECOMMENDED INTAKE					
Men:			>3,000	>90	>4,700
Women:			>2,310	>75	>4,700

*International units.

Data from USDA National Nutrient Database for Standard Reference.

The Nutrition Rainbow

Strive to eat a variety of colors of fruits and vegetables. Different colors offer different kinds of the health-protective phytochemicals that are linked to reducing the risk of cancer and heart disease (table 1.4).

TABLE 1.4 Fruits and Vegetables by Colors

Color	Fruits	Vegetables
Red	Strawberries, watermelon, cherries	Red peppers, tomatoes*
Orange	Mangos, peaches, cantaloupe	Carrots, sweet potato, pumpkin
Yellow	Pineapple, star fruit	Summer squash, corn
Green	Kiwi, grapes, honeydew melon, avocado	Peas, spinach, broccoli, kale
Blue or purple	Blueberries, grapes, prunes	Eggplant, beets
White	Banana, pear	Garlic, onion

*Technically, tomatoes are a fruit.

Here are tips for enjoying a more colorful diet. For breakfast, drink orange or pomegranate juice, add frozen blueberries to your cereal, or whip together a peach smoothie. For lunch, include a handful of baby carrots, crunch on peppers instead of pretzels, or choose a vegetable or tomato soup. For a snack, keep dried apricots or pineapple in your desk, or sip on V8 or carrot juice. For dinner, smother pasta with tomato sauce, order pizza with extra peppers or broccoli, or choose a Chinese stir-fry with extra veggies.

Dairy and Calcium-Rich Foods

Dairy foods such as milk, yogurt, and cheese are not only quick and easy sources of high-quality protein but also rich in vitamin D (if fortified) and calcium, a mineral that is particularly important not only for growing children and teens but also for women and men of all ages. A diet rich in calcium and vitamin D helps maintain strong bones, reduces the risk of osteoporosis, and protects against high blood pressure.

Dairy products are not the only natural sources of calcium, but they tend to be the most concentrated and convenient sources for people who

Eating Vegan to Save the Planet?

Some athletes choose plant-based foods and beverages as a way to help save the environment. Beef cattle and dairy cows (and other farm animals) produce methane, a greenhouse gas (GHG) that contributes to climate change. But the GHG emissions from animal agriculture comprises only 4 percent of global GHG emissions. (This number includes the carbon footprint of animals from birth to being consumed.) This is far less than the 28 percent from burning coal, oil, and natural gas (fossil fuels) to make electricity and the 28 percent of GHG emissions from transportation and the 22 percent from industry. If everyone were to eat a vegan diet every day, GHG emissions might drop by only 2.6 percent (although every little bit helps.) (Environmental Protection Agency 2016; White and Hall 2017).

If you are concerned about the environment, the biggest impact you can make is to reduce food waste. Up to 40 percent of the food we produce is wasted; 43 percent of that happens in our homes. Producing and transporting that wasted food to your supermarket (and landfill) needlessly consumes a lot of energy. Wasted food makes up 21 percent of all waste in U.S. landfills and, as it rots, creates GHG. To reduce food waste, shop carefully and use leftovers. Restaurants, college cafeterias, and other high-volume food producers need to figure out how to find meaningful homes for leftovers, such as by donating to food pantries.

eat on the run. If you prefer to limit your consumption of dairy products because you are lactose intolerant or are biased against dairy, you may have difficulty consuming the recommended intake of calcium from natural foods. For example, to absorb the same amount of calcium that you would obtain from one glass of milk, you'd need to consume either 3 cups of broccoli, 7 cups of spinach salad, 2 1/2 cups of white beans, 6 cups of pinto beans, 6 cups of sesame seeds, or 30 cups of unfortified soy milk. Calcium-fortified foods such as calcium-enriched soy milk, orange juice, almond "juice" (milk), other plant-based milk alternatives, and breakfast cereals such as Total can help you reach your calcium goals. Table 1.5 lists a few of the most common calcium sources and the amount of the source that provides a serving of calcium (300 mg). The table also provides the amount of vitamin D supplied by these sources.

TABLE 1.5 Calcium Equivalents

Calcium-rich foods	Amount needed for 300 mg calcium*	Vitamin D (IU**) Target intake = 400-600 IU
DAIRY SOURCES OF CALCIUM		
Milk, fortified	1 cup (240 ml)	100
Milk powder	1/3 cup dry (40 g)	90
Yogurt	8 oz (230 g)	0-115
Yogurt, Greek	9 oz (260 g)	0
Cheese, cheddar	1.5 oz (45 g)	10
Cottage cheese	2 cups	0
Frozen yogurt, soft serve	1 1/2 cups	10
Pizza, cheese	2 slices	0
Whey protein powder, EAS	6 scoops	0
PROTEIN-RICH SOURCES OF CALCIUM		
Soy milk, enriched	1 cup (240 ml)	40-120
Tofu	5 oz (150 g)	0
Salmon, canned with bones	4 oz (120 g)	440
Sardines, canned with bones	3 oz (90 g)	160-300
Almonds	3/4 cup (90 g)	0
Chia seeds	1/4 cup dry (120 g)	0
VEGETABLE SOURCES OF CALCIUM		
Broccoli, cooked	3 cups (500 g)	—
Collard or turnip greens, cooked	1 cup (200 g)	0
Kale or mustard greens, cooked	1 1/2 cups (200 g)	0
Bok choy	2 cups (240 g)	0
FOODS FORTIFIED WITH CALCIUM		
Total cereal	1 cup (30 g)	40-70
Orange juice, calcium and D enriched	1 cup (240 ml)	140
Almond milk	2/3 cup (160 ml)	0

*300 milligrams is considered one serving of dairy food.

**International units.

Data from USDA National Nutrient Database for Standard Reference (2011).

Milk: Does It Really Do a Body Good?

I'm sure you've heard antidairy people inform you that cows' milk is for calves, not humans, and is bad for health. Here are my thoughts:

• Each person has an individual response to milk (as well as all foods). Just as some people can't tolerate strawberries or fish, some people can't tolerate milk. If you experience bloating or a rumbly tummy after consuming milk, experiment with reducing your dairy intake to see whether you feel better. If you do feel better, remember that your body still needs the nutrients from milk: calcium, vitamin D, protein, riboflavin, and so on. Learn how to get them from other sources. Lactose-free milk, A2 milk (different than standard milk, which contains both A1 and A2 protein), and soy milk are viable alternatives that can be easier to digest.

• If you think almond and other plant-based "milks" are an equal swap for dairy milk, think again. I refer to almond milk as *almond juice* because it is very low in protein and lacks the nutrient-dense profile of dairy milk. If you choose almond, rice, coconut, or other plant milks, be sure to get your protein elsewhere in your diet. The best nondairy alternative to cows' milk is soy milk.

• If you are concerned about saturated fat causing heart disease, choose low-fat or fat-free dairy foods. Use olive oil instead of butter.

• If you are concerned about hormones in milk causing early puberty, note that numerous hormones are found in both plant and animal foods. Protein-based hormones are digested in the stomach, which kills their ability for biological activity. No science-based conclusion supports the idea that hormones in dairy products cause early puberty.

• If you are concerned about antibiotics in milk, rest assured, every tank of milk is tested for antibiotics and rejected if any are found. Today's farmers use antibiotics responsibly to heal sick cows. The historic use of antibiotics to prevent illness is an added cost for farmers, and by 2020 will be totally phased out in the United States, under the directive of the Food and Drug Administration (FDA).

Milk (dairy or soy) and other foods rich in calcium and vitamin D should be an important part of your diet throughout your lifetime. Because your bones are alive, they need calcium and vitamin D daily. Children and teens need calcium for growth. Adults also need calcium to maintain strong bones. Although you may stop growing by age 20, you don't reach peak bone density until age 30 to 35. The amount of calcium stored in your bones at that age is a critical factor in your susceptibility to fractures as you grow older. After age 35, bones start to thin as a normal part of aging. A calcium-rich diet, in combination with adequate protein, resistance exercise and strong muscles, can slow this process.

Nonfat, Low Fat, or Full Fat? Dairy foods offer a package of life-sustaining vitamins, minerals, and protein, but they also contain saturated fat (unless they are fat-free or skim-milk products). Saturated fat has been linked with heart disease, though some researchers question that link (Chowdhury 2014)—and whether or not *sat-fat is bad-fat* applies to milk and other dairy foods. Questions remain unanswered: Does limiting the amount of saturated fat address the health issues? Should we be looking at what comes with the saturated fat (refined sugar, as in cookies)? Are processed foods rich in saturated fat (ice cream, pastries, sausage, bacon, salami) the bigger culprit than the fat in milk, yogurt, and cheese?

To date, the *2015-2020 Dietary Guidelines for Americans* recommends a healthy eating pattern that limits saturated fat to less than 10 percent of calories (22 g saturated fat for a person who eats 2,000 calories a day).

FACT OR FICTION

A calcium supplement is an easy alternative source of calcium for people who don't like to drink milk.

The facts: Calcium supplements are incomplete substitutes for calcium-rich dairy or fortified soy products. Low-fat milk and yogurt offer a full spectrum of important vitamins, minerals, and protein; a calcium supplement offers only calcium (and maybe vitamin D). Dairy milk, for example, is rich in not only calcium and vitamin D but also potassium and phosphorous—nutrients that work in combination to help your body use calcium. Milk is also one of the best sources of riboflavin, a vitamin that helps convert the food you eat into energy. Active people, who generate more energy than their sedentary counterparts, need more riboflavin. If you avoid dairy products, your riboflavin intake is likely to be poor.

Granted, taking a calcium supplement is better than consuming no calcium, but I highly recommend a nutrition consultation with a registered dietitian to ensure appropriate calcium intake from your daily food choices. This nutrition professional can help you optimize your diet so you get the best balance of all the nutrients you need for good health and optimal sports performance. (See the Dietitian section in appendix A for information on finding a registered dietitian in your area.)

An 8-ounce (240 ml) glass of whole milk contains 4.5 grams of saturated fat. A 1 1/2-ounce serving of cheddar cheese contains 8 grams of saturated fat. Both can fit into your healthy eating pattern. Until we have more research, I will choose to spend my saturated fat on 2-percent fat milk with my breakfast cereal and then eat minimal butter, ice cream, or fat-filled processed foods. What's your preference?

How Much Is Enough?

As you can see in table 1.6, calcium needs vary according to age; growing teens need four servings of calcium-rich foods, and most adults need three servings. This may seem like a lot if you are not a milk drinker, but even weight-conscious athletes can easily consume the recommended daily minimum of three servings of low-fat dairy foods for only 300·calories. Try to get at least half, if not all, of your calcium requirements from food.

Some people have trouble digesting milk because they lack an enzyme (lactase) that digests milk sugar (lactose). These lactose-intolerant people still need calcium and can often tolerate yogurt (particularly Greek yogurt), hard cheeses such as cheddar and Parmesan, or even small amounts of milk taken with a meal. They can also drink soy milk, A2

TABLE 1.6 Calcium Requirements

Age	Calcium target (mg)	Number of servings
CHILDREN		
1-3 years	700	2.5
4-8 years	1,000	3.5
TEENAGERS		
9-18 years	1,300	4
WOMEN		
19-50 years	1,000	3
>50 years (postmenopause)	1,200	4
Amenorrheic athletes	1,200	4
Pregnant or breastfeeding	1,000-1,300	3-4
MEN		
19-70 years	1,000	3
>70 years	1,200	4

Data from Institute of Medicine Food and Nutrition Board, 2011, *Dietary Reference Intakes for Calcium and Vitamin D*. Washington DC: National Academies Press. Available: www.iom.edu/Reports/2010/Dietary-Reference-Intakes-for-Calcium-and-Vitamin-D.aspx.

Boosting Your Calcium Intake

Here are tips to help you boost your calcium intake to build and maintain strong bones:

- For breakfast, enjoy cereal with 1 cup of dairy or soy milk.
- Cook hot cereal in milk, or mix in 1/3 cup (40 g) of powdered milk. Top with slivered almonds.
- Make shakes and smoothies using kefir as the base.
- Add extra milk (instead of cream) to coffee, and enjoy lattes.
- Take powdered milk to the office to replace coffee whiteners.
- Munch on an apple, precut low-fat cheese, and crackers.
- Eat lots of broccoli, collard greens, kale, and bok choy.
- Add tofu to Asian soups or stir-fried meals. *Note:* Choose brands of tofu processed with calcium sulfate, otherwise, the tofu will be calcium poor.
- Chug chocolate (soy) milk for a postworkout recovery food.
- Add grated cheese, canned salmon (with bones), tofu cubes, or almonds to a salad.
- Add cheese to a sandwich or wrap.
- Enjoy crackers topped with canned salmon or sardines with bones for an easy lunch option.
- In a blender, mix soft tofu or plain yogurt with salad seasonings for a calcium-rich dressing.
- Drink dairy or soy milk with meals.
- Snack on a handful of almonds to curb your afternoon appetite.
- Treat yourself to milk-based hot cocoa in place of coffee.
- Make a yogurt parfait (yogurt, granola, berries) for a dessert or snack.
- Snack on fruit-flavored yogurt rather than ice cream.
- Make pudding with milk for a tasty calcium-rich treat.

milk, or lactose-free milk. As I mentioned before, rice, almond, and other nut milks are not nutritionally viable alternatives to dairy or soy milk.

Top Choices

To consume the amount of calcium you need to build and maintain strong bones (1,000 to 1,300 mg per day), you should plan to include a calcium-rich food in each meal. Evenly distributing your calcium intake throughout the day enhances calcium absorption.

- **Milk, fortified with vitamin D, from cows or soy.** Dairy or soy milk is an excellent source of calcium and protein. A glass of whole cows' milk (3.5 percent fat) has the same amount of fat as two pats of butter, but skim milk (0 percent fat) has almost no fat. Choosing reduced-fat milk, yogurt, and cheese seems a wise choice if you are concerned about your weight.

- **Yogurt, regular or Greek.** While plain yogurt is one of the richest food sources of calcium, Greek yogurt offers more protein. The active cultures in yogurt enhance calcium absorption. Note that frozen yogurt (and ice cream for that matter) is only a fair source of calcium. I consider both types of treats sugar-based foods that contain only a little milk. One cup of soft-serve frozen yogurt equals 1/3 cup (40 ml) of milk in terms of calcium, but it comes with twice as many calories.

- **Cheese.** Added to sandwiches, pasta, chili, and other vegetarian meals—or enjoyed as a snack with an apple or whole-grain crackers—cheese is a tasty way to boost calcium and protein. Because it's easy to consume your day's allotment of saturated fat from cheese, you might want to enjoy the reduced-fat options. Soy cheese is also a calcium option.

- **Dark green veggies.** Broccoli, bok choy (a vegetable common in Chinese cookery), and kale are among the best vegetable sources of calcium. Spinach, collard and beet greens, and Swiss chard also contain calcium, but your body can absorb very little of it because these veggies contain high levels of oxalic acid that binds the calcium and hinders absorption.

Protein-Rich Foods

Protein from plant sources (soy, beans, nuts, and legumes) and animal sources (meat, seafood, eggs, and poultry) is important in your daily diet, but you should eat protein as the accompaniment to the wholesome carbohydrate found in fruits, vegetables, and grains. If one-quarter to one-third of your plate at each meal is covered with a protein-rich food, you can consume the right amount of the amino acids you need to build and repair muscles. By choosing darker meats with iron and zinc (lean beef, chicken thigh), you reduce the risk of iron-deficiency anemia.

How Much Is Enough?

Athletes tend to eat either too much or too little protein, depending on their health consciousness, awareness of nutrition principles, or lifestyle. Some athletes fill up on too much meat. Others proclaim themselves veg-etarian, yet because they neglect to replace the beef with beans, they are often protein deficient.

Although slabs of steak and huge hamburgers have no place in any ath-lete's diet—or anyone's diet—an adequate amount of protein distributed evenly throughout the day is important for building muscles and repairing tissues. The purpose of this section is to highlight quick and easy protein choices. See chapter 7 for sport-specific protein needs.

For most people, including athletes, a daily total of 5 to 7 ounces (150 to 200 g) of protein-rich food plus the protein you get in two or three servings of dairy or soy milk, yogurt, or cheese (which you consume for calcium) offers adequate protein. Five ounces for a day is much less than the por-tions most Americans eat in one meal: 10-ounce (300 g) steaks, 6-ounce (180 g) chicken breasts, or slabs of roast beef. Many athletes polish off their required protein by lunchtime and continue to eat one to two times more than they need. Excess protein is not converted into bulging muscles.

Other people, however, miss out on adequate protein when they eat a meal that contains only fruit, veggies, or grains such as having a banana for breakfast, salad for lunch, and quinoa with roasted veggies for dinner. Dieters, in particular, who dine exclusively on salads and vegetables com-monly neglect their protein needs.

Top Choices

All types of protein-rich foods contain valuable amino acids. See table 1.7 for a comparison of popular protein-rich foods. The following choices can enhance your sports diet:

• **Beans.** Vegetarian refried beans (in a burrito), hummus (as a dip with baby carrots), and canned garbanzo or kidney beans (added to a salad) are three easy ways to boost your intake of plant protein—as well as carbo-hydrate. If you tend to avoid beans because they make you flatulent, try eating them with Beano, a product available at many health food stores and pharmacies that helps take the gas out of vegetarian diets.

TABLE 1.7 Comparing Protein Content of Commonly Eaten Foods

Food sources	Protein (g)
ANIMAL PROTEIN	
Egg white, 1	3
Tuna, 1 can (5 oz)	22-26
Beef, roast, 4 oz (120 g) cooked	30
Chicken breast, 4 oz (120 g) cooked*	30
PLANT PROTEIN	
Nuts, 1 oz (1/4 cup or 30 g)	6
Soy milk, 1 cup (240 ml)	7
Hummus, 1/2 cup (125 g)	8
Edamame, 1/2 cup	8
Peanut butter, 2 tbsp	9
Tofu, 4 oz (120 g)	11
Boca burger, 2.5 oz (75 g)	13
DAIRY PRODUCTS	
Yogurt, 6 oz (170 g) tub	6-7
Cheese, cheddar, 1 oz (30 g)	7
Milk, 1 cup (240 ml)	8
Greek yogurt, 6 oz (170 g) tub	18
Cottage cheese, 1/2 cup (113 g)	15
BREADS, CEREALS, GRAINS	
Bread, 1 slice	2
Cold cereal, 1 oz (30 g)	2
Rice, 1/3 cup dry (65 g) or 1 cup cooked	4
Oatmeal, 1/2 cup dry (40 g) or 1 cup cooked	5
Pasta, 2 oz (60 g) dry or cooked	8
STARCHY VEGETABLES**	
Peas, 1/2 cup cooked	2
Carrots, 1/2 cup cooked	2
Corn, 1/2 cup cooked	2
Beets, 1/2 cup cooked	2
Potato, 1 small	2

*4 oz (120 g) cooked (approximately the size of a deck of cards) = 5 to 6 oz (150 to 180 g) raw.

**Whereas starchy vegetables contribute a little protein, most watery vegetables (and fruits) offer negligible amounts of protein. They may contribute a total of 5 to 10 grams of protein per day, depending on how much you eat.

- **Chicken and turkey.** Poultry generally has less saturated fat than red meats, so it tends to be a more heart-healthy choice. Just be sure to buy skinless chicken or discard the fatty skin before cooking. Cooked until crispy, poultry skin can be a calorie-dense temptation.

- **Fish.** Fresh, frozen, or canned fish provides not only a lot of protein but also the omega-3 unsaturated fat that protects your health. The American Heart Association's recommended target is at least 7 ounces (200 g), or two servings, of canned or fresh fish per week. The best choices are the oilier varieties that live in cold ocean waters, such as salmon, mackerel, albacore tuna, sardines, bluefish, and herring, but any fish is better than no fish. Chapter 2 offers more information on fish.

- **Lean beef.** A lean roast beef sandwich made with two thick slices of whole-grain bread for carbohydrate is an excellent choice for protein as well as iron (prevents anemia), zinc (needed for muscle growth and repair), and B vitamins (help produce energy). Top round (such as you'd buy at a deli), eye of round, and round tip are among the leanest cuts of beef. A lean roast beef sandwich is preferable in terms of heart health to a grilled-cheese sandwich or chicken salad sandwich because of the lower fat content and, in terms of iron content, is preferable to yet another turkey sandwich. Limiting your intake to 12 to 18 ounces of beef per week will also minimize the risk of colon cancer (and think twice before routinely eating processed meats like ham, bacon, salami, hot dogs, and sausages).

- **Peanut butter and other nut butters.** Although nut butter by the jarful can be a dangerous diet breaker, a few tablespoons on whole-grain bread, an apple, or a banana for a snack or a quick meal offers protein, vitamins, and fiber. Nut butters are a good source of health-protective poly-unsaturated fat. People who eat at least two servings of peanut butter (or peanuts) per week tend to have a lower risk of heart disease (Kris-Etherton et al. 2001). Enjoy it regularly!

The all-natural peanut butter brands are the preferable choice. If you or your family dislikes the oily greeting when you open the jar of an all-natural brand, simply store the jar upside down. You can then more easily stir in the oil that separates out.

- **Tofu.** Tofu is an easy addition to a meatless diet because you don't have to cook it. It has a mild flavor, so you can easily add it to salads, chili, spaghetti sauce, stir-fry dishes, and casseroles. Look for tofu in the vegetable section of your grocery store. Buy firm tofu for slicing or cutting into cubes and soft or silken tofu for blending into smoothies or dips.

Even athletes who don't cook can easily incorporate adequate protein into a day's diet. Easy options from the grocery store include turkey breast from the deli counter; rotisserie chicken; tub of hummus; canned lentil soup; foil pouches of tuna, salmon, or chicken; almonds; and frozen edamame.

Fat and Oils

Sports dietitians used to say "Eat less fat," but today our message is "Eat the right kinds of fat." In particular, do the following:

• **Limit your intake of hard saturated fat.** These include beef lard and stick margarine. The *2015-2020 Dietary Guidelines for Americans* encourage us to develop a healthy eating pattern that offers less than 10 percent of total calories from saturated fat and instead emphasizes unsaturated fat. The American Heart Association recommends less than 6 percent for individuals with elevated LDL cholesterol levels. That 6 percent equates to about 120 calories (13 g) of saturated fat per 2,000 calories, or about 3 teaspoons per day.

• **Choose more soft or liquid mono- and polyunsaturated fats.** These include tub margarine, olive oil, and canola oil. That means more olive oil and less butter, more oily fish and less greasy meat. Minimize partially hydrogenated fats in commercially prepared foods such as crackers, cakes, cookies, chips, and pastries.

How Much Is Enough?

The *2015-2020 US Dietary Guidelines for Americans* no longer put a limit on total calories from fat. Yet, some athletes eat way too much saturated fat—buttered toast for breakfast, salads with lots of bacon bits and cheese for lunch, and pepperoni pizza for dinner. If you tend to choose foods high in saturated fat at each meal, strive to trade the bad fats for good ones. That is, spread peanut butter instead of butter on toast, add avocado and olives instead of bacon bits to a salad, and put peppers instead of pepperoni on pizza. If you eat enough wholesome foods at meals, you might also curb your appetite for snacking on highly processed chips, cookies, and other nutrient-poor, high-fat foods.

Top Choices

The following forms of fat are a positive addition to your sports diet because they knock down inflammation and are health enhancing.

- **Almonds, walnuts, and other nuts.** Because they are protective against heart disease, nuts (and nut oils, such as walnut oil) are a fine addition to cereal, salads, cooked vegetables, and even pasta meals.
- **Avocado.** Nutrient dense and rich in mono- and polyunsaturated fats, avocados are a positive addition to a sports diet. Mashed into guacamole, sliced in a turkey wrap, or diced and sprinkled on a salad, enjoy this green fruit with smoothies, snacks, and meals. It is a healthy alternative to mayonnaise and creamy salad dressings.
- **Chia and flaxseed (ground).** Both chia and flax contain alpha-linolenic acid (ALA), a health-protective omega-3 fat. Sprinkle ground flaxseed on cold cereal, blend it into shakes, and add it to pancake batter. Add chia to smoothies and soup for a thickener.
- **Olive oil.** This monounsaturated fat is associated with a low risk of heart disease and cancer. Use it for salads, a dip for bread, and keeping pasta from sticking together. If you use olive oil for its health-giving properties, buy unrefined extra-virgin olive oil (despite its higher cost). Extra-virgin olive oil offers more phenolic compounds—powerful antioxidants that can reduce inflammation.
- **Peanut butter and other nut butters.** All-natural brands are best because they are less processed, but even Skippy, Jif, and other commercial peanut butters offer predominantly health-protective fat.
- **Salmon, tuna, and oily fish.** Just two servings a week (a total of 7 to 12 oz, or 200 to 360 g) offers the health-protective omega-3 fats called EPA and DHA that protect against heart disease.

Sugars and Fun Foods

Even a well-balanced diet can include sweets and fun foods; the key is moderation. The plan is to first fill up on wholesome foods, and then, if desired, choose something sweet for a small treat. That is, there is little wrong with enjoying a bit of dark chocolate after a lunchtime sandwich. But there is a lot wrong with eating chocolate bars for lunch. I recommend that athletes follow the *2015-2020 Dietary Guidelines for Americans* to limit their intake of added sugars to 10 percent of calories. The American Heart Association suggests a limit of 100 calories of sugar for women and 150 calories of sugar for men. That's the amount in 16 to 24 ounces (480 to 720 ml) of a sport drink. Not much!

ORGANIC FOODS: ARE THEY BETTER?

Many of my clients wonder whether they should spend their food budgets on organic fruits and vegetables. Are organic foods better, safer, and more nutritious? According to a statement from the American Academy of Pediatrics (Forman et al. 2012), the simple answer is that organic foods can reduce exposure to pesticides and antibiotic-resistant bacteria, are better for the environment, are safer for farmers, and support small farms. Without question, pesticides are a danger to the environment and the farmworkers who are routinely exposed to high levels of toxic chemicals. Organic foods are not significantly better in terms of nutritional value. Simply eating a larger portion of a nonorganic counterpart would more than compensate for any nutrient discrepancy.

Whether consuming an organic diet leads to improved health or lower risk of disease has yet to be proven (Bradbury et al. 2014; Smith-Spangler et al. 2012). That said, infants and young children are most vulnerable to potential harm, including a possible link to lower IQ (CSPI 2012). The debate over organic versus conventional farming goes beyond nutrition and health and into politics and personal values. Here's a closer look at the story as I understand it to date.

To start, the term *organic* refers to the way farmers grow and process fruits, vegetables, grains, meat, poultry, eggs, and dairy products. The food label terms *natural, hormone free,* and *free range* do not necessarily mean organic. Only foods that are grown and processed according to U.S. Department of Agriculture (USDA) organic standards can be labeled as organic. Organic farmers do not use chemical fertilizers, insecticides, or weed killers on crops. Nor do they use growth hormones, antibiotics, or medications to enhance animal growth and prevent disease. Organic also does not mean pesticide-free; several synthetic pesticides are allowed in organic food production. Pesticides can also drift from nearby nonorganic farms.

Organic fruits and vegetables can cost more than standard produce by 30 percent or more. Are they worth the extra cost? In terms of taste, some athletes claim that organic foods taste better. In terms of nutrition, the differences are very small (Winter and Davis 2006).

One reason to choose organic relates to reducing the pesticide content in your body and therefore the potential risk of cancer and birth defects. Watchdog groups remind us that small amounts of pesticides can accumulate in the body, potentially increasing cancer risks, disrupting hormones, hindering reproduction, and contributing to birth defects. It remains unclear

Buying Locally Grown Food

Reasons other than health for buying locally grown (preferably organic) foods are to help sustain the earth and replenish its resources and to support small farms and help farmers earn a better living. Otherwise, farmers can easily be tempted to sell their land for house lots or industrial parks—and there goes more unpolluted beautiful open green space that we would otherwise enjoy when biking, running, and playing outside.

When you buy fruits and vegetables from a large grocery store chain, take note of where the produce is grown and evaluate the whole picture. Transporting produce from Asia and Africa consumes fuel that raises greenhouse gas emissions and contributes to climate change. Does this really fit the goal of establishing a sustainable environment? The compromise is to buy any kind of locally grown produce whenever possible.

as to how much we can tolerate without being harmed. Pesticides may be of particular concern during vulnerable periods of growth, such as early childhood. Some people question whether they contribute to learning disabilities and hyperactivity.

The U.S. Environmental Protection Agency (EPA) has established standards that require a 100- to 1,000-fold margin of safety for pesticide residues. It has set limits based on scientific data that indicate the level at which a pesticide will not cause "unreasonable risk to human health." A 2016 survey of 10,365 food samples (fresh, frozen, and canned) revealed that only 48 foods showed pesticide residue exceeding the tolerance (USDA Pesticide Data Program 2016).

According to experts at the watchdog Environmental Working Group (2018), the government's levels of allowable pesticides are too liberal. They agree, however, that the health benefits of eating more fruits and vegetables outweigh the known risks of consuming pesticide residue. So what's a hungry, but poor, athlete to do?

- Eat a variety of foods to minimize exposure to a specific pesticide residue.
- Carefully wash and rinse fruits and vegetables under running water; this can remove 99 percent of pesticide residue (depending on the food and the pesticide).

- Peel foods such as apples, potatoes, carrots, and pears (but keep in mind that this also peels off important nutrients).
- Remove the tops and outer portions of celery, lettuce, and cabbage.
- Buy organic versions of the foods you eat most often, such as apples if you are a five-a-day apple eater.
- When buying the fruits and vegetables that are known to have the highest amounts of pesticide residue (although they are still within the EPA's limits), choose organic: strawberries, spinach, nectarines, apples, grapes, peaches, cherries, pears, tomatoes, celery, potatoes, and bell peppers.
- To save money, choose conventionally grown fruits and vegetables known to have little or no pesticide residue (or nonedible skins that will be removed): avocado, sweet corn, pineapple, cabbage, onion, frozen sweet peas, papaya, asparagus, mango, eggplant, honeydew melon, kiwi, cantaloupe, cauliflower, and broccoli.

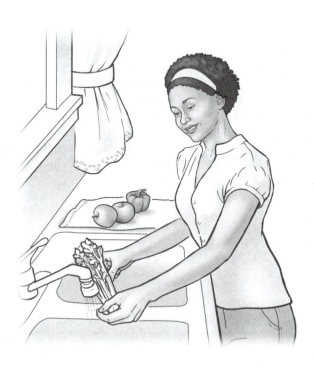

Obesogens and Processed Foods

By choosing more organic and all-natural foods, you likely end up eating fewer highly processed foods, some of which contain *obesogens*. Obesogens are chemical compounds that may contribute to more and bigger fat cells. Obesogens, which are found in some packaged foods, drugs, and industrial products (such as plastics), alter metabolic processes, disrupt hormonal balance, and can predispose some people to gain weight. Exposure to these chemicals in utero may explain, in part, why childhood obesity is on the rise, why even thin people are fatter than they used to be, and why morbid obesity, type 2 diabetes, and sex reversal in fish species (a sign of hormone disruption) are on the rise (Hollcamp 2012; Schwartz et al. 2017).

We need more research on the role of obesogens and on ways to reduce their presence in the environment. They are found in plastic, canned goods, and nonstick cookware (as well as some air fresheners, laundry products, and personal care products). Until more is known, this is another reason to choose foods in their natural state, with less processing and less packaging. For more information, see the Obesogens section in appendix A.

By eating more natural foods, you also reduce your intake of ultraprocessed foods (Cheetos, instant soup mixes, ramen noodles, Twinkies, and so on) that contain numerous additives that enhance the flavor, color, texture, and shelf life. These additives, as well as chemical byproducts released during heating of the ultraprocessed foods, might be associated with an increased risk of cancer (Fiolet et al. 2018). With more research, we can better understand how ultraprocessed foods affect our bodies. Until then, focus on creating a healthy eating pattern that includes more of the best foods and less of the rest.

EATING SHOULD BE ONE OF LIFE'S PLEASURES

Many athletes go to great extremes to eat healthfully. While the definition of healthful eating varies from person to person, it can, unfortunately, often take on a negative tone. Zealous "healthy eaters" tend to have many (well-intentioned) food rules, including the following:

- No refined sugar, gummy candy, soda pop, or sweets
- No potato chips, corn chips, cheese puffs, or salty snacks

- No doughnuts, pastries, pancakes, or Pop-Tarts
- No McDonald's, Burger King, pizza, or hot dogs
- No cookies, desserts, birthday cake, or holiday treats
- No highly processed foods in wrappers

While eliminating these "unhealthy" foods in their efforts to "eat clean" and put premium nutrition into their body's engine, these questions arise:

- Do you really need to eat a *perfect* diet to have an *excellent* diet? No.
- Does enjoying a hot dog or a candy bar once in a blue moon negate all of the "good stuff" you routinely eat? No.
- Is eating cake on your birthday cheating? Heavens no!

Fun foods, in moderation, can have their place in a balanced sports diet.

BUILD A STRONG SPORTS DIET

Now that you have read this chapter, you know which foods are the best choices. The trick is to assemble the best foods into wholesome meals and snacks. I recommend that you try to choose from at least three of the five food groups at each meal. Table 1.8 shows how this might work.

Foods made from a combination of ingredients can create a well-balanced meal in one dish. For example, whole-wheat pizza topped with peppers, onions, and mushrooms is far from junk food. It offers calcium-rich dairy (from the low-fat mozzarella); vegetables rich in potassium, beta-carotene, and vitamin C (from the tomato sauce and vegetable toppings); and carbohydrate-rich grain foods in the crust. A dinner of thick-crust pizza with a foundation of carbohydrate better fits into a sports diet than does a chicken Caesar salad that is mostly fat and protein.

You can consume the recommended intake of the vitamins, minerals, amino acids (the building blocks of protein), and other nutrients you need for good health within 1,200 to 1,500 calories if you wisely select from a

TABLE 1.8 Eating Multiple Food Groups Within a Meal

Food group	Meal 1	Meal 2	Meal 3
Grain	Oatmeal	Whole-wheat wrap	Pasta
Fruit	Raisins	Avocado	Fruit salad
Vegetable	(Canned) pumpkin	Salsa	Tomato sauce
Dairy/calcium	Low-fat (soy) milk	Low-fat cheese	Low-fat yogurt
Protein	Almonds	Turkey	Turkey meatballs

variety of wholesome foods. Because many active people consume 2,000 to 5,000 calories (depending on their age, level of activity, body size, and gender), they have the chance to consume abundant amounts of vitamins and other nutrients. Dieters, on the other hand, tend to take in fewer calories, so they need to carefully select nutrient-dense foods—foods that offer the most nutritional value for the least amount of calories—to reduce the risk of consuming a nutrient-deficient diet.

To determine whether your daily food intake is balanced and adequate, you can track your diet at websites listed in appendix A in the Dietary Analysis and Nutrition Assessment section.

Eating well need not be a major task. The following chapters offer additional tips to help you choose a sports diet that will invest in good health and high energy for sports, exercise, and a nourishing life. You "simply" need to do the following:

- Eat a variety of wholesome foods to consume a bigger variety of health-protective nutrients. Target at least three kinds of food per meal (and two kinds per snack, which I will address in chapter 5).

- Choose more of the best foods and less of the rest.

- Take mealtimes seriously, and use food to help you progress from being not just a good athlete but hopefully to being a great one. Do not underestimate the effectiveness of a well-planned sports diet!

CHAPTER 2

EATING TO STAY HEALTHY FOR THE LONG RUN

According to the Centers for Disease Control and Prevention, life expectancy is about 78.5 years for the average American. If you are going to live a long life, you might as well live a health-filled life. You'll have a lot more fun.

Good health starts will fully appreciating the power of food in the prevention and treatment of the so-called diseases of aging, which are, in reality, diseases of inactivity and poor nutrition. No single medicine is as powerful as a healthy diet combined with an active lifestyle. Luckily, the wholesome foods you need to protect your health are the same foods that should be part of your sports diet. A high-quality sports diet helps to ward off illness, reduce inflammation, heal injuries, and keep you off the bench.

Confusion abounds about foods that are "good" or "bad" for your health. My clients repeatedly ask me, "What foods should I avoid?" My standard answer is that the only "bad" foods are foods that are moldy or poisonous (or create an allergic response in your body); all other foods, in moderation, can be balanced into a healthy food plan.

Although there is no such thing as a bad food, there is a bad diet. Repeatedly eating meals and snacks of highly processed foods filled with saturated fat and refined sugars can indeed contribute to obesity, heart disease, cancer, hypertension, diabetes, kidney failure, inflammation, and other diseases associated with excessive eating. Yet, as outlined in chapter 1, choosing a menu based on wholesome grains, fruits, vegetables, nuts, beans, lean protein, and low-fat dairy or other calcium-rich foods—in addition to enjoying an active lifestyle—is clearly an investment in optimal health and sports performance. The purpose of this chapter is to help you make the best food choices for lifelong well-being.

DIET AND HEART HEALTH

Cardiovascular disease (CVD: cardio = heart, vascular = blood vessels) is the number one killer of both men and women in the United States. Two ways to reduce your risk of CVD are being physically fit and eating wisely. Yet, some active people believe they are exempt from the food rules about heart-healthy eating; they assume that being physically fit protects them from heart disease. Wrong! A friend of mine, a seemingly healthy 48-year-old marathoner, died suddenly of a massive heart attack. He'd run 2 hours and 10 minutes, stopped his watch, and was later found dead on the running path. Everyone was shocked.

Unfortunately, even the most health-conscious people can find themselves confused by the constant updates and changes regarding nutrition and heart health. This leaves us wondering what the real answers are to questions such as: Is beef bad? What about eggs? Should I use butter or margarine? The answers vary from person to person because we each have a unique genetic makeup. It won't be long before dietary recommendations will be based on genetic tests. But for today, here are suggestions for optimizing your diet based on the latest nutrition studies, so you can at least delay CVD if you cannot escape it.

Eat for Heart Health

The benefits of tweaking your daily food intake by making small heart-healthy choices can accumulate to make a big difference in the long run (table 2.1). The American Heart Association (AHA, www.heart.org) recommends enjoying a healthy eating pattern that is rich in vegetables, fruits, and whole-grain, high-fiber foods. You can enhance your eating pattern with the following diet and lifestyle choices to reduce your risk of cardiovascular disease:

- Reaching or maintaining a healthy weight
- Consuming at least 7 ounces (200 g) of oily fish per week
- Limiting your intake of saturated fat and partially hydrogenated oils
- Replacing saturated animal fat with healthy unsaturated fat from nuts, avocados, and plant oils
- Limiting your intake of beverages and foods with added sugars to control your weight
- Choosing and preparing foods with little or no salt
- Consuming alcohol in moderation (if at all)
- Making reasonably healthy choices when you dine away from home
- Being active for at least 30 minutes most days of the week

TABLE 2.1 Tweaking Your Menu for Heart Health

Standard food	Swap
White bagel with cream cheese	Whole wheat bagel with peanut butter
Omelet with full-fat cheese	Omelet with kale, mushrooms, and low-fat cheese
Potato chips with onion dip	Baked corn chips with guacamole
Turkey and cheese wrap	Turkey, tomato, and avocado wrap
Raw veggies dipped in blue cheese dressing	Raw veggies dipped in hummus
Salad with creamy dressing	Salad with olive oil dressing
6 oz (180 g) filet mignon	6 oz (180 g) salmon
Baked potato with butter	Baked potato with pesto

This book provides detailed information you can use to follow the AHA's guidelines.

Oatmeal and Heart Health

The type of fiber (soluble fiber) found in oats as well as in barley, lentils, split peas, and beans protects against heart disease. Find ways to include more of these foods in your diet. For example, trade toast or a bagel for a hearty bowl of oatmeal.

Research suggests that eating a bowlful of oatmeal (1 1/2 cups cooked) each day can help a person attain lower cholesterol levels, especially when eaten as part of a heart-healthy diet, and especially when the person has elevated cholesterol levels to begin with (Expert Panel on Detection, Evaluation, and Treatment of High Blood Cholesterol in Adults 2001).

If you don't have time to cook oatmeal at home, enjoy one or two packets of instant oatmeal for a midmorning or afternoon snack. Or do what I do—simply add raw oats (either instant or old fashioned) to your cold cereal. Wheaties and raw oats is an easy way to get two whole grains in one tasty bowl.

Eggs and Heart Health

Eggs are a nutrient-dense source of high-quality protein and offer beneficial carotenoids in the yolk that protect against age-related macular degeneration and cataracts. Historically, medical experts have told us that eating eggs is bad because of their high cholesterol content.

Newer studies suggest that egg cholesterol has little effect on blood cholesterol levels, especially when eaten as part of an overall healthy diet. Hence, the *Dietary Guidelines for Americans* no longer specify a limit on cholesterol intake for most healthy people. In a study of people with pre-diabetes or type 2 diabetes who were at high risk for CVD, no heart-health issues were reported when eating more than 12 eggs a week (about 2 eggs a day) for 12 weeks (Fuller et al. 2015). But use common sense. Eating six eggs a day might not be the wisest choice for everyone.

Losing excess body fat is a good way to lower your blood cholesterol, and nutrient-dense eggs can be a positive addition to a reducing diet. Eating two hard-boiled eggs alongside a bowl of oatmeal creates a satiating breakfast that can help curb your midmorning hankering for a doughnut. Whole eggs might not be so bad for breakfast after all!

Some eggs also offer omega-3 fat. Feeding chickens a special vegetarian feed that includes canola oil and flax can enhance the fat content of the egg yolk. Hence, "designer eggs" such as Eggland's Best offer double the omega-3 fat found in standard eggs. If you were to eat two omega-3 eggs, you'd get about 250 milligrams of omega-3 fat. Given the AHA recommends 1,000 milligrams (1 g) per day for people at risk of heart disease, and a serving of salmon offers 2,000 to 4,000 milligrams, I suggest you keep eating fish and use the eggs as a bonus!

Peanut Butter, Nuts, and Nut Butters and Heart Health

Many people try to stay away from peanut butter and nuts because they fear them as being fattening. Think again. People who frequently eat nuts are not fatter than nut avoiders (Flores-Mateo et al. 2013). Research on more than 260,000 people indicates that eating one serving of nuts or peanut butter five times a week can reduce the risk of heart disease by 50 percent (Kris-Etherton et al. 2001). Research also indicates that eating nuts can reduce the risk of type 2 diabetes by about 25 percent (Jiang et al. 2002). Nuts are rich in monounsaturated fat (as well as folate, niacin, thiamin, magnesium, fiber, and other health-protective nutrients). Adding walnuts to oatmeal, peanut butter to a bagel, sliced almonds to a salad, and mixed nuts to dried fruit for trail mix are just a few simple ways to include these health-protective foods in your daily diet—to say nothing of enjoying a good old peanut butter sandwich for lunch.

The trick with nuts and peanut butter is to keep the portion within your calorie budget. For 170 calories, you can enjoy a scant two tablespoons of nut butter or 1 ounce (30 g) of nuts: about 22 almonds, 28 peanuts, 20 pecans, 45 pistachios, 10 walnuts, or 1/4 cup of sunflower seeds. The good news is that nuts are very satisfying, and 1 ounce (or less) can curb your hunger for a while. Dieters can lose weight and keep it off when they include nuts, peanut butter, other nut butters, and other sources of healthy fat in their daily diets (McManus, Antinoro, and Sacks 2001).

Cooking Oils and Heart Health

When it comes to selecting heart-healthy fat for cooking, the rule of thumb is the softer, the better. That is, soft (liquid) vegetable oils have a higher percentage of unsaturated fat than does harder (solid) fat such as stick margarines and butter. Olive oil and canola oil are the two preferred types of fat to include in a heart-healthy diet. These oils are rich in monounsaturated fat and are considered better choices than safflower, corn, sunflower, and other polyunsaturated vegetable oils. Use olive and canola oils with salads, pesto, and pasta and when sauteing. Just be sure to use only moderate amounts if you want to lose body fat. Their calories, although preferable to the calories from saturated fat, still count and add up quickly.

Cooking with olive and canola oil is far healthier than using butter, coconut oil, bacon grease, lard, salt pork, or animal fat, which are all solid at room temperature.

Which Is Better: Butter, Olive Oil, or Coconut Oil?　Thanks to marketing, many athletes believe that coconut oil is a healthy fat. The American Heart Association (AHA) disagrees. Here's why. Coconut oil, like butter, beef fat, and palm oil, elevates the bad LDL cholesterol. Coconut oil also contains a significant amount of lauric acid, which is associated with raising the good HDL cholesterol. Because the AHA no longer considers high HDL to be a direct link to reducing the risk of heart disease, the group advises against using coconut oil as a preferred fat (Sacks et al. 2017).

To date, we lack research that measures the direct effect of coconut oil on CVD. We do know that dietary fats are mostly triglycerides, comprised of three fatty acids. Fatty acids come in short, medium, and long chains, as well as odd and even chains. Fatty acids can be saturated (no double bonds), polyunsaturated (many double bonds), or monounsaturated (one double bond), and the double bonds can be in a cis (same side) or trans (opposite side) position. These different configurations cause different metabolic effects. To get a better picture of how different kinds of fat affect heart health, we need to look at fatty acid content and the context in which a fat is processed and consumed. That is, does the saturated fat in processed red meat (bologna, hot dogs) increase the risk of heart disease more than red meat (lean roast beef) itself? Are fermented dairy foods, such as yogurt and cheese, heart healthier than butter? What is the impact of your fitness level, microbiome, and genetics on your personal response to dietary fat? (Forouhi et al. 2018; Stanhope et al. 2018).

There's not a simple answer to which is better: butter, olive oil, or coconut oil. As with any food, the dose is the poison. My advice is to eat a small amount of butter or coconut oil, if desired, and be more generous with the olive oil, a known heart-healthy choice. Pay attention to the amount of saturated fat in the other foods in your diet and choose a healthy eating style that adheres to the *2015-2020 Dietary Guidelines for Americans* recommendation to consume less than 10 percent of calories from saturated fat.

Fish and Heart Health

If good health is your wish, get hooked on fish. Research indicates that fish may guard against not only heart disease but also hypertension, cancer, arthritis, asthma, and who knows what else. The omega-3 fatty acids, the special polyunsaturated fat found in fish oil, block many harmful biochemical reactions that can cause blood to clot (predisposing you to heart attack and stroke) and the heart to beat irregularly (as occurs during a heart attack). Some researchers believe that fish oils can prevent heart disease rather than merely having a beneficial effect after the onset of the disease.

The AHA recommends eating at least 7 ounces (200 g) of oily fish per week (one large or two small fish servings) to provide the recommended amount of fish oil and reduce your risk of heart disease. Eating fish for dinner not only contributes fish oil to your diet but also simultaneously displaces the saturated fat in the meat you might have otherwise eaten. The following list can guide your fish choices so you select fish that are good sources of omega-3 fat, low in environmental contaminates such as mercury and polychlorinated biphenyl (PCB), and good for the environment because they are fished in a sustainable way.

Best Sources of Omega-3

Albacore tuna (troll- or pole-caught)

Freshwater coho salmon (farmed)

Oysters (farmed)

Pacific sardines (wild caught)

Rainbow trout (farmed)

Salmon (wild caught, from Alaska)

Good Sources of Omega-3

Arctic char (farmed)

Barramundi (farmed, from the United States)

Dungeness crab (wild caught, from California, Oregon, and Washington)

Longfin squid (wild caught, from the U.S. Atlantic)

Mussels (farmed)

Source: Monterey Bay Aquarium Seafood Watch, www.montereybayaquarium.org.

Just be sure that your fish is not fried or broiled in butter. If you shy away from cooking fish, simply take advantage of ready-to-eat cans or foil pouches of tuna, salmon, and sardines, or choose a fish-based entree when you eat in a restaurant.

Be careful about eating too much fish, however. Unfortunately, the fish highest in omega-3 fatty acids also deliver a dose of methylmercury from industrial pollution of the oceans. Long-term consumption of mercury can contribute to neurological and cardiovascular problems in adults, as well as cause significant damage to the developing brains of infants and children. If you are into sport fishing, eating sushi, or having tuna every day for lunch—and enjoy high-mercury fish several times a week—take heed. The mercury can accumulate in your body and create health problems (numbness and tingling in hands and feet, fatigue, muscle pain).

Yet, the U.S. Food and Drug Administration still advises pregnant women to enjoy up to 12 ounces (360 g) of fish a week because fish oil is important for normal brain development. The 12 ounces includes a large safety margin, but pregnant women should avoid shark, swordfish, king mackerel, and tile fish and limit their intake of albacore tuna to no more than one 6-ounce (180 g) can per week. Because these fish are long-lived and large, they accumulate mercury in their tissues over time by eating a lot of smaller mercury-containing fish. The safest fish are wild salmon from Alaska, canned salmon (chinook, chum, coho, pink, and sockeye species), pollock, catfish, shrimp, and canned light tuna. To calculate your potential mercury intake, go to www.gotmercury.org.

Lean Beef and Heart Health

Athletes commonly shun beef, believing it to be an artery clogger. Although that might be true for greasy burgers and hot dogs, small portions of lean beef aren't so bad for your health after all. (I addressed environmental concerns in chapter 1.) In terms of nutrients, lean beef is an excellent source of iron, zinc, and other nutrients athletes need. However, fatty beef tends to have more artery-clogging saturated fat than chicken or fish. Saturated fat is hard at room temperature. For example, hard beef fat differs from soft (less saturated) chicken fat.

If you need to lower your cholesterol, the AHA recommends that you consume less than 6 percent of your calories from saturated fat (the average intake in the United States is about 11 percent). For example, if you are on a 1,800-calorie reducing diet, 6 percent (14 g) is just about the amount of saturated fat you'd consume in a McDonald's Quarter Pounder With Cheese. If you are very active and require 3,000 calories per day, 6 percent of calories from saturated fat equates to about the amount in a

FACT OR FICTION

If you do not enjoy eating fish, you can simply take a fish oil supplement.

The facts: The American Heart Association does not consider fish oil capsules to be a sufficient alternative to eating fish. Fish eaters acquire health benefits not seen in fish oil pill poppers. A review of 22 well-controlled studies in which those in control groups took placebos suggests that fish oil pills fail to generate any protective effect against heart disease (including stroke, heart attack, death from irregular heartbeats, and heart failure) (Smith 2012). These well-controlled studies differ from previous observational studies that suggested health benefits from taking fish oil pills. Unfortunately, observational studies do not show cause and effect; they show that people who took fish oil pills likely had healthier lifestyles. This is a good example of why we need to focus on the whole diet, and not just one component.

That said, the newer 2018 VITAL Study (Manson 2019) reports that people who routinely eat less than one and one-half servings of fish per week reduced their risk of heart attack by taking daily 1 gram (1,000 mg.) omega-3's. Hence, if you are a non-fish eater, you might be wise to take a supplement. But also be sure to include in your daily diet omega-3 fat packaged in wholesome foods. Non-fish ways to ingest omega-3 fat is from plant sources such as flaxseed oil, walnuts, tofu, soy nuts, chia, canola oil, and olive oil. Vegetarians can take an algae-based omega-3 supplement. Plant sources offer a less potent type of omega-3 fat called alpha-linoleic acids (ALA), but any omega-3 fat is better than none. Omega-3 enriched foods, such as some eggs, milks and juices, are other options. Grass-fed beef also offers a trivial amount of omega-3s.

---

burrito bowl (with steak, cheese, and sour cream) with chips and guacamole from Chipotle.

Not all beef is fatty. The healthfulness of beef and other meats has improved because today's farmers have learned how to raise leaner animals and because butchers are trimming more of the fat from the meat found in stores. You can easily fit beef (and pork and lamb) into a heart-healthy sports diet if you select lean cuts, such as eye of round, rump roast, sirloin tip, flank steak, top round, and tenderloin and eat smaller portions, limiting yourself to a piece of lean protein about the size of the palm of your hand (think 4 ounces of beef stir-fried with broccoli, instead of 16 ounces of steak!)

You can more easily consume lean beef when you are preparing meals at home than when you are in a restaurant that prides itself on juicy, tender (read as *loaded with saturated fat*) beef. (At restaurants, if you choose salmon instead of steak, you'll not only avoid the saturated fat but you'll also boost the heart-healthy omega-3 fats.) Some people enjoy buffalo meat (bison) as a lean alternative to beef.

Supplements and Heart Health

Many people wonder about the role of vitamin supplements in enhancing heart health. Living healthfully would be so much easier if we could just take a pill that could compensate for both suboptimal eating and suboptimal genetics. Unfortunately, studies of vitamins and antioxidants that looked for reductions in heart disease saw few benefits—and even potential harm—from taking high doses of beta-carotene, selenium, and vitamin E. The same goes for folate and other B vitamins; research results have been disappointing. Hence, the AHA highly encourages you to get your vitamins and antioxidants from fruits, vegetables, whole grains, and plant oils. The right foods can be powerfully health promoting! See chapter 11 for more information about vitamin supplements.

DIET AND HIGH BLOOD PRESSURE

High blood pressure, or hypertension, is a major risk factor for heart disease and the chief risk factor for stroke. Hypertension is more common in people who are African American, older than 55, higher weight, inactive, and smokers. By measuring your blood pressure, you can determine whether it is in a healthy range. Reducing blood pressure reduces your risk of heart disease.

What Causes Hypertension?

Risk factors that can predispose people to hypertension include obesity, smoking, high stress, poor kidney function, and poor diet. Most people who exercise regularly are not obese, do not smoke, and eat a healthier-than-average diet, thus eliminating several risk factors. Many athletes, in fact, have low blood pressure. But you cannot change additional predisposing factors—such as your genetics, age, and race—that can sometimes cause high blood pressure in spite of all your good health habits. You also cannot overlook the fact that blood pressure increases as we age; as many as 70 percent of people over age 65 have high blood pressure. In a study of people 30 to 54 years of age with borderline high blood pressure, those

---

FACT OR FICTION

Eating a high-salt diet causes high blood pressure, and eating less salt will lower your blood pressure.

The facts: Reducing salt intake does not always reduce blood pressure. Only 10 percent of high blood pressure cases in the United States have a known cause. In the remaining 90 percent, no one cause can be identified. Health professionals debate whether the broad recommendation to reduce sodium intake is necessary. Yet, in Finland, because of a consistent salt education campaign, people reduced their salt intake by about one-third over 30 years. This was associated with a large decrease in blood pressure and a dramatic 75 to 80 percent decline in deaths from heart disease and stroke in Finns younger than 65 years of age (Karppanen and Mervaala 2006). Reducing your daily sodium intake to reduce your risk of cardiovascular disease seems to be a wise investment for the long run.

---

who reduced their sodium intake for 10 to 15 years experienced 25 percent fewer heart attacks and other cardiovascular events compared with those who consumed their standard sodium-rich meals (Cook et al. 2007).

Athletes and Salt

Salt is composed of 40 percent sodium and 60 percent chloride. The sodium helps maintain a proper fluid balance between the water in and around your body's cells; thus, you can enjoy some sodium—about 2,300 milligrams per day. The vast majority of Americans, however, routinely consume more than 3,400 milligrams a day; about 70 percent comes from restaurant and prepackaged, processed foods—far less than the 5 to 10 percent that comes from the saltshaker. Enjoying home-cooked meals and fruit, nuts, and other whole foods for snacks can significantly reduce your sodium intake.

The *2015-2020 Dietary Guidelines for Americans* recommends consuming less than 2,300 milligrams of sodium per day (a teaspoon of salt is about 2,300 mg). For people with high blood pressure, diabetes, and chronic kidney disease; African Americans; and non-athletic adults over 51 years of age—about half the U.S. population—the recommendation is 1,500 milligrams per day. Although you lose sodium when you perspire heavily, and some athletes lose more than others, most active people can get adequate sodium from the amounts that naturally occur in foods. The average person needs only 180 to 500 milligrams per day of sodium to function properly.

If you will be exercising moderately hard for more than four hours in the heat, you should purposefully consume salty foods and fluids. You should also consume salt if you exercise intensely for shorter periods. For example, the sodium in the sweat of professional football players varied widely, from 1,500 to 11,000 milligrams during two-hour summer practices (Greene et al. 2007). See chapters 8 and 10 for information on replacing sodium lost in sweat.

The daily value for sodium seems low for sweaty athletes. Consuming a low-sodium diet (<2,300 mg/day) may be less of a priority if you routinely train hard and sweat heavily, have normal or low blood pressure, and have no family history of hypertension. If you don't sweat much, however, reducing your daily sodium intake is likely a wise health investment.

Reducing Your Salt Intake

If you want a diet that is conducive to low blood pressure, your best bet is to buy foods in their natural state, such as raw unsalted peanuts and fresh (not canned) vegetables. Plan to eat lots of fresh fruits, vegetables, low-fat dairy products, and lean protein. Table 2.2 compares foods in terms of sodium content.

Commercially prepared and restaurant foods are the biggest contributors to sodium in the diet, so eating more home-cooked, unprocessed foods

TABLE 2.2   Comparing the Sodium Content of Popular Foods

Food type	Average sodium content	Comments
Cereal (cold)	250 mg/oz (mg/30 g)	Read food label, varies by brand
Baked goods	250 mg/serving	Once a day, if at all
Cheese (low fat)	200 mg/oz (mg/30 g)	Moderate amounts, 1-2 oz/day (30-60 g/day)
Breads	150 mg/slice	Read food label, varies by brand
Milk, yogurt (low fat)	125 mg/8 oz (mg/240 ml or g)	Read food label
Meat, fish, poultry	80 mg/4 oz (mg/120 g)	Unprocessed, unsalted
Eggs	60 mg/egg	Unprocessed, unsalted
Butter, margarine	50 mg/pat	Unsalted butter; swap for olive oil
Vegetables	10 mg/serving	Fresh and frozen; if canned, rinse well
Fruit, juice	5 mg/serving	Naturally low in sodium

is the simplest way to lower your salt intake. (Fast-food eaters commonly consume more than 4,000 mg of sodium per day.) If you are higher weight, try to lose a little excess body fat to lower your blood pressure. Eating less of the following foods will also lower your sodium intake and may contribute to a greater reduction in blood pressure:

- **Commercially prepared foods and meals.** These include frozen dinners, canned soups, and instant meals unless they are labeled low sodium. Processed foods account for the vast majority of the sodium in the American diet. Hungry athletes who eat a lot of convenience foods can easily consume a lot of sodium. Here's how: 1 cup of Ragu spaghetti sauce contains 960 milligrams of sodium; one block of Maruchan Chicken Ramen Noodles contains 1,660 milligrams; a can of Campbell's chicken noodle soup contains 2,225 milligrams; and half of a Newman's Own Four Cheese Thin & Crispy Frozen Pizza contains 1,155 milligrams.

- **Table salt.** Remove the saltshaker from the table. Omit or reduce salt from cooking and baking. You can often leave it out without affecting the outcome. If you must add salt, add it right before serving, not during cooking, to keep it on the food's surface so it tastes saltier.

- **Salty snack foods.** These include salted crackers, chips, pretzels, popcorn, salted nuts, olives, and pickles. Buy low-sodium versions, if they're available.

- **Smoked and cured meats and fish.** These include ham, bacon, sausage, corned beef, hot dogs, bologna, salami, pepperoni, lox, pickled herring, and jerky. Choose low-sodium versions if you like these foods.

- **Cheeses.** In particular, limit processed and low-fat cheeses, some of which may be higher in sodium than the regular forms.

- **Seasonings and condiments.** These include ketchup, mustard, relish, Worcestershire sauce, soy sauce, steak sauce, MSG, and garlic salt.

- **Baking soda, seltzers, and antacids.** Also, some laxatives may be high in sodium.

To add flavor to your foods, experiment with herbs and spices. When you try a new seasoning, cautiously add a small amount. Following are some tried-and-true combinations:

- **Beef:** dry mustard, pepper, marjoram, red wine, sherry
- **Chicken:** parsley, thyme, sage, tarragon, curry, white wine, vermouth
- **Fish:** bay leaf, cayenne pepper, dill, curry, onion, garlic
- **Eggs:** oregano, curry, chives, pepper, tomato, pinch of sugar

The DASH Diet

To clarify the connection between blood pressure and diet, the U.S. National Institutes of Health funded a large study of dietary approaches to stop hypertension (DASH). The DASH diet requires twice the average daily servings of fruits, vegetables, and dairy foods; one-third the usual intake of beef, pork, and ham; one-half the typical use of fat, oils, and salad dressings; and one-quarter the ordinary number of snacks and sweets (Blackburn 2001). When more than 400 people followed the DASH diet for

Increasing Your Potassium Intake

If sodium is the bad guy that contributes to high blood pressure, then potassium is the good guy that helps lower blood pressure. Potassium is found in most whole foods: fruits, vegetables, whole-grain breads and cereals, lentils, beans, nuts, and protein foods. Refined or highly processed foods, sweets, and oily foods (e.g., salad dressing, butter) are poor sources of potassium. You can increase your potassium intake by eating the following kinds of foods:

- Whole-wheat, oatmeal, and dark breads instead of white bread and flour products.
- More salads and raw or steamed veggies cooked in only a small amount of water, because the potassium leaches into the water. Steaming removes only 3 to 6 percent of the potassium, as compared with 10 to 15 percent with boiling. Microwaving is best for optimal potassium retention.
- Potatoes more often than rice, noodles, and pasta.
- Natural fruit juices instead of fruit-flavored beverages or soft drinks.

The suggested daily intake for potassium is 4,700 milligrams a day for the average person. The typical American diet contains 4,000 to 7,000 milligrams of potassium. A small amount of potassium is lost in sweat; 1 pound (0.5 kg) of sweat loss may contain 85 to 105 milligrams. Most active people consume enough potassium-rich foods to replace the potassium lost in sweat, but they should still boost their potassium intake to invest in good health.

three months, their blood pressure dropped. The researchers concluded that a diet rich in calcium, potassium, magnesium, and fiber contributes to lower blood pressure. When people simultaneously reduce sodium intake, their blood pressure drops even more. Those consuming 1,500 milligrams of sodium a day experience a greater drop in blood pressure than those who eat 3,300 milligrams (a typical American intake). An updated version of the DASH Diet—the OmniHeart study—removed the fat restriction and allowed more olive oil, creating a Mediterranean-style DASH diet with the same health benefits (Appel et al. 2005).

The DASH study points out that blood pressure is affected by more than just sodium intake. The same fruits, vegetables, whole grains, and low-fat dairy products and meats that optimize your sports diet can also optimize your health. Eating a potassium-rich diet seems to guard against hypertension. Potassium helps make arteries stronger and better able to withstand the blood vessel damage that can occur with aging. Calcium may also offset the effect of too much sodium in the diet. Refer to tables 1.2 and 1.3 for the potassium content of popular vegetables and fruits and table 1.5 for a list of calcium-rich foods.

DIET AND CANCER

In the United States, cancer is the second most frequent cause of death, following heart disease. Cancer isn't one disease, however; it is many. Each has its own high-risk groups, its own incidence and cure rates, and its own causes. Despite the gloomy news that two out of every five of us will get cancer, the encouraging news is that dietary changes can prevent perhaps one-third of cancer deaths. For example, people who eat at least five servings a day of fruits and vegetables have a 40 percent lower risk for certain cancers (lung, colon, stomach, esophagus, and mouth) compared with people who eat two or fewer servings of fruits and vegetables. A fruit-filled, high-fiber, cancer-protective diet is also a top-performance sports diet. Indulge in good health for high energy.

Protective Nutrients

One key to the role of diet in preventing cancer may lie in antioxidative capacity, or a nutrient's ability to deactivate harmful chemicals in the body known as free radicals. Free radicals are formed daily through normal body processes. Environmental pollutants such as cigarette smoke, automobile exhaust, radiation, and herbicides also generate free radical precursors. These unstable compounds can attack, infiltrate, and injure vital cell structures. Fortunately, our bodies have natural control systems that deactivate and minimize free radical reactions within the cells. These natural antioxidant control systems involve many vitamins and minerals.

Although researchers at one time hoped that high intakes of antioxidants from pills would reduce the incidence of some types of cancer, the current evidence is disappointing. Several large studies have shown few health benefits from supplemental antioxidants. The studies that drove the hope that antioxidants would protect against cancer came from people who ate lots of fruits and vegetables (and had higher blood levels of antioxidants). Most health professionals today emphasize the importance of obtaining these nutrients from food, not from supplements. Here are food options that might protect against cancer.

• **Carotenoids.** These precursors of vitamin A are found in plants and then converted into vitamin A in the body. Beta-carotene, as well as the more than 40 other carotenoids found in orange and green fruits and vegetables, helps prevent the formation of free radicals. Some of the best sources are carrots, spinach, sweet potatoes, kale, apricots, and cantaloupe. (If you eat too many carotene-rich vegetables and fruits, your skin can turn yellow. If that happens, cut back!)

• **Vitamin C.** This vitamin guards against harmful reactions within the cells. Some of the best sources are kiwi, citrus fruits, broccoli, green and red peppers, and strawberries. The body's tissues become saturated with vitamin C at about 200 milligrams a day, an amount easily attainable by eating the recommended 4 cups of fruits and vegetables.

• **Vitamin E.** Vitamin E protects the cell walls from free radical damage. Be sure to include foods rich in vitamin E when balancing your daily calorie budget, but consume them carefully because they are calorie dense. The best sources are vegetable oils (and foods made with them, such as salad dressings), almonds, peanuts, sunflower and sesame seeds, wheat germ, flax, and whole grains (table 2.3). The recommended dietary allowance (RDA) for vitamin E is 15 milligrams.

• **Selenium.** Selenium protects the cell walls from free radical damage and enhances the immune system's response, resulting in increased resistance to cancer growth. The best sources of selenium are seafood such as tuna fish, meats, eggs, milk, whole grains, and garlic. Supplements are not recommended because of the danger of toxicity with long-term supplementation over 200 micrograms.

Other cancer preventers include foods rich in fiber. Although population studies suggest that people who eat a lot of fiber from grains, fruits, and vegetables have a lower risk of cancer, scientists are unclear about whether the fiber is the protective nutrient. In addition to the known vitamins

TABLE 2.3 Vitamin E in Foods

Food	Portion	Vitamin E (mg)
Wheat germ, oil	1 tbsp	20
Sunflower seeds	1/4 cup (30 g)	8
Almonds	1/4 cup (30 g)	7
Wheat germ	1/4 cup (30 g)	5
Spinach, cooked	1 cup (180g)	4
Peanuts	1/4 cup (30 g)	3
Peanut butter	2 tbsp	3
Oil, canola	1 tbsp	3
Oil, olive	1 tbsp	2
Avocado	1/4 large (60 g)	2
Kale, cooked	1 cup (130 g)	2

Note: The RDA is 15 mg.

National Institutes of Health Office of Dietary Supplements, http://ods.od.nih.gov/factsheets/vitaminE-HealthProfessional (2018).

and minerals in grains, fresh fruits, and vegetables, these fiber-rich foods contain hundreds, perhaps thousands, of other lesser-known substances called phytochemicals that may protect your health. That's why you want to put more energy into eating a varied diet than into wondering which fiber to choose.

Cancer Prevention

To date, a few specific dietary components (alcohol, more than 18 ounces of red meat per week, processed meats such as hotdogs and bologna, possibly charred meat, and excess calories that lead to excess body fat) are strongly linked to a higher risk of cancer. Sometimes studies show an association with a higher (or lower) risk of cancer but association does not prove cause of cancer. For example, people who drink green tea may have a lower risk of cancer. Is that because of polyphenols in the tea? Or because tea drinkers have a healthier lifestyle?

Cancer (and other health problems) can be affected by not only your diet but also your lifestyle. Relaxation, peace of mind, a positive outlook on life, a contented spirit, absence of envy, love of mankind, and faith are powerful health-promoting factors without which optimal health cannot be achieved. A holistic approach to cancer prevention and health protection

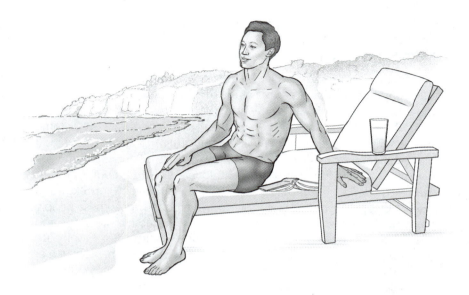

includes nourishing yourself with pleasant well-balanced meals, enjoying exercise as part of your daily routine, and taking time to smell the roses. Enjoying lots of broccoli, carrots, kale, sweet potatoes, and other colorful vegetables will do no harm, and no amount of supplementation will compensate for a stress-filled, health-eroding lifestyle. For people in recovery from cancer, the best outcomes come through honoring this healthy lifestyle approach, being physically active, and including conventional medical care (Johnson et al. 2018).

DIET AND DIABETES

An estimated 9.4 percent of the U.S. population has diabetes and another 34 percent have glucose levels high enough to be characterized as prediabetes (Centers for Disease Control and Prevention 2017). With the current epidemic of obesity that is plaguing the United States, a concurrent epidemic of diabetes is tagging alongside, not only in adults but also among children. Eating supersized fast foods and spending too much time in front of TV and computer screens instead of moving the body erodes health. Although one type of diabetes, insulin-dependent diabetes, is the result of the body's inability to produce adequate insulin to carry blood sugar into the cells, a second and more common type of diabetes, type 2, commonly occurs in people who are overweight and underfit. These

FACT OR FICTION

Eating lots of sugar causes diabetes.

The facts: Having excess body fat and being underfit are the big culprits that contribute to diabetes. In a study of 3,200 people (average age in the 50s) who were higher weight and had elevated blood glucose, both when fasting and after eating meals (a risk factor for diabetes), some of the subjects were given medicine (metformin) to lower their blood glucose. Others were instructed to exercise at least 150 minutes per week (five times a week for 30 minutes) and to lose weight (about 7 percent of their body weight, or about 11 lb for a 160-lb person, or 5 kg for a 73-kg person). And some were told to make no changes (these people made up the control group). The subjects who became more active and lost a little bit of weight dramatically reduced their risk of developing diabetes—by 58 percent. In contrast, the group that took medicine experienced a 31-percent drop during the almost three-year study (Knowler et al. 2002). By becoming active and staying active throughout your life, you'll greatly reduce your risk of developing adult-onset diabetes as well as other diseases of aging.

The best cure for diabetes is prevention. A balanced sports diet with even-sized meals eaten on a regular schedule can be a diabetes-preventing diet, particularly when it leads to an appropriate body weight. There's no need to eliminate carbohydrate; even people taking insulin can have 30 to 60 grams (120 to 240 calories) of carbohydrate per meal—or more, depending on how active they are. The trick is to spread them evenly throughout the day in the form of meals and snacks based on fruits, vegetables, whole grains, and wholesome starches (brown rice, quinoa, pinto beans) that are balanced with lean protein, low-fat dairy products, and healthy fats—as recommended in the *Dietary Guidelines for Americans*. For nonathletic people, a diet very low in sugars and starches may help control blood glucose levels, but the sustainability of such a restrictive eating style has yet to be determined by long-term studies. For more in-depth information about diabetes, see the resources in appendix A.

people need to lose weight, exercise more, get adequate sleep, and eat better-quality foods (or take medications). If not, the resulting high levels of blood glucose increase their risk of heart attacks, strokes, kidney disease, blindness, and limb amputation.

DIET AND BONE HEALTH

Bone health is determined by the building of strong bones in early life, followed by the rate of bone loss that comes with aging. Osteoporosis, or a thinning of the bones with aging, results in hunched backs and brittle bones; it is a serious health problem, particularly among older postmenopausal women. In a survey of more than 200,000 healthy women 50 years or older, 40 percent had osteopenia (reduced bone mass, the early stage of osteoporosis), and 7 percent had osteoporosis—and they didn't even know it. The women diagnosed with osteoporosis were four times more likely to fracture a bone within the next 12 months; those with osteopenia were almost two times more likely (Siris et al. 2001). Osteoporosis is also a major concern for men older than 70, so men need to take care of their bones in their earlier years as well. Cyclists and swimmers, because they participate in non-weight-bearing sports, also need to be concerned about their bone health.

Younger female athletes who have stopped having regular menstrual periods are at risk for low bone density that can develop into osteoporosis. Both amenorrheic and postmenopausal women lack adequate estrogen, a hormone that contributes to menstruation and helps maintain bone density. The good news is that osteoporosis is a preventable condition. It is not an inevitable result of old age. You can reduce your risk of developing osteoporosis by adopting a healthy lifestyle that avoids excessive alcohol and smoking and includes the following:

• **Calcium-rich diet.** A lifelong calcium-rich diet will help you build strong bones as well as maintain bone density by reducing the rate of calcium loss thereafter. To ensure the best protection, aim to consume 1,000 to 1,300 milligrams of calcium per day (see table 1.6). You should also consume 400 to 800 international units of vitamin D per day, which will help your body absorb the calcium you consume. If you are a parent, be sure your 11- to 14-year-old kids consume more milk than soda pop. Calcium is most important in the three years surrounding puberty and up to about age 30.

Unfortunately, the typical 25- to 40-year-old woman consumes only half the recommended intake of 1,000 milligrams of calcium. This may be one reason about 25 percent of women over 65 have osteoporosis (of whom 12 percent may die from medical complications of this condition). If you think taking calcium pills is the simple alternative to drinking milk, think again. Women who get their calcium from food sources tend to have stronger bones than those who rely on supplements (Napoli et al. 2007). Enjoying calcium-rich food at each meal (to evenly distribute your calcium intake throughout the day) can help you achieve the recommended intake. This is important not only for growing children but also for adults. As you get older, your body absorbs a smaller percentage of the calcium you consume.

- **Adequate protein.** Protein is important for bone health because it is an important structural component of bone. Some people have speculated a high protein diet weakens bones, purportedly by leaching calcium from bones to neutralize the acids generated by protein metabolism. While this may be a factor if the overall diet is low in calcium as well as fruits, vegetables, nuts, and seeds, which neutralize the acid, current research suggests that protein actually has a net positive effect. Protein strengthens bones by optimizing muscle mass. Muscle tugging on bones can improve bone density (Dolan and Sale 2018). See chapter 7 for information on adequate protein intake.

- **Regular exercise.** Participate in a regular exercise program that includes weight-bearing aerobic and muscle-building exercises. (If you are a swimmer or cyclist, you may want to cross-train by jogging, jumping rope, or doing other weight-bearing exercise to enhance bone strength.) Accompany these bone-strengthening exercises with adequate intakes of calcium, vitamin D, and protein.

- **Normal hormones.** Women with estrogen deficiencies have lower bone mineral densities despite high calcium intakes and participation in weight-bearing exercise programs. (That's one reason athletes with amenorrhea—absence of normal menses—are at high risk for stress fractures.) Athletes with amenorrhea commonly take the birth control pill, believing it will protect their bones, but research suggests that this may be ineffective (Gordon et al. 2017). The better bet for athletes with amenorrhea is to eat enough to support regular menses (see chapter 12 for more information).

- **Low sodium intake.** Because too much salt interferes with the retention of calcium (Sellmeyer, Schloetter, and Sebastian 2002), your best bet is to moderate your salt intake, especially if you have a genetic predisposition to osteoporosis.

Unfortunately, too many women follow too few of these guidelines. I once counseled a very thin 24-year-old group exercise leader with amenorrhea and the bones of a 60-year-old. She rarely drank milk (believing it to be a fattening fluid), ate a restrictive diet low in calories and protein, and was always trying to be thinner despite her obvious leanness.

Little did she know that her diet was contributing to the amenorrhea and that she was putting herself at risk of developing stress fractures, an early sign of poor bone health. She thought that exercise would keep her bones strong because she'd heard that exercise helps maintain bone density. Exercise does help, but calcium, estrogen, and adequate protein and calories are simultaneously essential.

Boosting Your Calcium Consumption

An excellent way to boost your calcium intake is to enjoy flavored milk (dairy or soy, chocolate, or vanilla) for a postworkout recovery food. You'll get not only calcium and vitamin D, but also fluid, electrolytes (including sodium), and high-quality protein. (See chapter 10 for more information about this popular recovery choice.) Note that almond and rice milks are really watery juices, and not dairy alternatives. Other than being fortified with calcium, they are nutrient poor. For example, almond milk offers only 1 gram of protein per 8 ounces (240 ml), as compared with 6 grams of protein in soy milk, and 8 grams in dairy milk.

Yogurt is a popular way to boost your calcium intake. Regular yogurt offers more calcium than milk (400 versus 300 mg per 8 oz, or 230 g); Greek yogurt has slightly less (230 mg.) Both contain probiotics—health-protective bacteria that boost your immune system and enhance digestion. When buying yogurt, look for "live and active cultures" on the label. Yogurt is especially helpful if you have had antibiotic treatment. Antibiotics kill both the good bacteria that live in your gut and the bad bacteria that cause health problems; yogurt helps replenish the good ones. The bacteria also digest most of the lactose (milk sugar) in yogurt, so many people who are lactose intolerant can enjoy yogurt as a milk alternative.

Because flavored yogurts can have a high sugar content—above and beyond the 12 grams of naturally occurring milk sugar in 8 ounces (240 ml) of milk—your best bet is to choose plain yogurt and add a teaspoon of honey or jam, or add plain yogurt to flavored yogurt. You'll come out way ahead in terms of sugar content. Remember, frozen yogurt has no active cultures and a high sugar content and marginal nutritional value. Don't fool yourself!

For athletes, yogurt is an easy-to-digest carbohydrate–protein combination that is a smart choice before and after exercise. A study of fatigued athletes suggests that those who regularly consumed yogurt had better immune function (Clancy et al. 2006). How about a postexercise fruit and yogurt smoothie?

Her doctor advised her to regain her menstrual period to protect her bone health. Because lack of menstruation is associated with inadequate nutrition, I recommended that she boost her energy intake by consuming more protein- and calcium-rich milk and yogurt. After two months of dietary improvements, she regained her menstrual period—a good step toward lifelong health. See chapters 12 and 17 and appendix A for more information about amenorrhea, relative energy deficiency in sport (RED-S), and osteoporosis.

FIBER FOR GOOD HEALTH

Fiber is a health-enhancing component that makes a carbohydrate "good." Fiber is found in foods such as whole grains, legumes, fruits, and vegetables. It is the part of plant cells that humans can't digest. Food processing—such as milling whole wheat into white flour and peeling skins—removes the fiber. So, to reach the target intake specified in the *2015-2020 Dietary Guidelines for Americans* of 25 to 38 grams of fiber per day (more specifically, 14 grams of fiber per 1,000 calories), try to eat foods in their natural state.

Fiber lowers blood cholesterol, promotes regular bowel movements, and improves blood sugar control. Fiber-rich foods form a strong foundation for a sports diet—as long as you don't eat too much fiber that leads to undesired "pit stops." Although it's difficult to tease out which health benefits are related to fiber and which to the other healthy components of fruits, vegetables, whole grains, beans, legumes, and nuts, you won't go wrong adding roughage to your diet.

Fiber was once thought to reduce the risk of colon cancer. Disappointing results from studies fail to show a protective benefit of fiber (Rock 2007). Yet, fiber's positive association with lowering the risk of heart disease, helping to control diabetes, aiding with weight control, and preventing and treating constipation offers more than enough reasons to stack your diet with fiber-rich foods. The health-protective microbes that live in your gut thrive on fiber.

You should try to eat a variety of fiber-rich foods daily because different foods offer different types of fiber with different health benefits. You should consume both of the two main types of fiber:

- **Insoluble fiber.** This type of fiber gives plants their structure. It does not dissolve in water. Common sources are wheat bran, vegetables, and whole grains. Insoluble fiber absorbs water, increases fecal bulk, and makes the stools easier to pass.

• **Soluble fiber.** This type of fiber forms a gel in water. It is found in oatmeal, barley, and kidney beans (as well as in pectin and guar gums, two fibers often added to foods and listed among the ingredients). Soluble fiber lowers blood cholesterol, particularly in people with elevated cholesterol. Soluble fiber can also help stabilize blood glucose levels, which is why fiber-rich snacks are a wise preexercise choice (assuming they settle comfortably

Fruits and Veggies Matter

No matter what your health concerns—preventing cancer, heart disease, diabetes, obesity, high blood pressure, whatever—the bottom-line message from every health organization (including the American Heart Association; the American Cancer Society; the National Heart, Lung and Blood Institute; and the USDA) is to eat more fruits and vegetables. Yet, more than 90 percent of Americans fail to consume the recommended amount.

Ideally, you should include a hefty portion of fruits or veggies in every meal and snack. Here are tips to help you boost your intake of these carbohydrate-rich foods that not only fuel your muscles but also protect your health:

• Whip together a fruit smoothie for breakfast: orange juice, mango, frozen berries.

• To your egg omelet, add diced peppers, tomato, and mushrooms.

• Add blueberries or sliced banana to pancakes; top with applesauce.

• No fresh fruit for your cereal? Use canned peaches, raisins, chopped dates, or frozen berries.

• Put leftover dinner veggies into your lunchtime salad or soup.

• Keep within easy reach grab-and-go snacks, such as small boxes of raisins, trail mix with dried fruit, frozen 100 percent fruit juice bars, cherry tomatoes, baby carrots, and celery sticks.

• Add shredded carrots to casseroles, chili, lasagna, meatloaf, or soup.

For additional tips and recipes using fruits and vegetables, see the recipes in part IV.

and don't make you "gas propelled"). Some sustaining preexercise snacks are oatmeal, lentil soup, and hummus, as tolerated.

You can increase your fiber intake to the 28 grams per 2,000 calories recommended by the *Dietary Guidelines for Americans* by taking the following actions:

- Enjoy fruits and vegetables at as many meals and snacks as possible.
- Choose a high-fiber cereal (with at least 5 grams of fiber per serving), or mix high- and low-fiber cereals. Top the cereal with berries and other fruits.
- Buy 100 percent whole-grain breads, cereals, and crackers with at least 2 grams of fiber per serving.
- Opt for brown rice, quinoa, farro, wheat berries, corn, and other whole grains.
- Add wheat germ, ground flaxseed, chia, nuts, or sesame seeds to yogurt, cereals, and baked goods.
- Eat more beans—in chili, sprinkled on salads, mixed with rice, made into hummus, and added to soups.
- Snack on popcorn (homemade air popped or using canola oil) or dried fruits and nuts.
- Read food labels. Unexpected foods, such as some brands of orange juice and yogurt, have added fiber.

The information in table 2.4 can help you choose the foods richest in fiber.

FACT OR FICTION

Fiber hastens the time it takes for food to pass through your system.

The facts: Fiber can increase fecal weight and the number of trips to the bathroom, but it usually does not increase transit time. Transit time varies for each person, but it normally averages between two and four days. This varies according to stress, exercise, and diet. Your best bet as an active person is to determine the right combination of fiber-rich foods that promotes regular bowel movements. You may need to restrict your fiber intake if exercise itself becomes a powerful bowel stimulant. See chapter 9 for more information on gut issues.

TABLE 2.4 Fiber in Foods

Cereal	Fiber (g)	Grain	Fiber (g)
Fiber One	14	Quinoa, 1 cup	5
All-Bran Extra Fiber, 1/2 cup	13	Popcorn, 3 cups	5
All-Bran, 1/2 cup	10	Brown rice, 1 cup	5
Kashi Go Lean, 1 cup	10	Triscuits, 7	4
Raisin Bran, Kellogg's, 1 cup	7	Multigrain bread, 1 slice	2
Cheerios, 1 cup	3	Spaghetti, 1 cup	2
Oatmeal, instant, Quaker, 1 packet	3	White rice, 1 cup	1
Vegetables	**Fiber (g)**	**Fruits**	**Fiber (g)**
Potato, 1 large with skin	7	Pear, 1 medium with skin	6
Brussels sprouts, 1 cup	4	Apple, 1 medium with skin	4
Spinach, 1 cup	4	Blueberries, 1 cup	4
Peas, 1/2 cup	4	Orange, 1 medium	3
Carrot, 1 medium	2	Banana, 1 medium	3
Corn, 1/2 cup	2	Kiwi, 1 medium	2
Lettuce, 1 cup	1	Raisins, 1/4 cup	2
Legumes	**Fiber (g)**	**Nuts and seeds**	**Fiber (g)**
Lentils, boiled, 1/2 cup	8	Flaxseed, 1 tbsp	3
Chickpeas, canned, 1/2 cup	7	Almonds, 1 oz (~23)	3
Kidney beans, canned, 1/2 cup	6	Peanut butter, 2 tbsp	2
Edamame, shelled 1/2 cup	5	Cashews, 1 oz (~18)	1

Data from USDA National Nutrient Database for Standard Reference (2018).

TO YOUR GOOD HEALTH

Whether you want to reduce your risk of cancer, heart disease, high blood pressure, or diabetes, health professionals agree that your best bet is a diet rich in fruits, vegetables, whole grains, and dairy products; moderate in lean protein; and reduced in sodium (fewer processed foods). So please, think twice before you dig your grave with your knife and fork. Keep in mind these basic messages:

- Plan one or two fruits or vegetables into every meal. Breakfast can easily include orange juice and a banana; lunch, a handful of baby carrots and an apple; dinner, a double portion of mixed vegetables.

- Boost your intake of "good fat" (within your calorie budget) by choosing olive and canola oils for cooking and salads. Enjoy more avocado, nuts, and nut butters.
- Enjoy smaller portions of lean meats and larger portions of beans and legumes (see chapter 7).
- By combining the best food choices with a regular exercise program, you can invest in your future well-being. Although genetics does play a strong role in heart disease, cancer, hypertension, and osteoporosis, you can help put the odds in your favor by eating wisely. As Hippocrates said, "Let food be thy medicine."

CHAPTER 3

BREAKFAST: THE KEY TO A SUCCESSFUL SPORTS DIET

Just as your car works better when it has fuel in its tank, your body and your brain work better when you give them adequate morning fuel. Yet, many people push their bodies through a busy day with empty fuel tanks. This is counter to your circadian rhythms and how you were designed to function. Food affects the internal clock that controls your circadian rhythms. Skipping breakfast, restricting daytime food, and eating in chaotic patterns disrupt normal biological rhythms. The result is low energy, cravings for sugary foods, a high intake of sweets and treats, and often-undesired weight gain—to say nothing of development of cardio-vascular disease, type 2 diabetes, and obesity (St-Onge et al. 2017). In this day and age of breakfast skippers, there remains little doubt in my mind that eating evenly spaced meals throughout the day—starting at breakfast—is important for your health and well-being, as well as your athletic performance. Eat up!

DON'T SKIP BREAKFAST

Of all the nutrition mistakes you might make, skipping breakfast is the biggest. Raiya, an early-morning exerciser at her local YMCA, learned this the hard way: She collapsed from low blood sugar after one of her morning workouts. She managed to struggle through the hour-long spin class (stationary cycling) but felt very light headed and dizzy, and she ended up in a heap on the floor, surrounded by the other frightened exercisers. She had blacked out because she had no fuel to feed her brain.

Raiya's story is a dramatic example of how skipping breakfast can hinder a morning workout. In comparison, a high-energy breakfast sets the stage for a high-energy day, with better recovery for morning exercisers and better workouts for afternoon exercisers (Clayton et al. 2015). Nevertheless, many active people come up with familiar excuses for skipping the morning meal:

I'm not hungry in the morning.

I don't have time.

I don't like breakfast foods.

I'm on a diet.

If I eat breakfast, I feel hungrier all day.

Excuses, excuses. If you skip breakfast, you're likely to concentrate less effectively in the late morning, work or study less efficiently, feel irritable and short tempered, or fall short of energy for your afternoon workout. If you are a breakfast-skipping parent, your kids are more likely to skip breakfast, too, and the result is more snacking, irregular eating patterns, and a poorer-quality diet—all of which can have a negative influence on their (and your) energy and weight (Affenito 2007). Plus, they likely won't be able to concentrate as well in the class before lunch (Wesnes, Pincock, and Scholey 2012). For every flimsy excuse to skip breakfast, there's an even better reason to eat it.

No Morning Appetite

If you are not hungry for breakfast, you probably ate too many calories the night before. I often counsel athletes who eat a huge dinner at 9:00 p.m., mindlessly munch through a bag of chips while watching TV at night, or devour a bedtime bowl of ice cream as their reward for having survived a busy day. These snacks can certainly curb a morning appetite. Unfortunately for your health, when evening snacks replace a wholesome breakfast, you can end up with an inadequate sports diet.

Mark, a 35-year-old computer programmer and runner, wasn't hungry for breakfast for another reason: His morning workout killed his appetite. However, by 10:00 a.m. his appetite came to life again. He'd try to hold off until lunchtime, but he raided the candy machine three out of five workdays. I recommended that Mark keep breakfast foods at work—energy bars, trail mix, packets of instant oatmeal. These nonperishable foods would be ready and waiting for a hassle-free yet nourishing meal.

For morning exercisers, a wholesome breakfast that combines carbohydrate with protein—cereal with milk, granola with Greek yogurt, toast with banana and peanut butter—promptly replaces the depleted glycogen stores and helps refuel and heal the muscles so they'll be refreshed for the next training session. The sooner you eat, the more quickly you'll recover. For more information on refueling after exercise, see chapter 10.

A recovery breakfast is particularly important if you do two workouts per day. I often talk with triathletes who say they're not yet hungry for breakfast after the first workout. They then skimp at lunchtime, afraid that a substantial meal might interfere with their afternoon workout. They end up dragging themselves through a poor training session. In this situation, I recommend eating breakfast, brunch, or an early lunch around 10:00 or 11:00. The food will be adequately digested in time to fuel the muscles that afternoon. If you feel thirsty but not hungry, refreshing liquids throughout the morning, such as apple cider, chocolate milk, or smoothies, can help refuel you as well as quench your thirst. You'll discover that you have more energy and a better second workout.

You Do Have Time for Breakfast

I just don't have time to eat breakfast. I get up at 5:30, go to the rink, skate for an hour, then dash to school by 7:45.

Obviously, this ice hockey player's morning schedule didn't allow him to relax and enjoy a leisurely meal. However, Nick still needed the energy to tackle his high school classes. I reminded Nick that breakfast doesn't have to be a sit-down, cooked meal. It can be a substantial snack after hockey practice while riding to school. I advised him to plan and prepare a

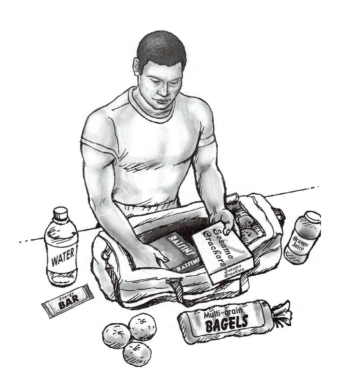

breakfast-to-go the night before. If he could make time to train for hockey, he could make time to eat right for training.

Nick discovered that his "duffle-bag breakfast" was indeed worth the effort. Two peanut butter and raisin sandwiches and a bottle of grape juice satisfied his ravenous appetite and improved his ability to concentrate at school. No longer did he sit in class counting the minutes until lunch and listening to his stomach grumble. Rather, he was able to concentrate on his class work and even improve his grades.

Maria, a nurse who was training for her first marathon, had the same excuse of no time for breakfast. She'd rise at 6:00 and be at the hospital by 6:45; she didn't want to eat breakfast at that early hour, claiming her stomach was not awake. However, by her break time at 10:00, she'd be grumpy, unable to focus on her work, and ravenously looking for doughnuts or cookies in the nurses' station.

I recommended that Maria eat something nutritious between 7:00 and 9:00 to curb the overwhelming 10:00 a.m. hunger that interfered with her ability to concentrate and be pleasant to her patients. Maria made the effort to do one of the following every day:

- Bring overnight oats to work to eat within four hours of waking. (See Oatmeal Suggestions in chapter 18.)
- Buy a bagel, egg, and cheese sandwich at the coffee shop.
- Take an earlier break and enjoy a hot breakfast at the cafeteria.
- Keep emergency food in her desk drawer: graham crackers, peanut butter, dried fruit.

She soon became a breakfast advocate, feeling so much better when well fueled rather than half starved.

If you lack creative quick-fix breakfast ideas, the following food choices can help you make a fast break to becoming a regular breakfast eater:

- **Yogurt.** Keep your refrigerator well stocked; add cereal and chopped nuts for crunch.
- **Banana.** Eat an extra-large one, spread with nut butter and chased by a large glass of milk.
- **Fruit smoothie.** Whip together juice or milk, frozen fruit, and dried milk (or protein powder) and pour it into a travel mug. (See chapter 25 for smoothie ideas.)
- **Trail mix.** Combine almonds, granola, and chopped dates (or any dried fruit), and prepack the mix in small plastic bags that you can tuck in your pocket.

- **Whole-wheat bagel.** Slap on two slices of cheese; then wash it down with orange juice.
- **Graham crackers.** Enjoy them as a crunchy "peanut butter sandwich" along with a latte made with low-fat milk.
- **Wrap.** Stuff it with hummus, cheese, sliced turkey, or other handy fillings.

BREAKFAST FOR DIETERS

Everyone who wants to lose weight knows that diets start at breakfast, right? Not so fast! Skipping breakfast to save calories can be an unsuccessful approach to weight loss. Some research suggests that dieters who skip breakfast tend to gain weight over time (Neumark-Sztainer et al. 2006). Other research suggests eating breakfast might contribute to weight gain for the average (non-athletic) person (Sievert 2018). I invite athletes to remember, if you are tempted to save calories by skimping on breakfast, you don't gain weight by eating this meal. You do gain weight if you skip breakfast, get too hungry (as can easily happen with people who exercise), and then overindulge at night. If you are going to skip a meal, skip dinner, not breakfast. Your goal should be to fuel by day and eat a little less at

FACT OR FICTION

Eating chocolate cake for breakfast will make you fat.

The facts: According to researcher Daniela Jakubowicz and colleagues (2012), routinely eating 300 calories of chocolate cake (or another dessert) along with 300 calories of wholesome breakfast foods might actually help you lose weight! She studied 193 obese, nondiabetic adults who ate either a 300-calorie low-carbohydrate breakfast or a 600-calorie breakfast that included protein plus chocolate cake (or another sweet dessert). Both groups were instructed to eat the same daily total amount of calories: 1,400 for the women and 1,600 for the men. By 32 weeks, the cake eaters had lost about 20 pounds (9 kg) more than their peers because they were better able to adhere to the diet plan.

Jakubowicz noticed that those who had cake for breakfast had fewer cravings for carbohydrate and sweets later in the day. By front-loading their calories, they were less hungry and less likely to stray from their food plans. They had curbed their cravings for sweets and treats, in comparison to those who ate the smaller breakfast.

night so that you lose weight when you are sleeping and not when you need to be fully functioning.

A survey of almost 3,000 dieters who lost more than 30 pounds (14 kg) and kept it off for at least a year reported that 78 percent of the dieters ate breakfast every day, and 88 percent ate breakfast five or more days a week. Only 4 percent reported never eating breakfast. The breakfast eaters also reported being slightly more active during the day. This study suggests that breakfast is indeed an important part of a successful weight-loss program (Wyatt et al. 2002). You can't go wrong with eating breakfast!

Time and again I advise dieters to fuel during the day and eat less at night. Time and again they look at me with fear in their eyes. As Pat, an at-home mom who wanted to lose weight, explained, "If I eat breakfast, I get hungrier and seem to eat more the whole day." Her breakfast was only two hard-boiled eggs, enough to get the digestive juices flowing, but not enough to satisfy her appetite. When she ate a substantial 500-calorie breakfast (1 1/2 english muffins with 2 eggs scrambled with a half cup of cottage cheese), she felt fine and didn't overindulge later in the afternoon. If you eat *enough calories* at breakfast, you will not be hungrier—especially if the breakfast contains 20 to 30 grams of protein (e.g., eggs plus cottage cheese). Although she initially couldn't believe that 500-calorie breakfasts would help her lose weight, she discovered that they did. Table 3.1 offers a few examples of 500-calorie breakfasts.

TABLE 3.1 500-Calorie Breakfasts

Food	Calories
BREAKFAST ON THE RUN	
Bagel, medium large	300
Peanut butter, 2 tbsp	200
Total	**500**
NONTRADITIONAL BREAKFAST	
2 slices of cheese pizza	500
Total	**500**
DESK-DRAWER BREAKFAST	
Instant oatmeal, 2 packets	250
Raisins, 1 small box (1.5 oz, or 45 g)	130
Almonds, 17	120
Total	**500**

CEREAL: A BREAKFAST FOR CHAMPIONS

My clients commonly ask what I recommend for breakfast. In general, my answer is any combination of wholesome choices from at least three, if not four, food groups. More specifically, my answer is cereal because it's a simple way to get four types of foods—whole grains, low-fat milk, nuts, and fruit—plus a host of other benefits. By eating a bowl of whole-grain cereal topped with fruit, you can get half of the recommended daily fruit and whole-grain servings before you even get out of your pajamas. Add a side of protein for greater satiety (hard-boiled eggs, cottage cheese, nuts, Greek yogurt).

What's So Great About Cereal?

I'm big on cereals because they have all of these positive characteristics:

- **Quick and easy.** People of all ages and cooking abilities can easily pour cereal into a bowl—no cooking or messy cleanup.
- **Convenient.** By simply stocking the cupboard, gym bag, or desk drawer, you can have a breakfast ready for the morning rush. A plastic bag of dry cereal is better than nothing. Toss in a handful of chopped walnuts and some dried cranberries, and you have a balanced meal—with no cooking or blending!
- **Rich in carbohydrate from whole grains.** Your muscles need carbohydrate for energy. Whole-grain cereal, a banana, and juice contribute nutrient-rich carbohydrates; milk offers a protein accompaniment. To boost the protein value of your carbohydrate-based cereal breakfast, add nuts, Greek yogurt, or one to two (hard boiled) eggs on the side, as desired.
- **Rich in fiber.** When you select bran and whole-grain cereals, you reduce your risk of becoming constipated, an inconvenience that can certainly interfere with your enjoyment of exercise. Fiber also has protective qualities that may reduce your risk of heart disease as well as curb your appetite and assist with weight loss.

    Bran cereals can provide far more fiber than most fruits and vegetables. High-fiber cereals with at least 5 grams of fiber per ounce (30 g) include Kashi Good Friends, All-Bran, Fiber One, Raisin Bran, Oat Bran, Bran Flakes, and any of the multitudes of cereals with *bran* or *fiber* in the name (table 3.2). You can also boost the fiber content of any cereal by simply sprinkling Kashi, All-Bran, or Fiber

TABLE 3.2 Nutritional Value in Commonly Eaten Cereals

Cereal	Amount	Calories	Sugar (g)	Folic acid (%DV*)	Fiber (g)	Sodium (mg)	Iron (%DV)
All-Bran Original	1/2 cup	80	6	50	10	80	25
Cap'n Crunch	3/4 cup	110	12	25	1	200	25
Cheerios	1 cup	100	1	50	3	160	45
Bran Flakes, Trader Joe's	3/4 cup	100	6	35	5	220	45
Corn Flakes, Kellogg's	1 cup	100	3	30	1	200	45
Fiber One	1/2 cup	60	0	25	14	105	25
Fruit Loops	1 cup	110	9	25	3	170	25
Frosted Flakes	3/4 cup	110	11	25	< 1	140	25
Frosted Mini-Wheats	21 biscuits	190	11	25	6	0	90
Golden Grahams	3/4 cup	120	10	25	2	140	25
Grape-Nuts	1/2 cup	200	5	50	7	290	90
Great Grains	3/4 cup	210	13	25	4	135	50
Honey Nut Cheerios	3/4 cup	110	9	50	2	160	25
Kashi Go Lean**	1 cup	140	6	0	10	85	10
Kashi Heart to Heart**	3/4 cup	120	5	0	5	85	10
Life Original	3/4 cup	120	6	100	2	160	50
Muesli, Alpen**	2/3 cup	210	8	0	6	15	15
Oatmeal Flakes, Trader Joe's	3/4 cup	110	7	50	3	190	50
Puffins**	3/4 cup	90	5	0	5	190	2
Quaker Oatmeal Squares	1 cup	210	9	100	5	190	90
Quaker 100% Natural**	1/2 cup	210	15	0	3	25	6
Raisin Bran, Kellogg's	1 cup	190	18	25	7	250	25
Rice Krispies	1 1/4 cup	130	4	50	< 1	190	50
Special K	1 cup	120	4	100	< 1	220	45
Total	3/4 cup	100	5	100	3	140	100
Wheaties	3/4 cup	100	4	100	3	190	45

*Daily value

**All natural, no added vitamins or minerals

Nutrition information from food labels, November 2018.

One on it, as well as chopped nuts, ground flaxseed, sunflower seeds, or chia seeds.

- **Rich in iron.** Vegetarians take note: By selecting fortified or enriched brands, you can easily boost your iron intake and reduce your risk of becoming anemic. Choose a brand that supplies at least 25 percent of the daily value (see table 3.2). Enjoy berries or another source of vitamin C with the cereal to enhance iron absorption from the cereal.

  If you prefer all-natural or organic cereals with no additives, remember that "no additives" means there is no iron added, as is often the case with Kashi, Puffins, granola, Shredded Wheat, puffed rice, and other all-natural brands. If you like, you can mix all-natural cereals with iron-enriched varieties (e.g., granola with Cheerios, Shredded Wheat with Wheat Chex), or you can choose iron-rich foods at other meals or take an iron supplement.

- **Rich in folic acid.** Folic acid is associated with a lower risk of certain types of birth defects. This B vitamin is found in only small amounts in grains but in higher amounts (100 to 400 micrograms, 25 to 100 percent of the daily value) in fortified foods such as breakfast cereals.

- **Rich in calcium.** Cereal is rich in calcium when it's eaten with low-fat milk or yogurt or calcium-fortified soy milk. Women and children in particular (but also men) benefit from this calcium booster that helps maintain strong bones and protects against osteoporosis. Plant-based milks are calcium fortified, but they commonly lack protein; the more nourishing nondairy alternative is soy milk.

Choose Wholesome Cereals

By "wholesome cereals," I mean those with sugar not listed among the first ingredients. (Ingredients are listed by order of weight, from most to least.) By reading the Nutrition Facts on box labels, you can learn the amount of sugar in a cereal. Simply multiply the grams of *Added Sugars* (listed under Total Carbohydrate) by 4 calories per gram to determine the calories of sugar per serving. Quaker Oatmeal Squares, for example, has brown sugar and sugar listed as the third and fourth ingredients. A 1-cup serving contains 9 grams of sugar (9 g sugar × 4 cal/g = 36 cal) in 210 calories. That means that about 17 percent of the calories are from added sugar.

(continued)

Given that 10 percent of daily calories can appropriately come from sugar, the 9 grams (36 calories) of sugar in Oatmeal Squares could certainly fit into your day's 200- to 300-calorie sugar budget. Sugar is a carbohydrate that fuels the muscles; it doesn't poison them. I invite you to focus more on a cereal's fiber and whole-grain content than on its sugar content. The overall healthfulness of a breakfast cereal can outweigh those few nutritionally empty sugar calories (figure 3.1).

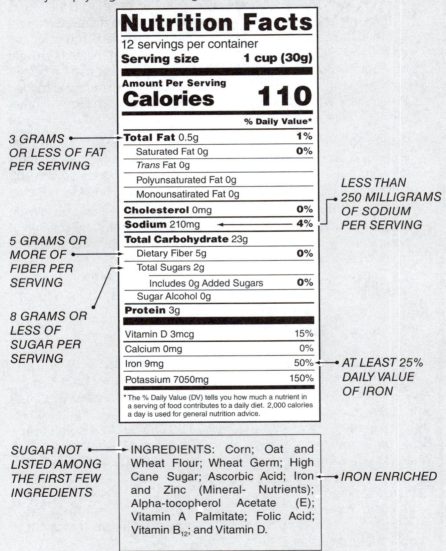

3 GRAMS OR LESS OF FAT PER SERVING

LESS THAN 250 MILLIGRAMS OF SODIUM PER SERVING

5 GRAMS OR MORE OF FIBER PER SERVING

8 GRAMS OR LESS OF SUGAR PER SERVING

AT LEAST 25% DAILY VALUE OF IRON

SUGAR NOT LISTED AMONG THE FIRST FEW INGREDIENTS

IRON ENRICHED

INGREDIENTS: Corn; Oat and Wheat Flour; Wheat Germ; High Cane Sugar; Ascorbic Acid; Iron and Zinc (Mineral- Nutrients); Alpha-tocopherol Acetate (E); Vitamin A Palmitate; Folic Acid; Vitamin B₁₂; and Vitamin D.

FIGURE 3.1 Check the Nutrition Facts label of your favorite cereals for these key elements. If it doesn't meet the criteria, combine it with others to achieve a healthy mix.

- **A good balance of carbs plus protein.** An effective sports breakfast offers three times more carbohydrate than protein. (Think 60 grams of carbohydrate to fuel muscles plus 20 grams of protein to build and repair muscles.) Raisin bran plus milk plus two eggs, or granola plus Greek yogurt plus berries can do a great job.

- **Versatile.** Rather than becoming bored by always eating the same brand, try mixing cereals to concoct endless varieties of flavors. I typically have 6 to 10 varieties in my cupboard. My friends laugh when they discover this impressive stockpile. I further vary the flavors by adding different mix-ins, such as diced apricots, dried blueberries, slivered almonds, chia, ground flax, pumpkin seeds, cinnamon, nutmeg, maple syrup, or vanilla extract.

OTHER POWER BREAKFASTS

Cereal may be a breakfast of champions, but it's not the only one. For you non-cereal eaters, rest assured that other breakfasts can fuel you for a high-energy day. See the recipes in part IV for wholesome breakfast breads and muffins you might want to enjoy with a glass of milk and fruit or 100-percent fruit juice.

For weight management, a high-protein breakfast can provide lasting advantages. Research indicates that people who ate a protein-rich breakfast (containing eggs) consumed fewer calories at dinner compared with those who had cornflakes with milk or a croissant and orange juice (Fallaize et al. 2012). Perhaps that's why Dimitri, a businessman and former collegiate soccer player, easily lost 20 pounds (9 kg) of fat when he started eating dinner-size portions of chicken, fish, and lean steak for breakfast along with a big bowl of fruit salad and whole-wheat toast. He then enjoyed cereal for dinner (and ate a colorful salad at lunch, to get his veggies for the day).

Breakfast To Go

If you are destined to eat breakfast at a quick-service restaurant, be sure to make wise food choices.

- Rather than highly processed bacon, sausage, croissant, or biscuit combinations, choose the egg and english muffin or wrap. Oatmeal, whole-wheat pancakes, cold cereal, veggie omelet with a side of potato, bagels (with peanut butter), english muffins, and fruit–yogurt–granola parfaits are other options.

- Because fresh fruits can be hard to find on the menu, remember to tuck an apple or orange into your pocket. Or, take a big swig of 100-percent fruit juice before you leave home.

- Treat yourself to a latte (with milk), instead of coffee with cream, for more protein and calcium.
- Find a deli with fresh bagels, fruit, juice, and yogurt.
- Skip the breakfast temptations (doughnuts, croissants) and bring a box of whole-grain cereal, slivered almonds, and craisins to the office. On your way to work, pick up some milk, along with your coffee, if desired. If you are traveling and staying at a hotel, you can save yourself time, money, and temptation by bringing your own cereal and dried fruit (and spoon). Bring powdered milk, or buy a small container of milk at the corner store. A water glass or milk carton can double as a cereal bowl.

Creative Breakfasts

If you skip breakfast because you don't like breakfast foods, just eat something else. Who said you have to eat cereal or toast? Any food you eat at other times of the day can be eaten at breakfast. I happen to love leftover pizza or Chinese food for a morning change of pace.

Maximizing Protein at Breakfast

For athletes who want to optimize muscle mass, the goal is to consume at least 20 grams of protein every three to four hours. The same goes for athletes who want to lose weight. Protein is satisfying and can curb the urge to snack. Here's how to add about 20 grams of protein to your breakfast:

- 3 eggs
- 3 cheese sticks or 3 ounces (90 g) low-fat cheese
- 3 to 4 ounces (90 to 120 g) deli ham or turkey
- 6 ounces (180 g) Greek yogurt
- 3/4 to 1 cup (240 g) cottage cheese

To create a protein-rich breakfast, include eggs scrambled with (cottage) cheese, Greek yogurt with high-protein granola, a fruit smoothie made with Greek yogurt, or yes, a side of last night's leftover chicken along with your bowl of cereal. See chapter 18 for additional protein-rich breakfast ideas, including high-protein oatmeal pancakes and protein-packed scrambled eggs.

You might even want to eat most of your treats at breakfast. One of my clients learned that by enjoying a chocolate croissant in the morning, she killed her desire for sweets the rest of the day. No longer did she want cookies for an afternoon snack. Rather, she enjoyed the bowl of cereal that seemed humdrum at 8:00 a.m.

Your goal is to eat one-quarter to one-third of your daily calories in the morning. Some acceptable choices are planned leftovers from dinner, a baked or microwaved (sweet) potato with cottage cheese, a peanut butter and honey sandwich, a yogurt "sundae" with sliced fruit and sunflower seeds, tomato soup with crackers, avocado toast with a hard-boiled egg, or even special holiday foods. Why not occasionally enjoy for breakfast a fun treat such as leftover birthday cake or Thanksgiving pie? You're better off eating them during the day and burning off their calories than holding off until evening, when you may succumb to overconsumption in a moment of weakness. The bottom line is that any breakfast is better than no breakfast, a bigger breakfast is preferable to a skimpy breakfast, and a hearty breakfast that includes wholesome grains, nuts, protein, and fruit or veggies is best for your health and performance.

COFFEE: THE MORNING EYE-OPENER

Coffee is a universally loved morning beverage. Every culture the world around enjoys some type of caffeinated beverage, be it tea in England and China, espresso in Italy, or a "coffee regular" in the United States. The average American consumes about 200 milligrams of caffeine per day, the equivalent of 10 to 12 ounces—a large mug, or 300 to 360 ml—of coffee.

FACT FOR FICTION

Coffee will raise your blood pressure, increase your risk of cancer, and increase your risk of heart disease.

The facts: Whether you drink caffeinated coffee or decaf, you are likely to live longer than coffee abstainers (Floegel et al. 2012). The health-protective benefits come not from the caffeine but from compounds in the coffee bean, such as polyphenols or magnesium. To date, no obvious negative connection has been made between caffeine and heart disease, cancer, or blood pressure. On the positive side, coffee drinkers might actually have a lower risk of diabetes and Parkinson's disease. And we know that preexercise coffee can enhance athletic performance (see chapter 9).

About 10 percent of Americans ingest more than 1,000 milligrams of caffeine per day and sustain themselves on the cream and sugar in coffee (plus a few cigarettes alongside). For them, heart disease is indeed more common—and linked to the poor diet and unhealthy lifestyle.

In addition to smokers, those who should abstain from caffeine are ulcer patients and others prone to stomach distress. (Caffeine stimulates gastric secretions and may cause "coffee stomach.") Athletes with anemia should also avoid a high intake of caffeine. Substances in coffee and tea can interfere with the absorption of iron. If you have anemia and routinely drink coffee or tea with meals or up to one hour after a meal, you might be cheating yourself nutritionally. A cup of coffee consumed with a hamburger can reduce by about 40 percent the absorption of the hamburger's iron. However, drinking caffeinated beverages up to an hour before eating seems to have no negative effect on iron absorption.

The biggest health worries about coffee have to do with the following habits surrounding that beverage:

- Adding cream or coffee whiteners containing hydrogenated (saturated) fat that contributes to heart disease. At least switch to milk or powdered milk for whitening your coffee.
- Drinking coffee instead of eating a wholesome breakfast. A large coffee with two creamers and two sugars contains 70 nutritionally empty calories. Multiply that by three mugs, and you could have had a nourishing bowl of cereal for the same number of calories. Table 3.3 provides the fat content of common coffee beverages. Many people who say they "live on coffee" could easily drink much less if they ate a satisfying breakfast and lunch. Food is better fuel than caffeine.
- Drinking coffee to stay alert. A good night's sleep might be a better investment. You could also try drinking a tall glass of ice water to perk yourself up. Sometimes dehydration contributes to fatigue.

Questions abound about the role of coffee in a healthy diet. Here are answers to commonly asked questions.

What does coffee do to my body?

The caffeine in coffee is a mild stimulant that increases the activity of the central nervous system. Hence, caffeine helps you stay alert and enhances mental focus. Caffeine's stimulant effect peaks in about one hour and then declines as the liver breaks down the caffeine. If you are an occasional coffee drinker, you'll tend to be more sensitive to caffeine's stimulant effects than the daily coffee consumer who has developed a tolerance to caffeine.

TABLE 3.3 Gulp! It's a Calorie Cafe!

Think twice before routinely ordering a speciality coffee. Those liquid calories count!

Beverage	Calories	Fat (g)
Dunkin black coffee 16 oz (480 ml)	5	0
Dunkin Iced coffee with cream and sugar, 16 oz (480 ml)	120	6
Dunkin Caramel Swirl Iced Coffee, 16 oz (480 ml)	170	6
Dunkin Coffee Coolatta with skim milk, 16 oz (480 ml)	280	0
Dunkin Mocha Swirl Coolatta with cream, 16 oz (480 ml)	630	22
Dunkin Strawberry Fruit Coolatta, 16 oz (480 ml)	300	0
Starbucks Vanilla Chai, 12 oz (360 ml)	200	5
Starbucks Hot chocolate with whole milk, 12 oz (360 ml)	280	10
Starbucks Caffe Mocha with skim milk, 12 oz (360 ml)	250	9
Starbucks Strawberry Smoothie, 24 oz (720 ml)	300	2
Starbucks Latte with whole milk, 12 oz (360 ml)	180	9
Starbucks Latte with skim milk, 12 oz (360 ml)	100	0
Starbucks Coffee Frappuccino, 12 oz (360 ml)	180	2.5
Starbucks Coffee Frappuccino, 24 oz (720 ml)	350	5
Starbucks Java Chip Frappuccino with whipped cream, 16 oz (480 ml)	470	18
Starbucks Matcha Green Tea Frappuccino with whole milk, 16 oz (480 ml)	430	16

Nutrition information from www.dunkindonuts.com and www.starbucks.com, November 2018

Although a little coffee offers enjoyable benefits of alertness, enhanced performance, and a happier mood, if you drink too much coffee, you start to experience adverse effects: caffeine jitters, acid stomach, and anxiety. Drinking more than 32 ounces (1 L) of coffee or 64 ounces (2 L) of tea per day is pushing the limits of "reasonable intake" (CSPI 2006b).

Do people get addicted to coffee?

Although coffee has been a popular beverage for centuries, its sustained popularity fails to classify it as "addictive." Coffee is not associated with the behaviors found with hard drugs (such as a need for more and more coffee, antisocial behavior, and severe difficulty stopping consumption). If you are a regular coffee drinker who decides to cut coffee out of your diet, you may develop headaches, fatigue, or drowsiness. The solution is to gradually decrease your caffeine intake rather than eliminate coffee cold turkey. And be aware, if you should get a headache caused by caffeine withdrawal, that caffeine-containing medicines such as Anacin and Excedrin will foil your efforts to reduce your caffeine intake.

Switching to tea reduces caffeine intake. Other ways to reduce your caffeine include drinking more of the following caffeine-free alternatives: decaffeinated coffee, decaffeinated tea, green and herbal teas, hot water with a lemon wedge, low-sodium broth or bouillon, hot cocoa, Ovaltine, other hot milk-based drinks, mulled cider, and hot cranberry or apple juice. Without a doubt, the best caffeine-free alternative to an eye-opening cup of coffee is exercise. A quick walk and fresh air might be far more effective than a cup of brew.

How much caffeine is in espresso?

Ounce for ounce, espresso is about twice as strong as coffee (35 versus 17 mg of caffeine per oz—but a Starbucks gourmet espresso has 65 mg of caffeine per oz). Because a serving of espresso is small, however, you end up with less caffeine: 35 to 65 milligrams from one shot (1 ounce) of espresso versus 135 milligrams from an 8-ounce (240 ml) cup of standard coffee.

Are there concerns about women who consume caffeine?

Pregnant women should prudently limit their caffeine to less than 300 milligrams per day (less than 15 oz, or 445 ml, of coffee). Caffeine readily crosses the placenta and, in excess, may be associated with premature birth. Women who are breastfeeding should also limit their intake. Caffeine crosses into breast milk and can make babies agitated and poor sleepers. Women who are trying to get pregnant might want to limit their caffeine intake to less than 200 or 300 milligrams of caffeine a day. Women who are worried about getting osteoporosis may have heard

FACT OR FICTION

Coke and Pepsi are loaded with caffeine.

The facts: A 12-ounce (360 ml) can of cola averages 35 to 50 milligrams of caffeine. This is far less than the typical 12-ounce mug of coffee, which averages 200 milligrams of caffeine. Even Red Bull has "only" 80 milligrams of caffeine per 8.4-ounce can. The real kick from soft drinks and energy drinks comes from sugar, not caffeine.

that caffeine is linked to low bone density. They can address that issue by adding more milk to their coffee or enjoying lattes to boost calcium intake to the recommended level.

If I drink too much alcohol, will coffee help me sober up?

No. This is a common misconception. Coffee will just make you a wide-awake drunk. Coffee does not speed the time needed for the liver to detoxify alcohol. But coffee does get some water into your body, and that can have a positive effect, but you will still need a designated driver.

Does coffee count toward my daily fluid needs?

Yes. All fluids count—plain water, juice, soup, watermelon, and even coffee. The rumor that coffee dehydrates people lacks scientific support (Armstrong 2002). Yes, coffee might make you urinate more in 2 hours, but not in 24 hours. Even during exercise in the heat, athletes can consume coffee and not be concerned about dehydration.

For information about coffee and performance, see chapters 9 and 11 and appendix A.

CHAPTER 4

LUNCH AND DINNER: AT HOME, ON THE RUN, AND ON THE ROAD

Relaxing lunches and dinners—nicely prepared, attractively served, and shared with family and friends—are rare occurrences for many active people and sports families. Instead, they rapidly devour hit-or-miss meals on the fly. Yet, when life is full, stress is high, and schedules are crazy, eating well-balanced meals on a predictable schedule can provide the energy you need to better manage stress and prevent fatigue. This chapter provides meal management tips so you can care for your health while balancing work, workouts, and family and managing stress.

THE LUNCH BUNCH

For active people who should be in a continuous cycle of fueling up for workouts and refueling afterward, lunch is the second most important meal of the day. Breakfast remains number one. Lunch refuels morning or noontime exercisers and offers fuel to those preparing for afternoon sessions. Given that active people tend to get hungry every four hours (if not sooner), if you eat breakfast at 7:00 or 8:00 a.m., you are certainly ready for lunch at 11:00 or 12:00. But if you eat too little breakfast (as commonly happens), you'll be hungry for lunch by 10:00 a.m.—and that throws off the rest of the day's eating schedule.

The solution to the "I cannot wait until noon to eat lunch" predicament is simple: You can eat a bigger breakfast that sustains you until noon, eat a midmorning snack (more correctly, the second half of your too-small breakfast), or eat the first of two lunches, one at 10:00 and the other at 2:00.

For a nation of lunch skippers, eating two lunches may seem like a wacky idea. But why not? Ideally, you should eat according to hunger, not by the clock. After all, hunger is simply your body's request for more fuel.

If you've eaten only a light breakfast or have exercised hard in the morning, you can easily be ready for lunch-1 at 10:00 a.m. and lunch-2 at 2:00 p.m. That's what I do, and this system keeps me evenly fueled and helps me arrive home agreeably ready for dinner, but not starving.

In general, when you plan your intake for the day, you should try to divide your calories evenly. Given the tendency to become hungry every four hours, active people can appropriately eat 25 percent of their calories at each of four meals (breakfast, lunch-1, lunch-2, and dinner); this covers a 16-hour time span. If you are a grazer, each food bucket covers four hours; eat your "balanced meal" within that time block. Alternatively, you can eat one-third of your calories from each of three food buckets within six-hour time blocks (breakfast plus snack, lunch plus snack, dinner plus snack). By experimenting with this concept of evenly sized and evenly spaced meals, you'll likely eradicate your afternoon sweet cravings or after-dinner dietary disasters. You won't be eating more total calories; you'll just be trading snacks for an additional healthier meal.

Despite the importance of lunch, logistics tend to be a hassle. If you pack your own lunch, what do you pack? If you buy lunch, what's a healthy bargain? If you're on a diet, what's best to eat? Here are helpful tips to improve your lunch intake.

Packing Your Cooler

If you pack your lunch, the what-to-pack dilemma quickly becomes tiring. Ideally, you find the time to shop for and prepare enough food on weekends to last the week. Otherwise, most people tend to pack more or less the same food every day and end up with yet another turkey sandwich, salad, or frozen meal. As long as you're content with what you choose, fine. But if you're tired of the same stuff, consider these suggestions:

- Strive for at least 500 calories (even if you are on a reducing diet) from at least three (preferably four) types of food at lunch. This means sesame crackers +Greek yogurt +(soy) nuts +a banana or salad +turkey +cottage cheese +quinoa. Just yogurt or just a salad is likely too little fuel and too little protein, carbohydrate, vitamins, and minerals.

- Pack planned leftovers from dinner and heat them in a microwave oven. They're preferable to the highly processed cup of noodles or frozen lunches that cost more than they're worth.

If you're lucky enough to have a cafeteria at work or to participate in a business lunch, take advantage of the opportunity to enjoy a hot meal. Eating a dinner at lunch does the following:

- Fuels you for a high-energy after-work exercise session.

- Simplifies the "what to eat for dinner" routine because you'll feel less hungry and may be content to enjoy a bowl of cereal or a sandwich.
- Reduces the hungry horrors that you might otherwise have to fight if you skip lunch or hold off until dinner. You are going to eat the calories eventually, so you might as well honor your hunger and eat now.

Lunch for Dieters

Because many Americans regard meals as fattening, dieters tend to skip or skimp on lunch. As one higher-weight walker confided, "I'm fat, so I don't give myself permission to eat much lunch because I should be dieting. I don't want anyone to see me eating a real meal." That sad statement is common in our society. I urged her to take better care of herself and at least eat enough "diet foods" to keep her metabolism going and fuel her muscles for her walking program. Once she started to have a turkey and cheese wrap and an orange for lunch, she discovered the benefits of eating this meal. She was more effective at work, less hungry in the afternoon, less likely to raid the refrigerator the minute she arrived home, and better able to lose weight. She learned that lunch works.

Super Salads

Salads are a popular lunch and a super way to boost your intake of vegetables. In just one big bowlful you can get your 2 1/2 cups (five daily servings) of vegetables—if not more. Yet lunchtime salads can be either good news or bad news, depending on the salad.

If you are a dieter who deems salads an appropriate lunch, take heed. A meager salad offers too few calories. You'll likely end up visiting the

FACT OR FICTION

Peanut butter is fattening; don't eat it for lunch!

The facts: Although a peanut butter sandwich may have more calories than a turkey sandwich, it is more satisfying and may help you avoid the afternoon cookies and snacks that would otherwise sneak into your intake for the day. Peanut (or any nut) butter is an outstanding sports food—even for dieters—because it's satisfying and health promoting and helps you stay fueled for the whole afternoon. I enjoy two peanut butter and honey sandwiches almost every day—lunch-1 and lunch-2— and I'm not fat! People who frequently eat nuts are actually leaner than nut avoiders.

vending machine that afternoon. I suggest that dieters have a salad for dinner but eat a substantial meal at lunch. If you take full advantage of a brimming salad bar, also take heed. A typical salad bar meal can easily contain 1,000 calories, with 45 percent of those from fat (salad dressing). This is not a diet meal.

To create a high-energy sports salad that is the mainstay of your lunch or dinner, include enough carbohydrate- and protein-rich foods to make it substantial, but limit the fat to control the calories. Here are six tips to help you get the most in your salad bowl.

Tip 1: Choose a Variety of Dark, Colorful Veggies

Include red tomatoes, green peppers, orange carrots, leafy greens (such as arugula, kale, and baby spinach), and dark lettuces in your salad. Colorful vegetables nutritionally surpass paler lettuces, cucumbers, celery, and radishes. For example, a salad made with spinach has seven times the vitamin C as one made with iceberg lettuce; one made with dark romaine has twice the vitamin C. Plus, colorful vegetables are brimming with the antioxidant nutrients and phytochemicals that protect your health. Yes, white is also a color; white cauliflower is a good source of vitamin C (70 mg per cup, raw) and the cancer-fighting nutrients found in the cruciferous vegetable family to which it belongs.

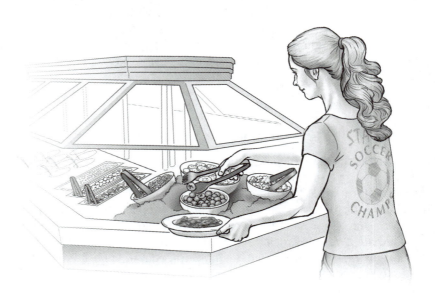

Tip 2: Pile on the Potassium-Rich Vegetables and Fruits

Potassium is an electrolyte that gets lost in sweat. Potassium also helps protect against high blood pressure. Enjoying abundant potassium-rich vegetables and fruits, in addition to limiting salt, is a wise choice if you or others in your genetic family have high blood pressure. You should try to get at least 3,500 milligrams of potassium every day, an easy task for salad lovers. Some of the vegetables richest in potassium are romaine lettuce, broccoli, tomatoes, and carrots (refer to table 1.2 in chapter 1). Some fruits rich in potassium that blend nicely into a salad include dried apricot bits, chopped dates, and avocado (refer to table 1.3 in chapter 1).

Tip 3: Include Adequate Protein

Add protein to your salad by topping it with cottage cheese; flaked tuna; canned salmon; diced hard-boiled egg; or sliced turkey, chicken, or other lean meats. For plant-based protein, toss in diced tofu, chickpeas, kidney beans, edamame (green soybeans), walnuts, sunflower seeds, soy nuts, slivered almonds, or peanuts. Athletes who eat just the greens and neglect the protein often end up anemic, injured, and chronically sick with colds or the flu.

Tip 4: Include Adequate Carbohydrate

It is a good idea to pack your salad with carbohydrate-rich options that fuel your muscles and offer more substance than just a crunch from leafy greens.

- Carbohydrate-dense vegetables such as corn, corn relish, peas, beets, and carrots
- Beans and legumes such as chickpeas, kidney beans, hummus, and lentils
- Cooked rice, pasta, quinoa, and (sweet) potato chunks
- Orange sections, diced apple, dried cranberries, and sliced strawberries
- Toasted croutons (limit your intake of buttered croutons that leave you with greasy fingers)
- Accompany the salad with a thick slice of whole-grain bread.

Tip 5: Remember the Calcium

For calcium (and protein), add cheese (blue cheese bolsters your micro-biome); cubes of tofu; dressing made from plain yogurt seasoned with oregano, basil, and other Italian herbs; a scoop of cottage cheese (although cottage cheese is actually a better source of protein than of calcium); a

Salad Toppings: Nuts and Seeds

Some athletes top their salads with nutrient-rich nuts and seeds. Table 4.1 shows how 1/4 cup (two spoonfuls or a large handful) of these add-ins contribute important nutrients, but also a lot of calories. If you are weight conscious, note that adding a cup of cottage cheese to the salad would give you much more protein (30 grams) for the same or fewer calories. Vegetarians take note: You'll get a small protein boost (5 to 10 grams) from the nuts and seeds, but you should also include beans and tofu to reach the target of at least 20 grams of protein per meal.

TABLE 4.1 Nutritional Value of Nuts and Seeds

Seed, nut 1/4 cup, 30 g	Calories	Protein (g)	Fiber (g)	Calcium (mg)	Iron (mg)
Chia seeds	140	5	10	180	8
Flaxseed, ground	150	5	8	70	1.5
Hemp hearts	220	12	2	30	3
Pumpkin seeds	170	9	2	50	2
Sesame seeds	200	6	4	350	5
Sunflower seeds	190	6	3	20	1
Walnuts	190	4	2	30	1
		Target per meal: ~20-30 g	Daily target: 25-35 g	Daily target: 1,000 mg	Daily target: 8 mg men, 18 mg women

sprinkling of sunflower or sesame seeds. Drink a (decaf) latte along with the salad, or have yogurt for dessert. Don't try to live on lettuce alone!

Tip 6: Enjoy Healthy Fats

Avocado, chopped nuts, olives, and olive oil are heart-healthy fats that can appropriately fit into a balanced sports diet, as long as you can afford the calories.

Remember that even fat-free dressings have calories—15 to 45 per 2 tablespoons—and should be used sparingly. Light dressings can have 30 to 80 calories per 2 tablespoons. Two tablespoons is not much for a big salad, so double or triple that for a more honest estimate!

At restaurants, always request that the dressing be served on the side so you can control the amount you consume. Add the dressing sparingly, or dip a forkful of salad into the dressing before each bite. A few innocent ladles of salad dressing can transform a potentially healthy salad into a high-fat nutrition nightmare. Even olive oil, a "healthy" addition to a sports diet, can offer excess calories. (Vinegar is "free"; oil is not.) On a large salad, a hefty dousing of dressing can easily add 800 to 1,000 calories. On even a small side salad, a dressing can drown the salad's healthfulness in 400 calories of fat. These fat calories appease the appetite and add to your waistline—but fail to fuel the muscles with carbohydrate. I often advise my clients to educate themselves about salad dressing calories by measuring out the amount of dressing they normally use on a salad. Using the food label on the bottle of salad oil or prepared dressing, they can then estimate the calories, and they tend to be shocked!

To reduce the fat and calories from salad dressing, choose low-fat dressings or simply dilute a regular dressing with extra vinegar, lemon juice, water, or milk in creamy dressings. By using only small amounts of this diluted version, you'll get lots of flavor and moisture with fewer calories. You might also want to venture into using a variety of vinegars. Balsamic is one of my favorites.

DINNER AT HOME AND ON THE ROAD

In the United States, dinners are commonly the biggest meal of the day— the reward for having survived yet another busy, stress-filled day. I invite you to start putting dinner at the bottom of your meal priority list and placing more focus on breakfast and lunch. That way, you'll have more energy to cope with daytime stresses, enjoy a better workout, and feel less in need of high-calorie rewards at night. Yes, you can and should still enjoy a pleasant evening meal—but you won't need a humongous feast, followed by endless snacks.

Active people commonly eat huge dinners because they eat too little during the day. If this sounds familiar, experiment with reorganizing your good-nutrition game plan so you put more emphasis on breakfast and lunch (or lunches) to fuel up and remain fueled throughout the busy day. Use the evening meal as a time to relax—without overeating—and, whenever possible, keep dinner relatively smaller so it ends up equal in size to the heartier breakfast and lunch (or lunches).

As Gretchen, a kindergarten teacher, said, "I used to stuff myself at night as a reward for having survived a hectic day. I'd arrive home starved, stressed, and tired, and then overeat and feel lousy. Now I eat a truly satisfying breakfast and lunch 1. I have a lot more energy for my students during the day. I eat my second lunch when school ends, and this gives me more energy for my family in the evening. By eating a lighter dinner, I sleep much better and feel better overall."

Dinner at Home

When dinner is home based, you need a game plan to assemble a team of nutritious foods. Some people take advantage of meal kits and effortlessly cook up the preassembled ingredients. Others plan for and create wholesome dinners without much time or effort—with little or no cooking. The following tips, plus the recipes in part IV, offer tried-and-true menu suggestions to help you enjoy both dinner and dinnertime.

Tip 1: Don't Arrive Home Too Hungry

One prerequisite for successful nighttime dining is to eat a hearty lunch plus a second lunch or afternoon snack. Irina, a busy stockbroker, experimented with my suggestion to eat a heartier lunch plus a second lunch at 4:00 before her 5:30 p.m. kickboxing class. In one day, she discovered that this food enhanced her energy for exercise plus transformed her 7:00 I'm-too-hungry-to-cook bowl of ice cream for dinner into a bowl of soup. A substantial lunch (or two) lessens fatigue in the afternoon, fuels higher-quality afternoon workouts, provides the physical and mental energy you need to prepare a nourishing supper, and helps you cope with the day's stresses.

Tip 2: Plan Time to Shop for Food

Good nutrition starts in the grocery store. By stocking your kitchen shelves and freezer with a variety of wholesome foods that are ready and waiting, you will be more likely to eat a better dinner. Kirsten, a 24-year-old dental assistant, used to spend most of her food budget in restaurants on the way home from work because at home she faced bare cupboards and an empty refrigerator. Although she liked to cook, she rarely did so because she simply didn't plan the time to grocery shop. Plus, she got discouraged by meats and vegetables that often spoiled before she got around to cooking them.

I advised Kirsten to schedule a specific day and time to shop for food either at the grocery store or online and delivered to her house. She kept that appointment and was then able to stock her freezer with individually

FACT OR FICTION

Freezing destroys a food's nutritional value.

The facts: Freezing retains a food's nutritional value. Frozen broccoli can provide far more nutrients than, let's say, the wilted, five-day-old stalks you might drag from your refrigerator. Frozen foods provide quick nutrition with less fuss and waste than fresh items do.

wrapped chicken breasts, lean hamburger patties, turkey burgers, and frozen vegetables—particularly vitamin-rich broccoli, spinach, and winter squash. Once she had stocked her kitchen with frozen foods and other staples, Kirsten discovered that she preferred to come home for dinner.

I always stock basic foods that won't spoil quickly. On days when I arrive home to an empty refrigerator, I can either pull together a no-cook meal or quickly prepare a hot dinner.

Following are some of my standard meals:

- English muffin pizzas
- Whole-grain crackers, peanut butter, banana, and milk
- Lentil soup with extra broccoli, leftover rice, and a cup of yogurt
- Refried beans (heated in the microwave oven), salsa, and (cottage) cheese rolled in a tortilla or wrap
- Tuna sandwich with vegetable soup
- Oatmeal cooked with milk and topped with chopped dates and slivered almonds

Some standard ingredients you might want to stock include the following:

Cupboard

Spaghetti	Oatmeal	Soups (lentil, minestrone)
Spaghetti sauce	Almonds	
Rice, brown	Peanut butter	Bananas
Potatoes, white	Salsa	Raisins
Potatoes, sweet	Tuna	Canned peaches
Graham crackers	Canned salmon	Dates
Triscuits	Kidney beans	
Popcorn kernels	Refried beans	

Refrigerator

Shredded mozza-
rella cheese

Low-fat cottage
cheese

Low-fat Greek
yogurt

Low-fat milk

Eggs (omega-3)

Hummus

Seasonal fruit

Orange juice

Baby carrots

Red and green
peppers

Cherry tomatoes

Tortillas

Freezer

Whole-grain breads

Bagels

English muffins

Strawberries

Blueberries

Winter squash

Broccoli

Chicken breasts

Ground turkey

Extra-lean
hamburger

When creating a meal from these staples, you want to choose items from at least three, if not four, of the five food groups, using carbohydrate–protein combinations with each meal. Table 4.2 shows four 650-calorie, 60 percent carbohydrate, well-balanced meals that require no cooking. The portions are appropriate for an active woman who needs 2,000 to 2,400 calories per day; a hungry man may want more.

TABLE 4.2 650-Calorie Meals

Food group	Menu 1: Crackers with tuna	Menu 2: Peanut butter and raisin sandwich
1. Grain	12 Triscuits	2 slices oatmeal bread
2. Protein	1 5-oz can tuna with 1 tbsp light mayo	2 tbsp peanut butter
3. Fruit	1 cup berries	1/4 cup (30 g) raisins
4. Vegetable	8 cherry tomatoes	10 baby carrots
5. Dairy	1 cup (230 g) yogurt (+ berries)	1 cup (240 ml) low-fat milk
Food group	**Menu 3: Pizza**	**Menu 4: Burrito**
1. Grain	2 english muffins	2 tortillas
2. Protein	Almonds (appetizer)	1 cup (250 g) vegetarian refried beans
3. Fruit	1 cup (240 ml) orange juice	1/2 cup (120 g) canned peaches
4. Vegetable	3/4 cup (180 g) spaghetti sauce	1/4 cup (60 g) salsa
5. Dairy	1/2 cup (120 g) grated mozzarella cheese	1 cup (230 g) low-fat cottage cheese

Tip 3: Plan Time for Food Prep

Lauren, a 53-year-old high school teacher, enjoyed preparing meals on the weekends when she had the time to cook. She always created a big batch of something on Sunday so it would be waiting for her when she arrived home tired and hungry after work and workouts. She preferred convenience to variety and thrived on beans and rice for a week, then lasagna the next week, split pea soup the third, and so on. When Lauren couldn't face another repetitive dinner, she cooked something else and put the leftovers in the freezer.

Meatless Meals

When menu planning, how about including Meatless Mondays (if not for more days of the week)? Although lean meat is not bad for your health (fatty meat can be the culprit), the environment benefits from less meat consumption. Animals raised for meat create greenhouse gas emissions that contribute to global warming. If we all were to eat a little less meat, we would help reduce our carbon footprint. Easy, meatless entrees that even nonvegetarians will enjoy include rice and beans; pasta with white beans, olive oil, and garlic; bean burritos; a mushroom and onion omelet; minestrone soup with a hummus wrap; and pizza (preferably homemade with a whole-wheat crust and lots of veggie toppings).

A meatless meal of pasta is popular and easy to cook. Although carbohydrate-rich pasta does provide muscle fuel for your body's engine, a bowlful of plain white pasta with butter or oil is a marginal source of vitamins and minerals—the "spark plugs" (enzymes that help convert food into energy) needed for top performance. Whole-wheat pastas offer only a little more nutritional value. Wheat (and all other grains, in general) are better sources of muscle fuel than vitamins. Even spinach and tomato pastas are overrated; they contain very little of the vegetables.

To boost pasta's nutritional power, combine it with vitamin-rich tomato sauce (fresh or from a jar), spinach and garlic sauce, pesto, or stir-fried vegetables (broccoli, spinach, or green peppers from the freezer), and be sure to add a side of protein (canned beans, cottage cheese, hummus, tofu).

Dinner Out

Some people eat in restaurants (or order take-out meals) because the cupboards are empty or they prefer not to cook. Others enjoy dining in restaurants with their friends. And some end up in restaurants because of business meetings. Whatever the situation, every active person who relies on restaurants for a balanced sports diet faces the challenge of choosing healthy meals among all the rich temptations. Unfortunately, many people select whatever's fast and happens to tempt their taste buds at the moment, particularly when they are tired, hungry, stressed, anxious, or lonely. Here are suggestions for what to eat when you are not the cook.

Healthy Choices

The most important first step to selecting healthy restaurant meals is to patronize the restaurants that offer nutrient-rich sports foods; don't go to a steak house if you're looking for pasta for muscle fuel. Study the menu on the Internet or outside the door before you sit down to see whether the restaurant offers rice, baked potatoes, bread, and other carbohydrate-based foods. Try to avoid the places that serve only fried items. Also, find out whether they allow special requests. If the menu clearly states "no substitutions," you might be in the wrong place.

When you're in an appropriate restaurant, choose your foods wisely. In general, you should request foods that are baked, broiled, roasted, or steamed—anything but fried. Low-fat poultry and fish items tend to be better choices than items naturally high in fat, such as a juicy steak, spareribs, cheese, and sausages. Keep the following foods in mind as you peruse a menu:

- **Appetizers.** Shrimp cocktail, fruit cup, or hummus make great starters for your meal.
- **Breads.** Unbuttered rolls and breads are great––particularly if they are whole grain. If the standard fare is buttered (as in garlic bread), request some plain bread also, and enjoy the buttery bread in moderation. Dip the plain bread in a little olive oil, rather than smother it with butter.
- **Soups.** Broth-based soups (such as vegetable, chicken and rice, miso, and Chinese soups) and hearty minestrone, split pea, navy bean, and lentil soups can be good sources of carbohydrate and are healthier than creamy chowders and bisques. They are also a source of fluids.
- **Salads.** Enjoy the greens and veggies but, if you are watching your weight, limit the high-calorie toppings (cheese, bacon bits, buttery croutons, olives, nuts, seeds, avocado). Always request that the dressing be served on the side so you can control how much you use.

- **Seafood and poultry.** Request chicken or fish that's baked, roasted, steamed, stir-fried, or broiled—and don't forget sushi. Because many chefs add a lot of butter when broiling foods such as fish, you might want to request that your entree be broiled dry (cooked without this extra fat). If the entree is sauteed, request that the chef saute it with very little butter or oil and add no extra fat before serving.

- **Beef.** Many restaurants pride themselves on serving huge slabs of beef or 12-ounce (360 g) steaks. If you order beef, plan to cut this double portion in half and take the rest home for tomorrow's dinner, share it with a companion (who has ordered accordingly), or simply leave it. Trim all the visible fat, and request that any gravy or sauce be served on the side so you can use it sparingly, if at all. Your goal is to eat meat as the accompaniment to the meal, not as the focus. Your muscles will perform better if two-thirds of your plate is covered with carbohydrate-based potatoes, vegetables, and bread. How about stir-fried beef with lots of rice, a beef fajita, or even a veggie burger instead of a slab of steak?

- **Potatoes.** Baked potatoes—both white and sweet—are a great source of carbohydrate. Don't let the chef load them up with butter or sour cream; request that these toppings be served on the side so you can control how much you eat. Better yet, trade those fat calories for more carbohydrate. Add moisture by mashing the potato with milk (special request). This may sound a bit messy, but it's a delicious, low-fat way to enjoy what might otherwise be a dry potato.

- **Pasta.** Pick pasta served with tomato sauces (carbohydrate) rather than the high-fat cheese, oil, or cream sauces. Also be cautious of cheese-filled lasagna, tortellini, and manicotti. These choices often offer more fat than carbohydrate.

- **Rice.** In a Chinese restaurant, you'll be better off filling up on an extra bowl of plain rice, another good source of carbohydrate, than on egg rolls or other fried appetizers. Brown rice is preferable to white rice, when available.

- **Vegetables.** Request plain, unbuttered vegetables with any special sauces (hollandaise, lemon butter) served on the side.

- **Asian food.** Steamed brown rice with stir-fry combinations such as chicken with green beans or shrimp with Asian veggies are the best choices. Ask for extra vegetables. You can also request that the food be cooked with less oil. Be cautious at buffets; the chefs tend to add extra oil so the food is less sticky.

- **Dessert.** Sorbet, frozen yogurt, angel food cake, and berries are among the best choices for your sports diet. Fresh fruit is often available, even if it isn't listed on the menu. If you can't resist a decadent dessert, be sure to enjoy it after you have eaten plenty of carbohydrate to fuel your muscles. That is, don't eat a carbohydrate-poor salad for dinner to save room for high-fat cheesecake for dessert.

When you are faced with a meal that's mostly protein and fat that fills your stomach but leaves your muscles unfueled, top it off with your own high-carbohydrate after-dinner snacks that you keep handy, such as fig bars, animal crackers, or dried pineapple. However, also try to make special requests. Remember, you are the boss when it comes to restaurant eating. The restaurant's job is to serve you the high-quality sports foods that enhance your health and your performance. Bon appetit!

Gas Station Nutrition

If you are among the many athletes, referees, coaches, athletic trainers, and support crews—including parents, partners, and siblings—who spend too much time on the road, traveling from one sporting event to the next, you are likely familiar with "gas station nutrition." The following tips can help you eat reasonably well from a gas station or vending machine—or at least, eat better than if you have no plan at all. But first, for the purposes of this section, you need to understand the definition of *well-balanced sports diet*—and note that well balanced applies to your entire day's eating, not just one meal or snack. Hence, a good breakfast, lunch, and dinner can help offset suboptimal midnight treats.

As I talked about in chapter 1, a well-balanced sports diet includes foods from at least three—ideally four—of these food groupings:

1. *Fruits and vegetables* for vitamins and minerals to boost your immune system and help keep your body healthy.
2. *Grain-based foods* to fuel your muscles and your brain.
3. *Protein-rich foods* to build and repair your muscles.
4. *Calcium-rich foods* such as dairy, to enhance bone health and also offer high-quality protein for muscles.

Balance also includes calorie balance. Be sure to read the calorie information on food labels and eat only the portion that fits into your calorie budget: 600 to 800 calories per meal for active women and 800 to 1,000 calories per meal for active men.

Table 4.3 lists typical gas station snacks and groups the foods according to nutrient profile. Your job is to choose one food from at least three of the four groups. Using this template, you can manage to pick a somewhat balanced, halfway decent sports meal when you are on the road (or at a vending machine).

TABLE 4.3 Typical Gas Station Snacks

1. Fruits and vegetables	2. Grain-based foods	3. Protein-rich foods	4. Calcium-rich foods and dairy*
100% fruit juice	belVita biscuits	Almonds	Cheese sticks
Apples	Cereal cups (Raisin	Canned tuna	Flavored milk: chocolate,
Applesauce	Bran)	Clif Builder's Bar	strawberry, vanilla
Bananas	Clif Bars	Egg, hard boiled	Milk, dairy or soy
Canned fruit	Corn chips, Sunchips	Jerky (beef, turkey)	Presliced cheese (indi-
Dried fruit	Graham crackers	KIND Bar	vidually wrapped)
Orange juice	Granola bars	Milk	Yogurt, regular or Greek
Oranges	Muffin (bran, corn)	Mixed nuts	
Raisins	Peanut butter crackers	Peanuts	
Salsa	Popcorn, SmartFood	Sunflower seeds	
V8 juice	PowerBars	Trail mix	
	Pretzels	Yogurt, cheese	
	Triscuits, Wheat Thins		

*If you are lactose intolerant, cheddar cheese is a lactose-free dairy option—but you likely want to travel with Lactaid Pills. Nondairy calcium-rich foods such as soy milk or calcium-fortified orange juice can be difficult to find on the road.

Your "balanced diet" might resemble these "tasty" (ha!) meals:

Orange juice, popcorn, protein bar, and yogurt

Salsa, corn chips, almonds, and milk

Banana, peanuts, Wheat Thins, and a cheese stick

Fruits and vegetables are the most difficult foods to find when you are on the road. Because your body stores vitamins in the liver, your diet can be low in fruits and veggies for a week or so and you will not suffer from malnutrition. (A healthy person's liver stores enough vitamin C to last at least three weeks.) But you will want to restock your liver's diminished supply when you get back home by consuming fruit smoothies, colorful salads, and generous portions of fresh fruits and vegetables.

Traveling With a Cooler

A wise alternative to "dining" at gas stations is to travel with a minicooler and refreezable ice packs. Stock the cooler with sandwiches (peanut butter and jam, hummus and cheese), beverages, and wholesome sports foods appropriate for fueling up while traveling to the event and refueling afterward. A pretrip food-shopping spree at a large supermarket can save you (and your teammates) a lot of money. Here are suggestions:

- **Perishable items:** clementines, bananas, baby carrots, peppers (eat them like apples), Greek yogurt, cheese sticks, chocolate milk, deli turkey, hard-boiled eggs, hummus, wraps, mini bagels
- **Nonperishable items:** tuna in a pouch, peanut butter, almonds, granola bars, graham crackers, energy bars, applesauce, dates, V8 juice (for sodium in hot weather)

Quick-Service Choices

Eating at a quick-service restaurant can spell sports diet disaster if you choose a Fat City venue. You'll have an easy opportunity to select items that are high in saturated fat and calories, but low in carbohydrate, fiber, fruits, and vegetables. Although the occasional burger-and-fries meal is of less concern after an event, fast foods as a common part of your diet need to be balanced with wholesome grains, fruits, and vegetables. Fortunately for our health, most of today's quick-service restaurants offer healthy options. Table 4.4 suggests ways to shave the fat and calories from grab-and-go meals.

Travelers, in particular, need to learn how to fuel themselves wisely, even if on a budget. If you are a 150-pound (68 kg) athlete who needs 2,700

TABLE 4.4 Tweaking the Fat and Calories in Fast Foods

By making slightly different choices, you can save yourself a significant amount of calories and saturated fat—yet still have a satisfying meal.

Instead of this:	Calories	Fat (g)	Try this:	Calories saved	Grams of fat saved
Sausage Egg McMuffin	450	27	Egg McMuffin	150	15
Big Mac	550	29	2 small hamburgers	50	13
Filet-O-Fish	390	19	Grilled chicken wrap	130	10
BK Whopper	670	40	Whopper, no mayo	160	17
Domino's 14 in. (34 cm) MeatZZa pizza, 2 slices	740	34	Domino's 14 in. cheese pizza, 2 slices	160	14
KFC extra-crispy chicken breast, 1 piece	530	35	KFC original recipe chicken breast, 1 piece	150	14
Taco Bell taco salad, beef	760	39	Taco Bell Express taco salad	180	13

*Nutrition information from websites, October 2018.

to 3,000 calories a day, the cheapest way to stave off hunger is to fill up on fatty foods—such as tempting value meals. Bad idea. These high-fat meals not only clog the arteries and bulk up the waistline but also fail to adequately fuel the muscles. A better bet is to carry carbohydrate-rich foods with you. Some easy-to-tote choices are bagels, energy bars, fig cookies, pretzels, dry cereals (such as Toasted Oatmeal Squares or granola), dried fruits (such as dates, apricots), and 12-ounce (350 ml) bottles of 100 percent fruit juice.

The following menu ideas can help you healthfully navigate the world of fast foods:

- Any way you look at them, burgers and french fries have high fat content. You'll be better off going to an eatery that offers more than just burgers. Find a menu that offers grilled chicken sandwiches or hummus wraps accompanied by soups (brothy or beany ones). Other options are rotisserie, roasted, or grilled chicken meals with mashed potatoes, rice, and vegetables, and salad bars complete with kidney beans, chickpeas, and multigrain breads.

- If you order a burger, request a second roll or extra bread (or napkins). Squish the grease into the first roll (or napkins), and then replace it with another roll.

- Boost carbohydrate intake with beverages such as juices, smoothies, and low-fat shakes. Pack supplemental carbohydrate, such as craisins or granola bars.

- Shy away from value meals. You'll be better off having a burger and milk than having your money "go to waist" by choosing a meal deal with fries.

- Beware of chicken sandwiches topped with special mayonnaise-based sauces, which can make them as fatty as fried chicken sandwiches. Request that the server hold the sauce, or scrape off the mayo yourself.

- If you order fried chicken, get the larger pieces, remove all the skin, and eat just the meat. By removing the skin and breading from the original recipe KFC breast, you remove 200 calories and 17 grams of fat. Order extra rolls, corn bread with honey or jam, corn on the cob, and other vegetables for more carbohydrate.

  Even though roasted and rotisserie chickens are preferable to fried, be aware that the crispy skin is still fatty. Additionally, many of the accompaniments to chicken meals glisten with butter; however, any vegetable tends to be better than no vegetable. Ask whether unbuttered, steamed vegetables are an option.

FACT OR FICTION

A fast-food salad is preferable to a burger.

The facts: Many salads come loaded with dried fruits, nuts, avocado, corn, sunflower seeds, and beans. Nutritious ingredients, yes, but caloric—especially if lots of cheese is sprinkled on top, along with a flood of salad dressing. Table 4.5 shows some salads that can be higher in calories and sodium than a fast-food burger.

TABLE 4.5 High-Calorie Salads

Entree	Calories	Fat (g) total	Fat: % of calories	Sodium (mg)
Big Mac	550	30	50%	1,000
Olive Garden: Grilled Chicken Caesar Salad	600	40	60%	1,230
Panera: Southwest Chile Lime Ranch Salad with chicken	670	35	45%	800
Whopper	670	40	50%	970
Wendy's: Spicy Chicken Caesar Salad	720	40	55%	1,760
Applebee's: Oriental Grilled Chicken Salad without dressing	1,050	65	55%	2,150
Cheesecake Factory: Grilled Chicken Tostada Salad	1,150	65	55%	2,150
Applebee's: Oriental Grilled Chicken Salad with dressing	1,300	85	60%	2,240

- Resist the temptation to choose baked potatoes smothered with high-fat toppings. Your best bet is to order an additional plain potato and split the broccoli and cheese topping (14 g of fat) between the two. That way, you end up with a hearty 800-calorie, high-carbohydrate meal, with only 15 percent of the calories from fat. For additional protein, drink low-fat milk.

- Order pizza with thick crust rather than extra cheese. More dough means more muscle fuel. A slice of Domino's thick-crust pizza has 9 more grams of carbohydrate than a slice of the thin-crust pizza. Pile on vegetables (green peppers, mushrooms, onions), but stay away from the pepperoni, sausage, and ground beef. Don't be shy about using a napkin to blot the fat that cooks out of the cheese.

- Seek a deli that offers wholesome breads. Request a sandwich that emphasizes the bread rather than the filling. A large wrap (preferably whole wheat) provides ample carbohydrate. Hold the mayo, and add moistness with hummus, light salad dressings (if available), mustard, or ketchup. The lowest-fat fillings are turkey, ham, and lean roast beef.
- Hearty bean soups accompanied by crackers, bread, or corn bread provide a satisfying carbohydrate-rich, low-fat meal. Chili, if not glistening with a layer of grease, can be a good choice. For example, a Wendy's large chili with eight crackers provides a satisfying 350 calories, and only 20 percent of those calories (7 g) are from fat.

You can find an energizing sports diet even if you are eating on the road. You simply need to eat before you get too hungry so that you do not succumb to the high-fat options that satisfy your hunger but leave your muscles poorly fueled.

Team Dinners

Once upon a time, the team dinner was pasta with meatballs. Today, the team likely includes athletes who are vegetarian (if not vegan), cannot eat wheat or dairy, and are allergic to peanuts. To simplify team dinners, think about having "make your meals" with a buffet that includes gluten-free, lactose-free, and meat-free options. Each athlete can put together his or her own grain bowl, burrito, salad bowl, or taco. Organized chaos, for certain, but fun for all. Meals are a time to enjoy each other's company, no matter what the dietary limitations are.

CHAPTER 5

BETWEEN MEALS: SNACKING FOR HEALTH AND SUSTAINED ENERGY

Most of my clients undereat meals and overeat snacks; they are forever seeking a quick energy fix, and snacks commonly make up 20 to 50 percent of their total calories. If you are a big-time snacker, I encourage you to redefine snacks as meals so you are less likely to choose cookies, candy, caffeine, and other typical snack foods. In fact, I generally eliminate the word *snack* when counseling clients. I teach them to think *two lunches* instead of *lunch and afternoon snack*. That way, they end up choosing wholesome foods (such as banana and peanut butter) and not typical snacks (such as candy and chips) in the afternoon.

WISE SNACKING

Although some people try not to snack because they believe that eating between meals is sinful and fattening, the truth is that snacking is important. Active people tend to get hungry at least every four hours, so if you have lunch at noon, your body will want a snack (or a second lunch) by 4:00 p.m., if not sooner. If you will be exercising in the afternoon, you need added fuel to energize your workout. Snacking is good for you and your workouts, and you should make it part of your sports diet, preferably with a *second lunch* instead of *afternoon sweet treats*. A planned wholesome snack is a far better option than a stimulant drink such as Red Bull or 5-Hour Energy (see chapter 8).

Fast Snacks

When you are eating on the run and grabbing snacks instead of real meals, be sure to choose wholesome foods that combine protein with carbohydrate. You can make wise choices from among many nutritious and conveniently available items. Here are popular suggestions. The information in parentheses offers an additional option.

- A whole-grain english muffin with peanut butter and a (decaf) latte
- A slice of (whole-wheat) thick-crust pizza with green peppers
- Hummus, pita, and baby carrots
- Rye toast topped with mashed avocado and sliced hard-boiled eggs
- Grape-Nuts with (Greek) yogurt and (frozen) blueberries
- Chinese takeout—stir-fried chicken with vegetables and steamed (brown) rice
- Instant oatmeal made with low-fat milk and slivered almonds

Note that each of these mini-meals includes foods from three food groups. Ideally, you'll choose foods from different groups to balance your diet. That way, even if you graze throughout the day, you will consume a variety of the nutrients you need for good health and top performance. The following list provides additional ideas for snacks and grazing at home and on the road:

- **Dry cereal.** Mix your favorite cereal with raisins, dried fruits, cinnamon, or nuts.
- **Instant oatmeal.** Microwave the oatmeal with dairy or soy milk instead of water to boost its nutrition power. Sprinkle with craisins, chopped dates or any fresh or dried fruit, and chopped nuts.
- **Popcorn.** Eat it plain or sprinkled with spices such as chili powder, garlic powder, onion powder, or soy sauce. If you like, use olive oil spray so the spices stick.
- **Pretzels.** If you wish to reduce your salt intake, knock the salt off or buy salt-free pretzels.
- **Crackers.** Graham, sesame, bran, and whole-grain, low-fat brands are good choices.
- **Muffins.** Homemade with canola oil are best; wholesome bran or corn muffins are preferable to those made with white flour (see the recipes in part IV). If store bought, choose small muffins, or cut a huge one in half and share it with a friend.

- **Bagels.** Whole-grain varieties with more vitamins and minerals are preferable to bagels made with white flour.
- **Fruits.** Choose bananas, apples, berries, or any fresh fruit. The more variety of colors, the better for your health. When traveling, pack dried fruit for concentrated nutrition.
- **Smoothies.** Whip together milk, yogurt, or juice; fresh or frozen fruit; and wheat germ, chia, or flax meal (see the recipes in chapter 25).
- **Frozen fruit bars.** You can slowly savor these pleasant treats in good health.
- **Yogurt.** Buy plain low-fat yogurt—make that Greek yogurt if you want extra protein—and flavor it with vanilla, honey, maple syrup, cinnamon, instant decaffeinated coffee, applesauce, (canned) fruit, or (frozen) berries.
- **Energy bars, breakfast bars, breakfast biscuits, granola bars.** Prewrapped and portable, these travel well in pockets and gym bags and can be very handy.

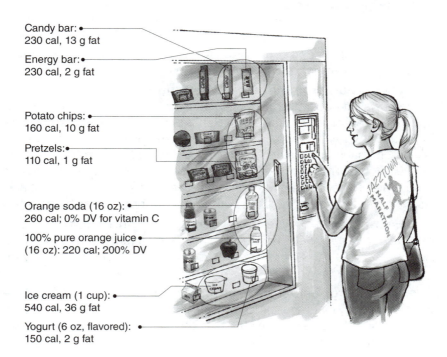

Candy bar:
230 cal, 13 g fat

Energy bar:
230 cal, 2 g fat

Potato chips:
160 cal, 10 g fat

Pretzels:
110 cal, 1 g fat

Orange soda (16 oz):
260 cal; 0% DV for vitamin C

100% pure orange juice
(16 oz): 220 cal; 200% DV

Ice cream (1 cup):
540 cal, 36 g fat

Yogurt (6 oz, flavored):
150 cal, 2 g fat

- **Nuts, seeds, trail mix.** Peanuts, walnuts, almonds, sunflower seeds, pumpkin seeds, soy nuts, and other nuts and seeds are excellent sources of protein, B vitamins, vitamin E, and healthy fat.
- **Sandwiches.** Sandwiches don't have to be just for lunch; they are great for snacks. Choose peanut butter, turkey, hummus, lean roast beef, or tuna (with light mayo).
- **Baked (sweet) potatoes.** Microwave ovens make these a handy snack. They're tasty warm or cold, a carbohydrate-rich choice for refueling your muscles after a hard workout. Try sweet potatoes with applesauce and a dash of nutmeg—mmm!

Energy Bars: Prewrapped Convenience

PowerBars, Luna bars, Clif Bars, Balance Bars—energy bars await you at every convenience store, each boasting its ability to enhance your performance. The following information will help you decide how much of your food budget to dedicate to these popular snacks. Ideally, you will have more banana peels than bar wrappers in your wastebasket.

- **Energy bars are portable.** You can easily tuck these compact, lightweight, and often vitamin-enriched bars into a pocket for "emergency food." Energy bars are handy for runners and bikers who want to carry a durable snack on a long run or ride, for dancers who want fuel without bulk, and for hikers who want a light backpack.
- **Energy bars promote preexercise eating.** Fueling before exercising is a great way to boost stamina and endurance. The energy bar industry has done an excellent job of educating us that preexercise eating is important for optimizing performance. The associated energy boost likely does not result from magic ingredients (chromium, amino acids) but from eating 200 to 300 calories. These calories clearly fuel you better than the zero calories in no snack. Note that calories from tried-and-true fig bars, graham crackers, bananas, and granola bars are also effective preexercise energizers.
- **Energy bars promote eating during endurance exercise.** Energy bars are also a great way to boost stamina and endurance during extended exercise, such as hikes and bike rides, so you don't have to rely only on what you eat before you exercise.
- **Most energy bars claim to be highly digestible.** One could debate whether energy bars are easier to digest than standard food because digestibility varies greatly from athlete to athlete. As with all sports snacks, you have to learn through trial and error during training which foods work

for your system and which foods don't. One key to comfortably tolerating energy bars is to drink plenty of water along with them. Otherwise, the product might settle poorly.

• **Some energy bars boast about high protein content.** While 10 or 20 grams of protein in a bar can be a convenient way to insert protein into your snacks, does your body really need the extra protein? (See chapter 7.)

• **Some energy bars boast about low carbohydrate content.** These are poor choices for athletes. You want to snack on carbohydrate because it is the best source of fuel for your muscles. And despite popular belief, carbohydrate is not fattening; rather, excess calories are fattening.

• **Energy bars are expensive.** You'll have to fork over at least one dollar, if not two, to buy most sports bars. The better value is to buy granola bars or breakfast bars from the supermarket at a lower price (table 5.1). A handful of raisins can also do a great job.

• **Energy bars have no magical ingredients.** They are simply a convenient source of calories (energy). They suit the needs of many hungry people who seek a prewrapped, hassle-free, somewhat nutritious snack.

TABLE 5.1   Energy Bars Versus Standard Food

If you are going to buy granola bars and energy bars, your most economical bet is to get them at a grocery store or in bulk at Costco or BJ's. If you buy them at a convenience store, the price will be much higher than the cost per 100 calories listed here, which is based on buying the bars at a grocery store. In general, unprocessed foods without wrappers (e.g., apples, dried fruit, nuts) are the preferable snacks.

Sports snack	Calories/ packet	Cost/100 calories	Cost/ unit
Fig Newtons, 2 oz packet	200	$0.27	$0.54
belVita Breakfast Biscuit, 1.8 oz packet	230	$0.32	$0.74
Nature Valley Granola Bar, Oats 'N Honey, 1.5 oz packet	190	$0.34	$0.66
Quaker Chewy Bar, chocolate chip 0.8 oz bar	100	$0.44	$0.44
Raisins, 1 oz box	90	$0.60	$0.57
Clif Bar, chocolate chip, 2.4 oz bar	250	$0.64	$1.59*
KIND Bar, nuts and dark chocolate, 1.4 oz bar	200	$0.75	$1.59*
RX Bar, chocolate chip, 1.8 oz bar	220	$1.22	$2.49*

*Clif, Kind, RX bars sold individually, not in a six-pack.

Note: Nutrition information from food labels. Prices based in Massachusetts, December 2018.

Is There a "Best" Bar?

If you are confused about which bar is the best bar, you are not alone. My clients commonly ask me which ones I recommend. My answer depends on their nutritional needs. The best bar is one that suits your health issues, food philosophy, and taste buds. For some people, the best bar is the one that is gluten free. For others, the best bar is made with organic ingredients. And for many, the best is simply the one that tastes the best.

To help you untangle energy bar confusion, here is a comprehensive, but incomplete, list of energy bars arranged by type. (It is just a list and not an endorsement of the products.) Perhaps this list will help you see how the industry markets to seemingly every possible niche. Try not to be swayed by a product's name; it might be more powerful than the sports food itself!

- **Additive free (that also means no added vitamins or minerals).** Clif Mojo and Nectar, Epic, Good Greens, Gnu, Honey Stinger Waffle, Kashi, KIND, Larabar, Optimum, Peak Energy, Perfect 10, PowerBar Nut Naturals, ProBar, Pure, Raw Revolution, Red Square Powerflax, RX, thinkThin, Trail Mix Honey-bar, Zing
- **Budget friendly.** Nutri-Grain, Nature Valley Granola, Kashi Chewy, Quaker Chewy
- **Caffeine containing.** Better Than Coffee; Clif CoolMint Chocolate; Clif Peanut Toffee Razz; Honey Stinger Caffeinated; Peak Energy Plus; Picky Bar Game, Set, Matcha; Verb
- **Dairy free (see also vegan).** Bonk Breaker, Bumble Bar, Clif Builder's and Nectar, Enjoy Life, GoMacro, KIND, Larabar, Perfect 10, Picky, RX, thinkThin Crunch, Vega Endurance
- **Enriched and fortified with added vitamins.** Balance, Zone-Perfect
- **Fiber, high (grams fiber).** Fiber One Chewy (5-6 g), Gnu Flavor and Fiber (12 g), NuGo Fiber d'Lish (12 g), Oatmega (7 g), Quest (13-14 g), thinkThin Protein and Fiber Bar (5 g)
- **Gut friendly, low FODMAP.** Fody, GoMacro Peanut Butter Protein Replenishment, EnjoyLife Dark Chocolate (and other flavors), GoodBelly, Happy
- **Gluten free.** Bonk Breaker, BumbleBar, Elev8Me, Enjoy Life, EnviroKidz Rice Cereal, Fody, Good Belly, GoMacro, Hammer,

KIND, Lara, Picky, PowerBar Protein Plus, Pure Protein, ProBar, RX, Quest, Raw Revolution, That's It Fruit, thinkThin, Truwomen, Zing, 88 Acres Seed and Oat

- **Gluten free and dairy free.** Bonk Breaker, Bumble Bar, Enjoy Life, Kind, Larabar, Picky, thinkThin
- **Low carb.** OhYeah! One, Pure Protein, Quest, Keto
- **Kosher.** GoMacro, Extend, Larabar, Pure Fit, ReNew Life Organic Energy, thinkThin, Truwomen
- **Nut free.** Don't Go Nuts, Enjoy Life, Freeyumm, Go Raw, Honey Stinger Waffle, Jumpstarter Bodyfuel, Luna Bar Lemon Zest, That's It, 88 Acres Seed and Oat
- **Organic.** Cascadian Farms, Clif, Pure, GoMacro, Red Square Powerflax
- **Peanut free.** Clif, Truwomen (some flavors), Enjoy Life
- **Protein bar (your choice of soy, whey, egg, or blended protein source) (grams protein):** Clif Builder (20 g), Gatorade Whey Protein Bar (20 g), GoMacro Protein Replenishment (10-12 g) Honey Stinger Protein (10 g), Lenny and Larry's Muscle Brownie (20 g), NuGo (10-12 g), Oatmega (14 g), PowerBar ProteinPlus (30 g), PowerCrunch (13 g), Pure Protein (20 g), Quest (21 g), RX (12 g), thinkThin Protein (20 g)
- **Raw.** Good Greens, Pure, Raw Revolution, Vega Whole Food Raw Energy Bar
- **Recovery bar (3-4 g carbohydrate to 1 g protein).** Clif, KIND Breakfast Protein, PowerBar Performance, Picky, RX
- **Soy free.** BumbleBar, Clif Nectar, Enjoy Life Chewy, GoRaw, KIND, Larabar, NuGo Fiber d'Lish, Oatmega, Picky, ProBar, Pure, Quest, Raw Revolution, Vega Endurance, Zing
- **Vegan (grams protein).** Clif (most flavors, 11 g), Clif Builder's (20 g), Go Macro (11 g), Good Greens (10 g), Hammer Vegan (15 g), Larabar (5 g), Picky (7 g), Pure Organic (4g), ProBar (8-11 g), thinkThin High Protein (some flavors are vegan, 13 g), Truwomen (12 g), Vega (10 g), 88 Acres Seed and Oat (6 g)
- **Women's bars (fewer calories; added calcium, iron, and folic acid).** Healthwarrior Chia, Iron Girl Energy, Larabar, Luna, PowerBar Pria, Truwomen
- **40-30-30 bars (40% carb, 30% protein, 30% fat)** Balance, ZonePerfect

SNACK ATTACKS

Snacks prevent not only hunger sensations but also cravings for sweets. Many of my clients complain about their constant cravings. They believe they are hopelessly, and helplessly, addicted to sugary snacks. I've helped many clients resolve their problematic sweet cravings easily and painlessly. The solution is simple: Eat before you get too hungry. When you are ravenous, you tend to crave sweets (and fat) and overeat. An apple won't do the job; you'll want apple pie . . . plus ice cream. When people get too hungry, they crave calorie-dense foods such as cookies, ice cream, chocolate—carbohydrate with fat (Gilhooly et al. 2007).

If you frequently experience uncontrollable snack attacks, examine the following case studies and solutions to learn how to tame the cookie monster within you. Remember, snack attacks, not snacks per se, are the problem.

Case 1: Predinner Snack Attack

I have the worst sweet tooth. I manage to fight sweet cravings until I get home, and then I inevitably attack the chocolate chip cookies. I feel as though I'm powerless and have no control over sweets. I hope you can put me on the straight and narrow.

—David, 47-year-old marathon runner, accountant, and father

Stories like David's are typical among my clients. He came to me feeling guilty about his lack of control over sweets. He required about 3,000 calories per day but ate zero calories at breakfast and barely ate lunch, only a 200-calorie yogurt, because he claimed he had no time. No wonder he was uncontrollably ravenous by the time he got home; he had accumulated a 2,800-calorie deficit! Nature took control by encouraging him to eat more than enough so that he would get adequate energy into his system.

I suggested that David eat his 1,600 cookie calories in the form of wholesome meals during the day. He started eating 800 calories for breakfast (cereal, milk, banana, and an english muffin with almond butter) and 1,000 calories of easy-to-eat snack-type foods for lunch and throughout the afternoon (two yogurts, two large bananas, two protein bars). Within one day he discovered that he wasn't a cookie monster after all. He could come home in a better mood, feel untempted by cookies, and have the energy to enjoy his family rather than be distracted by his need to eat cookies. This switch reduced his intake of saturated fat, improved the quality of his overall diet, helped him flatten the spare tire that had been inflating around his middle, and lowered his cholesterol—to say nothing of improving his quality of life.

Case 2: Premenstrual Snack Attack

I can easily tell the time of the month by my eating habits. Brownies and other premenstrual chocolate cravings do me in.

—Charlene, 21-year-old collegiate runner

Charlene, like many women, recognized that her eating patterns change with the stages of her menstrual cycle. In the week before her period, she has overwhelming cravings for fatty sugary foods (ice cream) or fatty salty foods (potato chips); the week afterward, she tends to crave more lower-fat foods or has very little appetite. Researchers have verified these eating patterns and report that a complex interplay of hormonal changes seems to influence women's food choices. High levels of estrogen may be linked to premenstrual carbohydrate cravings (Reed, Levin, and Evans 2008).

Women may also experience food cravings because they are hungrier. Before menstruation, a woman's metabolic rate may increase by 100 to 500 calories (Barr, Janelle, and Prior 1995). That addition would be the equivalent of another meal. But when Charlene felt bloated and fat because of premenstrual water weight gain, she, like most women, would put herself on a reducing diet. The result was double deprivation. She had a physiological need for extra calories just when she put herself on the calorie-deficient reducing diet. No wonder she experienced overwhelming hunger and craved sweets.

I told Charlene not to restrict calories, but instead, when she felt hungry in the week before her period, to give herself permission to eat up to 500 additional semi-wholesome calories. She started adding a hot cocoa to her standard breakfast, an oatmeal raisin cookie to lunch, and an afternoon snack of dark chocolate–covered almonds. She curbed the nagging hunger that had previously plagued her, and she was less irritable. Even her friends and family noticed a difference in her moods. She was thrilled to survive a menstrual cycle without gaining weight from evening brownie binges.

Chocolate in a Healthy Diet

Chocolate is made from cocoa, a plant food. It contains health-protective compounds called flavonoids that help relax and dilate blood vessels, reduce blood pressure, and increase blood flow to the brain. These flavonoids are also found in other plant foods, such as green tea, red wine, apples, and onions. Two tablespoons of natural cocoa powder (the kind used in baking) offers the same antioxidant power as 3/4 cup of blueberries or 1 1/2 glasses of red wine.

Of all the types of chocolate, dark chocolate (made with 70 percent cocoa) is the richest source of phytonutrients. Dark chocolate can help reduce blood cholesterol and offers heart-health benefits, specifically, improved blood vessel health and lower blood pressure (Taubert et al. 2007). Epidemiological surveys of large groups of people indicate that those who regularly consume chocolate take in more of these health-protective phytonutrients than do those who do not consume chocolate. This reduces their risk of heart disease. In the Netherlands, elderly men who routinely ate chocolate-containing products reduced their risk of heart disease by 50 percent and their risk of dying from other causes by 47 percent (Buijsse et al. 2006).

Despite all this good news about chocolate, it is still just a candy and not a life-sustaining food. Eat (dark) chocolate for pleasure; no excuses needed! Pure cocoa is bitter and unpalatable, so it needs a lot of added sugar to transform it into a delicious candy bar. The trick is to enjoy dark chocolate as part of the 150 to 200 discretionary sugar calories that can be part of your daily sports diet. There's little wrong with savoring a small piece of dark chocolate after a meal, when a little bit will do, and even this small amount has been shown to slightly reduce blood pressure (Taubert et al. 2007). As for me, I enjoy my dark chocolate during long hikes and bike rides. It tastes better to me than most commercial sports foods and nicely fuels both my body and my mind!

Case 3: Chocolate Snack Attack

Chocolate is my favorite food. I fight the urge to feed myself chocolate chip cookies for lunch, Hershey's Kisses for snacks, and chocolate ice cream for dinner.

—Jocelyn, 17-year-old high school basketball player

Some folks simply love sweets. They need no excuse to indulge in sugary goo. They eat sweets daily, three times if not more, starting with a chocolate chip muffin for breakfast, a big candy bar for lunch, sweet-and-sour pork for dinner, and then ice cream for dessert. Naturally, this high consumption of sweets results in a poor diet because sugar lacks vitamins and minerals.

As a healthy, active teen, Jocelyn had space in her diet to fit in sweets without jeopardizing her health. For people eating an overall wholesome diet, the *2015-2020 Dietary Guidelines for Americans* state that about 10 percent of the calories can come from refined sugar, if desired. Because Jocelyn required 2,800-plus calories per day, she could certainly fit in 280 calories of sugar, a reasonable amount.

Athletes who abuse sweets are more at risk for nutrition problems than those who routinely enjoy a small treat. Eating a pan of brownies for dinner is far different from eating one brownie as a fun food for dessert after a nourishing meal! Chocoholics who overindulge at night then commonly skip breakfast the next day because they're not hungry in the morning after having eaten too much chocolate the night before. They could nourish themselves better by eating a small chocolate dessert after dinner and then wake up hungry for a wholesome breakfast the next morning.

In Jocelyn's case the chocolate problem stemmed from having no time for breakfast, disliking school lunch, and having easy access to the vending machine. I encouraged her to eat breakfast on her way to school, which helped her consume fewer sweets during the day.

CHAPTER 6

CARBOHYDRATE: SIMPLIFYING A COMPLEX TOPIC

In this day and age of high-protein diets (to build muscle) and high-fat ketogenic diets (to lose weight), as well as chatter about *training low* (with depleted carbohydrate stores), confusion abounds about the role of carbohydrates in a sports diet. I constantly study the research and remain convinced that wholesome forms of carbohydrate are the best choices for both athletes and fitness exercisers for fueling your muscles and promoting good health. In this chapter, I will explain why.

People of all ages and athletic abilities will benefit from nourishing themselves with minimally processed carbohydrate-rich fruits, vegetables, beans, legumes, and whole-grain foods, along with the right balance of protein and healthy fats. But why do some athletes insist they feel better when they stop eating bread, cereal, and pasta? Carolyn, an avid triathlete, raved about how much better she felt after having cut out carbs. I asked, "What were you eating before you made this change?" Her answer indicated the Standard American diet (SAD), with skipped meals, abundant fast foods, and more junk snacks than high-quality meals. No wonder she felt better when she started eating better.

Other reasons for feeling so much better after giving up "carbs" might relate to food sensitivities. When you cut out a lot of foods, you eliminate the one or two items that might create feelings of unwellness. A registered dietitian can help you reach the same level of feeling great by working with you to figure out which foods contribute to the sensitivity.

Some athletes embrace a carb-free diet as a way to curb sugar binges that lead to eating too many carbs. An easier way to reduce carb binges is to prevent extreme hunger. Despite popular belief, carb binges are unlikely caused by being addicted to carbs, but rather caused by the physiological effects of hunger. Refer to chapters 5 (sweet cravings) and 16 (weight management).

The purpose of this chapter is to eliminate this confusion so you can make choices that best promote good health, appropriate weight, and optimal sports performance.

SIMPLE AND COMPLEX CARBOHYDRATES

The carbohydrate family includes both simple and complex carbohydrates. The simple carbohydrates are monosaccharides and disaccharides (single- and double-sugar molecules). Glucose, fructose, and galactose are monosaccharides, the simplest sugars, and can be symbolized like this:

The disaccharides can be symbolized like this:

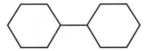

Four common sources of disaccharides are table sugar (sucrose), milk sugar (lactose, a combination of glucose and galactose), corn syrup, and honey.

Table sugar, corn syrup, and honey all contain glucose and fructose but in different amounts.

- Table sugar, upon digestion, breaks apart into 50 percent glucose and 50 percent fructose.
- High-fructose corn syrup (HFCS), commonly used in soft drinks, breaks down to about 55 percent fructose and 45 percent glucose. (HFCS is made using chemical processes that first convert cornstarch to corn syrup and then convert about 55 percent of the glucose in the corn syrup to fructose to make it taste sweeter.)
- Honey contains about 31 percent glucose, 38 percent fructose, 10 percent other sugars, 17 percent water, and 4 percent miscellaneous particles.

Your body eventually converts all monosaccharides and disaccharides to glucose, which travels in the blood (blood glucose) to fuel your muscles and brain.

Fruits and vegetables offer a variety of sugars in differing proportions. Because you absorb different sugars at different rates and by differing pathways, research indicates that consuming a variety of sugars allows for better absorption during exercise. This means that you should read the ingredient label on your sports drink to be sure it offers more than one type of sugar.

Honey has been mistakenly described as being superior to HFCS or refined white sugar. If you prefer honey because of the pleasant taste, fine. But it's not superior in terms of vitamins or performance. Sugar in any form—honey, maple syrup, corn syrup, brown sugar, raw sugar, or agave—offers insignificant nutritional value, and your body digests any type of sugar or carbohydrate into glucose before using it for fuel.

Another type of sugar that is found in many engineered sports foods is maltodextrins, also called glucose polymers. Maltodextrins are chains of about five glucose molecules. Sports drinks sweetened with maltodextrins can provide energy with rapid absorption and less sweetness than regular sugar provides. Sports fuels that use maltodextrins include Hammer Nutrition products.

Complex carbohydrates, such as starch in plant foods and glycogen in muscles, are formed when sugars link together to form long complex chains, similar to a string of hundreds of pearls. They can be symbolized like this:

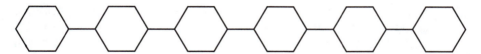

Plants store extra sugar in the form of starch. For example, corn is sweet when it's young, but it becomes starchy as it gets older. Its extra sugar converts into starch. In contrast to corn and other vegetables, fruits tend to convert starch into sugar as they ripen. A good example is the banana:

- A green banana with some yellow is 80 percent starch and 7 percent sugar.
- A mostly yellow banana is 25 percent starch and 65 percent sugar.
- A spotted and speckled banana is 5 percent starch and 90 percent sugar.

The potatoes, rice, bread, and other starches you eat are digested into glucose and then burned for energy or stored for future use. Humans store extra glucose mostly in the form of muscle glycogen and liver glycogen (but generally not as body fat). This glycogen is readily available for energy during exercise.

The Debate: Is Sugar Evil or OK for Athletes?

I'm sure you know people who avoid sugar like the plague. And you likely have friends who love the stuff and enjoy their daily sugar fix. While the antisugar folks report that sugar is health erosive, exercise scientists claim sugar is performance enhancing. That might leave you wondering: Should I eat sugar or avoid it? Here is information to help you better understand the two sides to the sugar debate: avoid sugar (DiNioloantonio and O'Keefe 2018) and allow sugar (Archer 2018).

Sugar: Just Say No

- Sugar is not an essential nutrient. Our bodies can make sugar (glucose) from the dietary fat and protein that we eat or by breaking down our body's muscle and adipose tissue.

- The average American eats about 100 pounds of sugar per year; that's 2 pounds a week and contributes abundant empty calories.

- Populations with a high intake of added sugars tend to have health issues. Reducing added sugar to less than 10 percent of total calories reduces risk of overweight, obesity, and tooth decay.

- Dietary sugar drives up blood sugar. Routinely consuming 150 sugar calories each day (e.g., one can of soda) increases the risk of developing diabetes by 1 percent. Much of this sugar is hidden in packaged foods.

- Metabolizing added sugar (with no nutritional value) requires vitamins and minerals. With very high sugar consumption (and low intake of other nourishing foods), one could become nutrient depleted.

- Trading empty sugar calories for nutrient-rich calories is a no-brainer. Limiting sugar intake does not harm anyone.

Sugar: OK for People Who Are Physically Fit

- Sugar consumption increased from less than 10 pounds per person per year in the late 1800s to about 100 pounds per person per year by World War II (1942) and remained relatively flat until 1980. Our health also improved between 1880 and 1980—so is it fair to say that the increase in sugar hurt our health?

- Sugar (and starch—a string of sugar molecules linked together) is in breast milk, dairy foods, fruit, honey, potato, wheat, corn, quinoa, and all grains. People around the globe have consumed these carbohydrates for years. So why now do sugar and starch suddenly become responsible for creating human obesity and diseases?

- The fear-mongering terms of *unhealthy*, *toxic*, and *poisonous* are simply unscientific. People who lack knowledge about physiology accept this antisugar rhetoric. But the fact is, no one food is *healthy* or *unhealthy*. You need to assess the whole diet.

- Poor health is not related to sugar, but to physical inactivity. Low levels of physical activity reduce the body's ability to metabolize sugar optimally, and that explains the true cause of obesity and metabolic diseases.

- In terms of diabetes, *blood* sugar, not *dietary* sugar, matters. The rise in blood sugar that occurs after eating is not pathological but rather the failure of the muscles and liver to take up the sugar. That is, it's not what you eat, but what your body does with what you eat. The bodies of physically active people readily take up sugar, unlike the bodies of inactive people.

- Physical activity affects appetite and energy intake. People who live a sedentary lifestyle tend to have a dysregulated appetite and can easily eat more calories than they burn. Lack of physical activity negatively affects health and sugar metabolism

Concluding Comments: One-Size Diet Does Not Fit All

Lack of physical activity, more so than sugar, is the greater threat to our health. Given that so many people are overfat and underfit, a diet low in sugars and starches is likely best for them. But for you—a sports-active, fit person with a reduced risk for heart disease, diabetes, and obesity—sugar and carbs are unlikely toxic, but rather a helpful way to enhance athletic performance (Lavie 2018).

No one is suggesting that athletes should eat unlimited amounts of sugar. Rather you should understand that, as an athlete, you want to embrace a healthy eating pattern that includes an appropriate balance of carbohydrate (sugars and starches) in each meal. The age-old advice to enjoy a variety of foods—with a bit of sugar, if desired—seems to be a reasonable goal.

Sugars and starches have similar abilities to fuel muscles but different abilities to nourish them with vitamins and minerals:

- The refined carbohydrate in sugary soft drinks provides energy but no vitamins or minerals.
- The highly processed carbohydrate in sports drinks, candies, and gels provides energy but no vitamins or minerals, unless the foods are fortified.
- The natural sugars and unrefined carbohydrate in fruits, vegetables, and whole grains provide energy, vitamins, minerals, fiber, and phytochemicals—the fuel and spark plugs that your body's engine needs to function best.

Is Carbohydrate Fattening?

Stacey, a personal trainer, wanted to eat bread, pasta, and other carbohydrate-rich foods for muscle fuel, but she also wanted to maintain a lean physique. Like many weight-conscious people who exercise, Stacey considered carbohydrate-based foods to be fattening, and she was frustrated. "I don't keep crackers, bread, cereal, or bagels in the house, because when they are there, I eat them—too many of them! I want to lose weight, not gain it from all that fattening carbohydrate."

The fact is, carbohydrate is not fattening in itself. Excess calories are fattening; in particular, excess calories from fat that accompanies the carbs—butter on bread, oil on pasta, mayonnaise on sandwiches, and cheese on crackers—are fattening. Fat provides 36 calories per teaspoon compared with 16 for carbohydrate. Additionally, the conversion of excess carbohydrate into body fat is limited because you preferentially burn carbohydrate when you exercise. Your body stores the excess dietary fat because the metabolic cost of converting excess carbohydrate into body fat is 23 percent of the ingested calories. Excess dietary fat, on the other hand, is easily stored as body fat; the metabolic cost of converting excess dietary fat into body fat is only 3 percent of ingested calories (Sims and Danforth 1987).

People often believe that carbohydrates are fattening because some carbohydrates can create a rapid rise in blood sugar, stimulate the body to secrete more insulin, and thereby promote fat storage. In fact, it is not so simple. Excess calories are fattening, not excess insulin. Insulin can, however, stimulate the appetite, as well as fat deposition, and that's where quickly digested carbohydrate gets a bad reputation. Choosing healthy eating patterns with slowly digested carbs (fiber-rich fruits, vegetables, and whole grains) generally means eating fewer refined foods, candies, and sweets that can easily add unwanted calories.

If you are destined to be gluttonous, your better bet is to overeat grapes (carbohydrate) rather than chips (fat). You'll fuel your muscles better, and the next day you'll enjoy a high-energy workout with muscles well loaded with carbohydrate. But be aware that a continuous intake of excess calories from carbohydrate will eventually contribute to weight gain. When your glycogen stores are filled, the excess calories are stored as body fat.

Rather than try to stay away from breads, bagels, and other grains, remember these points:

- Carbohydrate, preferably in the form of wholesome grains, fruits, and vegetables, is an important fuel for muscles during hard exercise.
- Excess calories, particularly from excess dietary fat, are the "enemy" in the battle of the bulge.
- When dieting to lose weight, plan to energize your workouts with wholesome carbohydrates such as whole-grain cereals and breads, pasta, and vegetables, but reduce your intake of the butter, oil, and mayonnaise that often accompany them.
- For added satiety, combine carbohydrate with protein, for example oatmeal with almonds, apple with peanut butter, and whole-wheat pasta with turkey meatballs.

If you tend to overindulge in carbohydrate sources such as bread and pasta, you should actually plan to eat your "trouble foods" more often, to make them less special. Carbohydrate binges commonly stem from feeling denied and deprived of these yummy foods. See chapter 16 for information on how to make peace with carbohydrate!

Quick and Slow Forms of Carbohydrate

Just as carbohydrate is referred to as *simple* or *complex* and *sugar* or *starches*, it can also be categorized as *quick* or *slow*. These terms refer to a complex system called the glycemic index (GI). The glycemic index is based on how 50 grams (200 calories) of carbohydrate (not counting fiber) in a food will affect blood sugar levels after an overnight fast. For example, white bread is a carbohydrate high on the glycemic index because it causes a rapid spike in blood sugar, whereas pinto beans are considered low on the glycemic index because they cause a more gradual increase in blood sugar levels.

The glycemic index was initially developed to help people with diabetes regulate their blood glucose levels. But people with diabetes generally eat foods in combinations (e.g., a sandwich with bread, turkey, and cheese), which can alter the glycemic index of the meal (Franz 2003). Athletes, however, commonly eat foods solo (e.g., a banana or a bagel). Hence, exercise scientists became curious about the possibility that quick and slow forms of carbohydrate might affect exercise performance differently because they affect blood glucose in different ways. Could athletes use this ranking system to determine what to eat before, during, and after exercise?

Low glycemic–index (low-GI) foods (apples, yogurt, lentils, beans, and other foods containing protein or fiber) provide a slow release of glucose into the bloodstream, and high-GI foods (e.g., sports drinks, jelly beans, and white bagels) quickly elevate blood sugar. Hence, low-GI foods might help endurance athletes perform better by providing sustained energy during long bouts of exercise. High-GI foods might be best to consume immediately after exercise to rapidly refuel the muscles in a tournament situation, when the athlete will be exercising hard within six hours.

Although this seems logical, the theory is not supported by research (Burdon et al. 2017). Hence, I tell my athletes to focus less on the glycemic index (table 6.1) and instead to enjoy carbohydrate-based foods that settle well and help them perform well. Too many factors influence a food's glycemic index, including where the food was grown, the amount eaten, added fat, the way the food is prepared, and whether the food is eaten hot or cold and in a fed or hungry body. To make the glycemic index even less meaningful, each of us has a daily glycemic response that can vary by as much as 43 percent on any given day (Vega-Lopez et al. 2007).

There is certainly no harm in eating slow-to-digest meals or snacks before embarking on a bout of endurance exercise, particularly if you are unable to consume fuel during the exercise session—if you are, say, a swimmer and have difficulty eating while exercising. You may find that the slow, steady release of energy offers a performance benefit (Moore et al. 2010). But consuming sports drinks, gels, fruit, or some form of carbohydrate during exercise offers a reliably stronger benefit. (Burke, Collier, and Hargreaves 1998). For sustained energy, your best bet is to simply eat an easily digested preexercise meal or snack and then, after the first hour, consume 200 to 350 calories of easily tolerated carbohydrate per hour of endurance exercise (Burke et al. 2011). See chapters 9 and 10 for more information about fueling before and during exercise.

For athletes who do double workouts or compete within four to six hours of the first session, choosing high-GI recovery foods to rapidly refuel

TABLE 6.1 Glycemic Index and Glycemic Load of Popular Sports Foods

Note the difference between a food's glycemic index (based on 50 grams of carbohydrate) and its glycemic load (based on a standard serving).

Food	Glycemic index (based on 50 g carbohydrate)	Glycemic load (based on 1 serving)	Size of 1 serving
Rice cakes	82	18	1 oz (30 g)
Cornflakes	81	20	1 oz (30 g)
Gatorade	78	12	8 oz (240 ml)
Wonder Bread	73	10	1 oz (30 g)
Bagel, white	69	24	2.5 oz (75 g)
Coca-Cola	63	16	8 oz (240 ml)
PowerBar, chocolate	58	24	2.3 oz (70 g)
Spaghetti	58	28	6 oz (180 g)
Snickers bar	57	18	1 oz (30 g)
Oatmeal, cooked	55	14	1 cup
Banana, underripe	47	11	4 oz (120 g)
Apple juice	44	13	8 oz (240 ml)
Orange	40	4	4 oz (120 g)
Chocolate milk (1.5% fat)	37	9	8 oz (240 ml)

Note: For a comprehensive list, visit www.glycemicindex.com.

Created from data in F.S. Atkinson, K. Foster-Powell, and J.C. Brand-Miller, "International Table of Glycemic Index and Glycemic Load Values: 2008," *Diabetes Care* 31, no 12 (2008) 2281-2283 and online-only tables at http://dx.doi.org/10.2337/dc08-1239.

is another practice that lacks scientific support (Brown et al. 2013). If you have to rapidly refuel from one bout of exhausting exercise to prepare for a second, eat *enough* easy-to-digest carbohydrate—at least 0.5 gram of carbohydrate per pound (1 g/kg) of body weight, or about 300 calories for a 150-pound (68 kg) person, every two hours for four to six hours. Also, enjoy a balance of healthy fat and protein to take care of all of your recovery needs, not just carbohydrate for glycogen. (See chapter 10 for more information about recovery.) If nothing else, a low-glycemic diet containing wholesome grains, fruits, and vegetables tends to offer the additional benefits of fighting inflammation and investing in your future well-being.

Sugar Highs and Lows

Some athletes claim to be sugar sensitive; that is, after they eat sugar, they report an energy spike followed by a crash. If that sounds familiar, the trick is to combine carbohydrate with protein or fat, such as bread plus peanut butter or an apple plus cheese. This changes the glycemic response of the carbohydrate. By experimenting with various types of snacks, you might notice that you perform better after eating 200 calories of oatmeal (a low-GI food) than you do after eating 200 calories of jelly beans (a high-GI food). Honor your personal response when choosing foods to support a winning edge for your body.

Keep in mind that most athletes don't get the blood sugar highs and lows seen in unfit people because well-trained muscles can readily take up carbohydrate from the bloodstream without much insulin. Athletes thereby have a reduced need for insulin compared to unfit people and are less likely to experience rebound hypoglycemia ("sugar crashes"). Because exercise is such a good way to keep blood sugar within a normal range, athletic people generally do not get the high blood sugar levels associated with type 2 diabetes, unless they are genetically high insulin secretors.

FACT OR FICTION

White bread is nutritionally worthless and a total waste of calories.

The facts: Although white bread fails to offer the whole-grain goodness found in whole-wheat, rye, or other hearty breads, it is neither a poison nor a bad food. It can be balanced into an overall wholesome diet. As I mentioned in chapter 1, the *2015-2020 Dietary Guidelines for Americans* state that at least half of your grains should come from whole grains. So if you have oatmeal for breakfast and brown rice for dinner, your diet can accommodate a sandwich made on white bread (or wrap) for lunch.

Most white breads are enriched with B vitamins and iron, so they are good sources of those nutrients. That's why it's OK for half your grains to come from enriched (refined) grains. If you were to eat only "100% natural" whole grains, you might not get enough of the B vitamin folate. Enriched white flour is a primary dietary source of folate for many people, particularly those who eat suboptimal amounts of fruits and vegetables (good sources of folate). See table 3.2 to learn about the difference in folate levels between enriched and all-natural breakfast cereals.

Athletic people who "crash" do so because they simply ran out of fuel. Megan, a weight-conscious high school runner, came to me complaining that she commonly felt light-headed, dizzy, and even nauseated during or after her hard runs. These symptoms of hypoglycemia (low blood sugar) stemmed from having consumed too little fuel at breakfast and lunch. She solved the problem by eating more at those meals, as well as enjoying a prerun snack of crackers and a low-fat cheese stick.

CARBOHYDRATE FOR GLYCOGEN

As mentioned, if you are trying to stay away from forms of carbohydrate such as bagels, potatoes, and breads because you mistakenly believe carbohydrate to be fattening, think again. They are not fattening, and you need them to fuel your muscles so that you can enjoy your exercise program.

The average 150-pound (68 kg) man has about 1,800 calories of carbohydrate stored in the liver, muscles, blood, and body fluids in approximately the distribution shown in table 6.2.

The carbohydrate in the muscles is used during exercise. The carbohydrate in the liver is released into the bloodstream to maintain a normal blood glucose level and feed the brain (as well as the muscles). These limited carbohydrate stores influence how long you can enjoy exercising. When your glycogen stores get too low, you hit the wall—that is, you feel overwhelmingly fatigued and yearn to quit. In a research study, cyclists with depleted muscle glycogen stores were able to exercise only 55 minutes to fatigue (as measured by an inability to maintain a specified pedaling speed on a stationary bicycle), as compared with more than twice as long—about 120 minutes—when they were carbohydrate loaded (Green et al. 2007). Food works!

In comparison to the approximately 1,800 calories of stored carbohydrate, the average lean 150-pound (68 kg) man also has 60,000 to 100,000 calories of stored fat—enough to run hundreds of miles. During low-level exercise such as walking, the muscles burn primarily fat for energy. During

TABLE 6.2 Carbohydrate Storage for a 150-Pound (68 kg) Man

Muscle glycogen	1,400 calories
Liver glycogen	320 calories
Glucose in plasma, body fluids	80 calories
Total	**1,800 calories**

light to moderate aerobic exercise, such as jogging, stored fat provides 50 to 60 percent of the fuel. When you exercise hard, as in sprinting, racing, lifting weights, or other intense exercise, you rely primarily on glycogen stores. Unfortunately, for competitive athletes, fat cannot be used exclusively as fuel because the muscles need a certain amount of carbohydrate to function well at high intensities, such as a surge up a hill or a sprint to the finish. Fitness exercisers can get away with a lower carbohydrate intake than elite athletes who push themselves to exhaustion can.

Biochemical changes that occur during training influence the amount of glycogen you can store in your muscles. The figures that follow indicate that well-trained muscles store 20 to 50 percent more glycogen than untrained muscles do (Costill et al. 1981; Sherman et al. 1981). This change enhances endurance capacity and is one reason a novice runner can't just load up on carbohydrate and run a top-quality marathon (table 6.3).

Because of the unfounded fears that carbohydrate is fattening or the belief that you need a high-protein diet to build muscle or a high-fat diet for endurance, many athletes today are skimping on carbohydrate foods. Some go on the paleo diet or keto diet; others go gluten free. The resulting low-carbohydrate intake can potentially hurt performance; it contrasts sharply with the diet of 2.5 to 4.5 grams of carbohydrate per pound of body weight (5 to 10 g/kg)—or 55 to 65 percent carbohydrate—recommended by most exercise and health professionals for people who train for one to three hours a day (table 6.4).

A case in point is ice hockey, an incredibly intense sport that relies on both muscular strength and power. During a game, carbohydrate is the primary fuel, and muscle carbohydrate (glycogen) stores decline between 38 and 88 percent. Muscle glycogen depletion relates closely to muscular fatigue. A motion analysis of elite ice hockey teams showed that the players with a high-carbohydrate (60 percent) diet skated not only 30 percent more distance but also faster than the players who ate their standard low-carbohydrate (40 percent) diet. In the final period of the game, which often determines whether a team wins or loses, the high-carbohydrate group skated 11 percent more distance than they did in the first period; the low-

TABLE 6.3 Muscle Glycogen per 100 Grams (3.5 oz) of Muscle

Untrained muscle	13 g
Trained muscle	32 g
Carbohydrate-loaded muscle	35-40 g

TABLE 6.4 Guidelines for Daily Carbohydrate Intake

Amount of exercise	Grams of carbohydrate per lb body weight per day	Grams of carbohydrate per kg body weight per day	Grams of carbohydrate per day for 120 lb (55 kg) athlete	Grams of carbohydrate per meal*	Grams of carbohydrate per day for 150 lb (68 kg) athlete	Grams of carbohydrate per meal*
Light exercise (<1 h/day)	1.5-2.5	3-5	180-300	45-75	225-375	55-95
Moderate exercise (~1 h/day)	2.5-3.0	5-7	300-360	75-90	375-450	95-110
Endurance exercise (1-3 h/day)	2.5-4.5	6-10	360-540	90-135	450-675	110-170
Extreme exercise (>4-5 h/day)	3.5-5.5	8-12	420-660	105-165	525-825	130-205

*By taking your daily carbohydrate needs and dividing them into four food buckets (breakfast, lunch 1, lunch 2, dinner), you can determine your carbohydrate target per section of the day.

Data from ACSM, AND, and DC Joint Position Statement: Nutrition and Athletic Performance, 2016

carbohydrate group skated 14 percent less. The researchers reached the following conclusions (Ackermark et al. 1996):

- Low muscle glycogen stores at the start of the game can jeopardize performance at the end of the game.
- Three days between games (with training on two of those days) plus a low-carbohydrate (40 percent) diet does not replace normal muscle glycogen stores (the players in the high-carbohydrate group had 45 percent more glycogen).
- The differences in performance between the well-fueled players and those who ate inadequate carbohydrate were most evident in the last period of the game.

Whether your sport is ice hockey, soccer, rugby, football, basketball, or any intense sport, remember to eat responsibly. Make carbohydrate the foundation of each meal and protein the accompaniment.

After exercise, it is important to consume carbohydrate to replenish muscle glycogen stores. In a landmark study, exercise physiologist J. Bergstrom and his colleagues (1967) compared the rate at which muscle glycogen was replaced in subjects who exercised to exhaustion and then ate either a high-protein, high-fat diet, or a high-carbohydrate diet. The subjects on the high-protein, high-fat diet (similar to an Atkins or other high-protein, low-carbohydrate diet with abundant eggs, chicken, beef, cheese, and nuts) remained glycogen depleted for five days (figure 6.1). The subjects on the high-carbohydrate diet totally replenished their muscle glycogen in two days. This result shows that protein and fat aren't stored as muscle glycogen and that carbohydrate is important for replacing depleted glycogen stores. Other research suggests that three sets of biceps curls (8 to 10 repetitions per set) reduce muscle glycogen by 35 percent (Martin, Armstrong, and Rodriquez 2005). With repeated days of low carbohydrate and high repetitions, the muscles of bodybuilders and marathon runners can soon become depleted. Hence, every athlete should eat meals in which two-thirds of the plate is dedicated to wholesome carbohydrates (grains, vegetables, fruits) and one-third to protein.

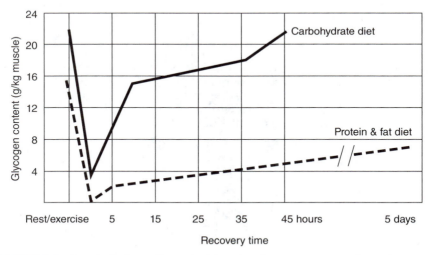

FIGURE 6.1 A carbohydrate diet replenishes the glycogen content of muscles more quickly than a protein and fat diet does.

Reprinted by permission from J. Bergström, L. Hermansen, E. Hultman, and B. Saltin, "Diet, Muscle Glycogen and Physical Performance," *Acta Physiologica Scandinavica* 71, no. 2-3 (1967); 140-150.

Train Low, Compete High?

Serious endurance and ultra-endurance athletes sometimes wonder whether they should train with poorly fueled muscles (low carbohydrate availability) to 1) teach the body to burn more fat so it spares the limited glycogen stores, and 2) drive up the metabolic adaptations that improve exercise capacity.

Training with low carbohydrate availability means exercising with low blood glucose or low muscle glycogen stores (or both). For example, this happens if you do a hard evening workout and eat just a salad with chicken for dinner (no bread or starches), and then exercise before eating breakfast the next morning. Or if you do double workouts and are "too busy" to eat enough before the second workout. When athletes exercise with depleted glycogen stores, they are unable to exercise at a very high intensity (Burke 2010). Hence, they should thoughtfully plan their high-intensity workouts for when they are fully glycogen loaded, so they can have a high-quality workout. On the one or two days a week when they train underfueled, they might want to consume preexercise coffee (or other sources of caffeine), eat extra protein (to help reduce muscle breakdown), and swish-and-spit a sports drink (to send positive signals to the brain) to make the workout less grueling (Bartlett, Hawley, and Morton 2015).

While training depleted might be advantageous for highly competitive endurance athletes (but also might increase risk of injury), I encourage recreational athletes to focus on the basic fueling practices that contribute to not only strong performance but also enjoyment of their exercise program. These include eating breakfast, getting enough sleep, following a healthy eating pattern, fueling up and refueling before and after workouts, and staying well hydrated. Until you master the basics, don't bother to delve into the fine-tuned practices for very competitive athletes.

WHAT ABOUT A VERY, VERY LOW-CARBOHYDRATE KETOGENIC DIET?

A keto diet is a very low-carbohydrate (less than 50 grams [200 calories] of carbohydrate per day) and very high-fat diet containing only a moderate protein serving at each meal. At least 70 percent of the calories come from fat, including butter, cream, olive oil, nuts, avocado, bacon, cheese, and pepperoni. The body switches from burning glucose as the primary fuel to burning fat (an uncomfortable transition). This generates a by-product called ketones. Ketones are an alternative fuel the body uses when glucose is in short supply. *Note:* A keto diet is *not* a high-protein diet. Protein can convert into glucose, which can take the body out of ketosis, the fat-burning mode.

Some athletes are attracted to a ketogenic diet as a means to manage their weight (see chapter 16 for more on this topic). Others, such as ultra-endurance runners, try the keto diet to reduce their need to consume fuel during extended exercise. And athletes with finicky stomachs try it to minimize intestinal distress.

More research is needed to determine whether or not the ketogenic diet is performance enhancing (Burke and Hawley 2018; McSwiney et al. 2018). If so, under what circumstances? Will it support long-term good health? Or does is involve a lot of restrictive eating for a questionable benefit? If the keto diet is calling to you, I encourage you to first consult with a registered sports dietitian who can suggest ways to tweak your current food intake to help you reach your performance and weight goals within the boundaries of a more easily sustained healthy eating pattern.

FUELING FOR ENDURANCE EXERCISE

If you are preparing for an intense endurance event that lasts more than 90 minutes—a competitive marathon, triathlon, cross-country ski race, or long-distance bike race—you should start the event with muscles that are fully loaded with carbohydrate. Although carbohydrate loading sounds simple (Just stuff yourself with pasta, right?), the truth is that many endurance athletes make food mistakes that hurt their performance. As one marathoner said after stuffing herself the night before her first marathon, "I woke up feeling very heavy and bloated . . . not the way I wanted to feel at the start of the race."

Wise athletes "carbo load" every training day, meaning they eat enough grains, fruits, and vegetables to fully refuel their muscles daily. (That is, unless they are elite athletes who choose to train depleted for carefully planned workouts, as explained in the earlier section, Train Low, Compete High.) Here are my nine tips to help all endurance athletes fuel optimally for their events.

1. **No drastic dietary changes.** Endurance athletes can train best with a daily carbohydrate intake of 2.5 to 4.5 grams of carbohydrate per pound of body weight (6 to 10 g/kg). This prevents chronic glycogen depletion and allows you to train hard, which means you can race hard on the day

of the event. The guidelines in table 6.4 can help you determine your daily carbohydrate needs based on where you are in your training (ramping up, tapering, off-season). Use table 6.6 later in this chapter, information on food labels, or food trackers to see how close you come to meeting your targets.

Preevent dietary changes can contribute to intestinal distress (diarrhea from too much fruit and fiber-rich whole grains, constipation from too much white bread and refined grains), so stick with your tried-and-true foods that have fueled your training sessions. If you will be too nervous to eat much the day before the event or are worried about undesired pit stops, you might want to boost your carbohydrate intake two or three days before the event to allow food adequate time to pass through your intestinal tract. As long as you don't exercise much, the glycogen will stay in your muscles. Then, the day before your competition, graze on crackers, chicken noodle soup, and other easily tolerated low-fiber foods.

2. **Taper your training.** Forget any plans for last-minute training sprees. Do your final high-volume endurance training and start tapering your training volume 8 to 14 days out. Although hard training builds you up, it also tears you down, and you need time to heal any damage that occurred during training and to completely refuel with carbohydrate. Exercise scientists suggest doing short-and-sweet high-intensity preevent workouts and reducing the weekly volume of exercise by 40 to 60 percent (Mujika 2010). For athletes in power sports, four days away from lifting weights improves peak force for the day of the event (Pritchard 2018).

Correct tapering requires tremendous mental discipline and control. Some athletes are afraid they will get out of shape because they are exercising less. Worry not. The proof will come when you perform better—perhaps 9 percent better. Swimmers, for example, maximized their performance when they tapered for two weeks (Costill et al. 1985). Again, the key is to reduce the training load, but maintain some high-intensity workout bouts (Mujika 2010).

Because you will be exercising less during the preevent taper, you do not need to eat hundreds of additional calories when carbohydrate loading. Simply maintain your standard intake (this should be grains, fruits, and vegetables as the foundation of every meal and snack, with protein as the accompaniment). The 600 to 1,000 or so calories that you generally burn during training will be used to give your muscles extra fuel. By saving the calories that you otherwise would have burned during training, you can approximately double your glycogen stores and will be able to exercise harder at the end of your event.

You'll know you have carbohydrate loaded properly if you gain 2 to 4 pounds (1 to 2 kg), which is mostly water weight. With each ounce (30 g)

Carbohydrate Loading Without Pasta

Not every athlete can carbohydrate load on pasta, breads, and cereals. About 1 percent of people in the United States and Canada have celiac disease, a disorder in which the body can't tolerate gluten, a protein found in wheat, rye, barley, and sometimes oats (if the oats are contaminated with wheat during processing). In these people, gluten triggers intestinal inflammation, damages the small intestine, and eventually can interfere with the absorption of nutrients, including iron and calcium. Gluten intolerance easily leads to anemia (if iron is not absorbed) and osteoporosis (if calcium is not absorbed).

Celiac disease can be difficult to diagnose because the symptoms vary from person to person. Some people experience diarrhea and cramping; others complain about constipation and bloating. I had a client who had no idea she had celiac disease—until she started getting stress fractures. Your best bet is to talk with your doctor if you are having intestinal problems or have other niggling health concerns, including unexplained fatigue, anemia, multiple stress fractures, infertility, and lactose intolerance. If you want to get tested for celiac disease, do so before you go on a gluten-free diet; this will capture the best test results.

For athletes, fueling without gluten is a surmountable obstacle. You can still carbohydrate load, however, on rice, corn, potatoes, yams, chickpeas, buckwheat, quinoa, bananas, fruits, vegetables, juices, and numerous other sources of carbohydrate. Look for "certified gluten free" on labels of packaged foods, because products made in a factory that processes wheat foods can be contaminated with gluten. See table 6.5 for a sample gluten-free carbohydrate-loading menu.

To help you with your gluten-free diet, I highly recommend that you meet with a local sports dietitian and read books on the topic, such as *Gluten-Free: The Definitive Resource Guide* (2016) by Shelley Case, RD. See appendix A for more sources.

of stored glycogen, you store about 3 ounces (90 ml) of water. This water becomes available during exercise and reduces dehydration.

3. **Eat enough protein.** Because endurance athletes burn some protein for energy, they should take special care to include some protein-rich food

in each meal. Even when carbohydrate loading, your diet should include 0.5 to 0.8 gram of protein per pound (1.2 to 1.7 g/kg) of body weight. Your body needs protein daily to prevent muscle breakdown and enable muscle repair.

4. **Do not fat load.** To achieve a carbohydrate-based diet containing about 4 grams of carbohydrate per pound of body weight (600 grams of carbohydrate for a 150-pound (68 kg) person, the equivalent of 2,400 calories of carbohydrate), you need to reduce your intake of calories from fat to make room for more carbohydrate. A little fat is OK, but don't fat load. For example, choose pasta with tomato (not Alfredo) sauce; trade the fat calories in two pats of butter and a dollop of sour cream for a second plain baked potato. When you trade fat for more carbohydrate, you need to eat a larger volume of food to obtain adequate calories. A 1-pound (480 g) box of spaghetti cooks into a mountain of pasta but provides only 1,600 calories. That's a reasonable calorie goal for a hefty meal before a challenging 100-mile bike ride, but it may be more volume than you anticipated. See table 6.5 for a sample carbohydrate-loading menu.

5. **Pay attention to your fiber intake.** Fiber-rich foods promote regular bowel movements and keep your system running smoothly. Bran cereal, whole-wheat bread, oatmeal, flax, fruits, and vegetables are good choices. If you carbohydrate load on too much white bread, pasta, rice, and other refined products, you're likely to become constipated, particularly if you are training less. Yet the day or two before an event, athletes who worry more about diarrhea than constipation prefer to eat very low-fiber diets. They carbohydrate load on juices, white bread, rice, pasta, and sherbet. Through trial and error, you'll learn what works for your body.

6. **Plan meal times carefully.** NYC Marathon queen Grete Waitz once said she never ate a very big meal the night before a marathon because it usually would give her trouble the next day. She preferred to eat a bigger lunch. You, too, might find that this pattern works well for your intestinal tract. That is, instead of relying on a big pasta dinner the night before the event, you might want to enjoy a substantial carbohydrate feast at breakfast or lunch. This earlier meal allows plenty of time for the food to move through your system—and reduces the stress of fretting about portable toilets. Plus, you also might sleep better. If you are a traveling athlete, you'll be more easily served at restaurants, which are often overcrowded at dinnertime.

You'll be better off eating a little bit too much than too little the day before the event, but don't overfeed yourself. Learning the right balance

TABLE 6.5 Sample Carbohydrate-Loading Menu—With or Without Pasta!

Even if you do not eat wheat, you can still carbohydrate load. The following 3,200-calorie high-carbohydrate diet provides about 3.5 grams of carbohydrate per pound of body weight (8 g/kg) for a 150-pound (68 kg) endurance athlete. (*Note:* If you cannot eat wheat, replace the two cups of pasta with two cups of rice.) The menu includes adequate protein (1 g/lb, or 2.2 g/kg) to maintain muscles.

For help assessing your own carbohydrate-loading menu using your favorite foods, use a food tracker (see appendix A).

Food	Calories	Carb (g)
BREAKFAST		
Oatmeal*, 1 cup (80 g) dry, cooked in milk, 1%, 16 oz (480 ml)	500	70
Raisins, 1.5 oz (45 g, small box)	130	35
Brown sugar, 1 tbsp	55	15
Apple cider, 12 oz (360 ml)	170	45
LUNCH		
Potato, large baked, topped with cottage cheese, 1% fat, 1 cup (230 g)	435	70
Baby carrots, 8, dipped in hummus, 1/2 cup	240	35
Grape juice, 12 oz (360 ml)	220	55
SNACK		
Banana, extra large	150	40
Peanut butter, 3 tbsp	270	10
DINNER		
Pasta, 2 cups cooked (or brown rice, 2 cups cooked)	430	90
Chicken, 5 oz (150 g), sauteed in olive oil, 2 tsp	330	—
Green beans, 1 cup	50	10
DESSERT		
Dried pineapple, 1/2 cup (2.5 oz, or 75 g)	220	55
Total	3,200	530

*People with celiac diseases should buy oatmeal that is certified "gluten free." Standard oatmeal can be contaminated with gluten if it is processed in a factory that processes wheat.

takes practice. Each long training session leading up to the endurance event offers the opportunity to learn which foods—and how much of them—to eat. You need to train your intestinal tract as well as your heart, lungs, and muscles. Remember to practice your preevent carbohydrate-loading meal during training so you'll have no surprises on the day of the event.

7. **Drink extra fluids.** To reduce your risk of starting the event dehydrated, be sure to drink extra water and juice. Abstain from too much wine and alcohol; they are not only poor sources of carbohydrate, but also dehydrating. Drink enough alcohol-free beverages to produce a significant volume of urine every two to four hours. The urine should be pale yellow, like lemonade. Don't bother to overhydrate to the extent that you have to urinate every half hour or several times during the night; your body is like a sponge and can absorb only so much fluid.

On the morning of the competition, drink another two or three glasses of fluid up to two hours before the event (to allow plenty of time to excrete the excess) and then another cup or two 5 to 10 minutes before race time. See chapters 8 and 10 for more information about proper hydration tactics.

8. **Be sensible about your selections.** Do not carbohydrate load on fruit only; you're likely to get diarrhea. Do not carbohydrate load on refined white bread products only; you'll likely become constipated. Do not carbohydrate load on beer; you'll have to exercise with a hangover. Do not do too much last-minute training; you'll fatigue your muscles. And do not blow it all by eating unfamiliar foods that might upset your system. Change your exercise program more than your diet.

9. **Eat breakfast on event day.** What you eat the day before the event is just part of the fueling plan. Eating enough breakfast before starting the endurance event is important; it will prevent hunger and help maintain normal blood sugar levels. Equally important is choosing food you're familiar with. As mentioned, you should practice preevent fueling with your long training sessions to learn which foods in what amounts work best for you and your intestinal tract.

Don't try new foods. That festive pancake breakfast may settle like Mississippi mud, and so may the unfamiliar sports food you've been saving for the occasion. See chapters 8, 9, and 10 for more information about preexercise fueling, as well as fueling during the event. With wise eating, you can enjoy miles of smiles.

BONKING

Carbohydrate is stored not only in muscle but also in the liver. Liver glycogen feeds into the bloodstream to maintain a normal blood sugar level essential for "brain food." Depleted liver glycogen can cause you to bonk, or crash. Despite having adequate muscle glycogen, an athlete may feel uncoordinated, light headed, unable to concentrate, and weakened because the liver is releasing inadequate sugar into the bloodstream. Athletes with low blood sugar tend to perform poorly because the poorly fueled brain curbs muscular function and mental drive. They also tend to be grumpy and easily irritated and have less fun. The solution is to eat before you exercise.

Gianni, a 28-year-old runner and banker, faithfully ate a carbohydrate-rich diet for three days before his first Boston Marathon. On the evening before the marathon, he ate dinner at 5:00 and then went to bed at 8:30 to make sure he had a good night's rest. But, as often happens with anxious athletes, he tossed and turned all night (which burned a significant amount of calories). Gianni got up early the next morning and chose not to eat breakfast, even though the marathon didn't start until 10:30. By that time, he had depleted his limited liver glycogen stores. He lost his mental drive about 8 miles (13 km) into the race and quit at 12 miles (19 km). His muscles were well fueled, but energy was unavailable to his brain, so he lacked the mental stamina to endure the marathon.

Gianni could have prevented this needless fatigue by eating oatmeal, cereal, or other forms of carbohydrate at breakfast to refuel his liver glycogen stores, as well as by starting to fuel soon after the start of the marathon. Athletic success depends on both well-fueled muscles and a well-fueled mind.

RECOVERY FROM DAILY TRAINING

Carbohydrate is important on a daily basis for those who train hard day after day and want to maintain high energy. If you habitually limit your intake of grains, fruits, and starchy vegetables, your muscles will feel chronically fatigued. You'll train, but not at your best.

Figure 6.2 illustrates the glycogen depletion that can occur when athletes eat an inadequate amount of carbohydrate and still try to exercise hard day after day (Costill et al. 1971). In this landmark study, on three consecutive days the subjects ran hard for 10 miles (16 km), at a pace of six to eight minutes per mile (1.6 km). They ate their standard meals, with too much protein and fat (and perhaps alcohol) and too little grain foods, fruits, and vegetables. The subjects' muscles became increasingly glycogen depleted. Had the runners eaten larger portions of carbohydrate (and smaller portions of protein and fat), they would have better replaced their glycogen stores and better invested in top performance.

This study emphasizes the need not only for daily grains, fruits, and starchy vegetables but also for recovery days with light or no training. If you are doing daily hard workouts, take heed: Your depleted muscles need at least one day, if not two, to refuel after exhaustive sessions. (If you are a casual exerciser who uses significantly less glycogen during, let's say, a half-hour walk or a gentle swim, recovery days are less essential.)

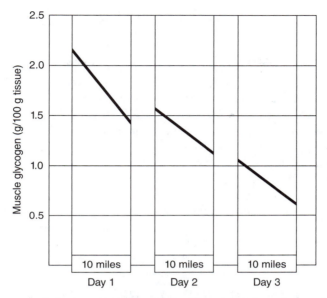

FIGURE 6.2 A carbohydrate-based sports diet is needed daily to prevent the cumulative effects of glycogen depletion that can occur when running 10 miles a day, day after day.

Adapted by permission from D.L. Costill, R. Bowers, G. Branam, and K. Sparks, "Muscle Glycogen Utilization During Prolonged Exercise on Successive Days," *Journal of Applied Physiology* 31, no. 6 (1971): 834-838.

Crystal, a 28-year-old nurse practitioner and dedicated exerciser, learned the importance of recovery days and adequate carbohydrate through a sports nutrition experiment. When she first came to see me, she insisted on training every day to get in shape for her first marathon. I recommended that she take one or two days off a week.

Crystal decided to experiment with her two-hour Sunday run to determine whether her running improved with running less and eating better. She discovered she could train at her best when she did little or no training the day before her long run (to rest her muscles), followed by a day off after her long run (to refuel). She stopped forcing herself to do the obligatory daily training run on days when her muscles felt fatigued. Instead, she planned two rest days per week and started focusing on *quality* training rather than *quantity* training. Her running improved, as did her mental outlook and enthusiasm for her sport. She ran a personal best in the marathon, cutting seven minutes off her time.

FACT OR FICTION

Athletes lose fitness on rest days.

The facts: You won't lose fitness on rest days; rather, such days enhance your strength and endurance by providing better-fueled muscles. Remember, the bad things happen when you exercise hard; the good things happen when you rest! Athletes who underestimate the value of rest and instead train relentlessly set the stage for injuries, chronic glycogen depletion, chronic fatigue, and reduced performance. These athletes often grab vitamin supplements, iron pills, and other enticing potions in the hope of boosting their energy. All they really need to do to perform better is exercise less.

If you are severely overtrained, you may need weeks, if not months, to recover. Don't underestimate the value of rest—as well as adequate sleep, calories, carbohydrate, and fluids.

CARBOHYDRATE-RICH FOODS

All too often, I talk with athletes who believe they eat a carbohydrate-rich diet when they really don't. Eric, a 33-year-old store manager and triathlete, intended to carbohydrate load the night before his first triathlon. Because of inadequate nutrition knowledge, he "carbohydrate loaded" with a pepperoni pizza with double cheese. Little did he know that of the 1,800 calories in the large pizza, 1,200 were from the protein and fat in the double cheese and pepperoni. Only 35 percent of the calories, from the thin crust and tomato sauce, were from carbohydrate (160 g). No wonder he felt sluggish during the event. I gave Eric a list of the carbohydrate content of common foods (table 6.6) to post on his refrigerator. With this tool he learned to select high-carbohydrate foods.

In addition, I taught Eric how to make better selections based on Nutrition Facts labels on food. You, too, can use these labels to guide your selections. Nutrition Facts labels list the number of grams of carbohydrate, protein, and fat (and alcohol, if present) per serving. To convert grams into calories, use this information:

1 gram carbohydrate = 4 calories

1 gram protein = 4 calories

1 gram fat = 9 calories

1 gram alcohol = 7 calories

TABLE 6.6 Carbohydrate Content of Common Foods

Food	Amount	Carbohydrate (g)
Raisins	1/3 cup	45
Banana	1 medium	25
Apricots, dried	10 halves	25
Apple, dried	1 medium	20
Orange	1 medium	20
Corn	1/2 cup	20
Winter squash	1/2 cup	15
Peas	1/2 cup	15
Carrot	1 medium	10
Broccoli	1/2 cup	5
Bagel, Starbucks	1	55
Grape-Nuts	2/3 cup	50
Raisin Bran, Kellogg's	1 cup	45
Tortilla (for burrito, wrap)	2.5 oz (55 g)	40
Granola bar, Nature Valley	2 bars (1 pkt)	30
Oatmeal, maple instant	1 packet	35
english muffin, Thomas'	1	25
Cheerios	1 cup	20
Bread, rye	1 slice	15
Graham crackers	2 squares	12
Grape juice	8 oz (240 ml)	35
Cran-raspberry juice	8 oz (240 ml)	30
Orange juice	8 oz (240 ml)	25
Milk, chocolate	8 oz (240 ml)	25
Gatorade	8 oz (240 ml)	20
Baked potato	1 large	65
Minestrone soup, Progresso	1 can (18.5 oz)	50
Macaroni and cheese, Annie's	1 cup	45
Pizza, frozen	2 slices	45

(continued)

TABLE 6.6 *(continued)*

Food	Amount	Carbohydrate (g)
Rice, cooked	1 cup	45
Lentils, cooked	1 cup	45
Spaghetti, cooked	1 cup	40
Quinoa, cooked	1 cup	40
Bean burrito, frozen	5 oz (150 g)	35
Refried beans, canned	1 cup	25
Frozen yogurt	1 cup	35
Fig Newton	2	20
Greek yogurt, vanilla	5.3 oz (150 g)	15
Honey	1 tbsp	15
Maple syrup	1 tbsp	15

Note: Nutrition information from food labels and the USDA National Nutrient Database for Standard Reference.

To determine the number of carbohydrate calories in a food item, multiply the number of grams of carbohydrate by four (calories per gram). Next, compare the carbohydrate calories to the total calories per serving to determine the percentage of calories that are from carbohydrate. For example, a 1/2 cup serving of a gourmet vanilla ice cream might have 200 total calories and 20 grams of carbohydrate.

20 grams of carbohydrate × 4 calories/gram
= 80 calories from carbohydrate

80 calories from carbohydrate ÷ 200 total calories
= 40% of calories from carbohydrate

Using food label information, you can determine that ice cream contains relatively fewer grams of carbohydrate than frozen yogurt does. For example, for every 100 calories of vanilla ice cream (1/4 cup; two spoonfuls), you get only 10 grams (40 calories) of carbohydrate. This is 40 percent of the total calories. On the other hand, for every 100 calories of frozen yogurt (1/2 cup; four spoonfuls), you get about 22 grams (88 calories) of carbohydrate—88 percent of total calories.

Your diet should provide carbohydrate as the foundation of each meal—more specifically, 2.5 to 4.5 grams of carbohydrate per pound (5 to 10 g/kg) if you train for one to three hours a day; fitness exercisers need less than endurance athletes (see table 6.4). Although you need not get obsessed about tracking grams of carbohydrate (unless that is of interest), you do want to choose more starches and grains and fewer high-fat foods. Replace muffins with bagels, salads with sandwiches, and Alfredo sauce with tomato sauce on pasta.

Learning about the composition of your training diet can be helpful. The Internet offers options for tracking your intake of carbohydrate (and other nutrients), which can be easier than gathering the information from food labels. (See the Food Trackers section in appendix A.) This can be particularly eye opening for people on the paleo diet, a gluten-free diet, or an Atkins-type low-carbohydrate diet, who do not eat grain foods. For example, Brian, a CrossFit fanatic, routinely snacked on handfuls of peanuts, almonds, and sunflower seeds. By measuring his food and recording his intake on MyFitnessPal, he quickly learned that he needed to boost his carbohydrate intake. He started combining the nuts and seeds with higher-carbohydrate items—craisins, dried apricots, and dates, as well as snacking on baked sweet potatoes. "You know, my training has improved since I made that switch. My muscles feel springier, and I have greater endurance. I feel better. I'm glad I learned this simple solution to my needless fatigue."

CHAPTER 7

PROTEIN: BUILDING AND REPAIRING MUSCLES

Traditionally, the (misguided) message has been clear: If you want to build muscles, you need to eat a lot of protein: six eggs for breakfast, a pound of deli turkey for lunch, and at least two, if not three, chicken breasts for dinner. The truth is that resistance exercises such as lifting heavy weight and doing push-ups—not eating excess protein—build and strengthen muscles. If you consume more protein than you need, you will simply burn more protein as a fuel source.

Confusion exists about the best sports diet. When you work out in the weight room at the gym, you likely hear that you need to consume lots of meat plus drink protein shakes between meals to be stronger. But when you hang around in the cardio area, you hear that carbohydrates should be the foundation of your meals. And you are left wondering, what's the right balance?

Carbohydrate-rich grains, fruits, and vegetables are indeed the best foundation for every type of training program. Even bodybuilders need a carbohydrate-based diet because carbohydrate is stored in the muscles for energy. You can't lift weights and demand a lot from your workout sessions if your muscles are carbohydrate depleted. Protein-based diets low in carbohydrate provide inadequate muscle fuel for you to perform the hard exercise required to build to your potential. As Alex, a fitness exerciser who tried to lose weight by eating a high-protein, high-fat diet, reported, "I just couldn't lift heavy weights as well when I cut out carbs."

The best sports diet contains ample, but not excessive, protein to build and repair muscle tissue, grow hair and fingernails, produce hormones, boost your immune system, and replace red blood cells. Most people who eat moderate portions of protein-rich foods daily get more protein than they need. Any excess protein is burned for energy or, as a last resort, stored as fat or glycogen. Humans do not store excess protein as muscle or amino acids (the building blocks of protein), so we need to consume adequate protein each day, and preferably distribute that protein evenly throughout the day. This is particularly important for dieters who are restricting calories, because they burn protein (from food and muscles) for energy when carbohydrate and calories are scarce.

The physiques of bodybuilders are not attributable to the excessively high amounts of protein they commonly consume but rather to their intense training. Bodybuilders work incredibly hard. They prefer a high-protein diet because protein not only builds and protects their muscles when they are cutting calories but also keeps them from feeling hungry—plus, lean protein is harder to overconsume than, let's say, pizza.

PROTEIN AND AMINO ACIDS

The need for protein is actually a need for amino acids. Proteins are made up of 20 amino acids that your body uses to build muscle tissue—hence,

Turning Protein Into Muscle

Just how do eggs, cottage cheese, and peanut butter turn into bigger muscles? Here are the steps to making muscle.

- When you eat protein (e.g., eggs, milk, meats, soy, beans), your stomach starts to digest it, and the intestines finish digesting the protein into individual amino acids. The amino acids are absorbed, sent to the liver, and then into the blood and to the muscles.

- Muscles use the amino acids to make more muscle, convert it to another type of amino acid (such as alanine and glutamine), or burn it for fuel. Leucine is the key amino acid that "turns on" the muscle-building process. Foods richest in leucine tend to be animal proteins (8 to 13 percent leucine) as compared to plant protein (6 to 8 percent leucine). Hence, vegetarian athletes want to eat generous amounts of plant proteins to boost their leucine intake (van Vliet, Burd, and van Loon 2015).

- The amount of protein that optimizes muscle building is about 0.12 to 0.15 grams of protein per pound (0.25 to 0.3 g protein/kg) of body weight within the first two hours after resistance exercise. Eating more protein provides only a very small benefit. So yes, you could eat twice as much, but you would not get much benefit in terms of bigger muscles.

- Most people can build only a few pounds of muscle in a month. That's far less than they dream!

their nickname "building blocks." Every tissue in your body is made up of some combination of them. Your body can make some amino acids itself, but eight of them are called essential amino acids and must come from the foods you eat.

While the amino acid leucine can *trigger* muscle building, your body needs all the essential amino acids to make new muscles. Natural protein-rich foods are the best sources of all the amino acids because they offer a complex and complete matrix that is more effective than processed proteins. For example, research on eggs highlights the benefits of protein from whole foods. A whole egg promotes 40 percent greater muscle protein synthesis in the five hours postexercise compared to eating just the egg white (van Vliet et al. 2017). Interactions among all the nutrients in foods facilitate a more robust response when compared to eating an isolated protein.

You can save yourself a lot of money by enjoying natural foods rather than expensive amino acid and protein supplements. Athletes have little need to buy supplements of leucine, or branched-chain amino acids. Contrary to what you might read in advertisements, standard foods rich in high-quality protein (dairy, fish, eggs, meats, soy), along with regular exercise, can help you achieve muscle growth.

WHAT'S THE RIGHT BALANCE?

When it comes to protein intake, athletes seem to fall into two categories. First are those who eat too much—the bodybuilders, weightlifters, and football players who can't seem to get enough of the stuff. Those in the second group eat too little—the runners, dancers, and weight-conscious athletes who rarely touch meat and trade most protein calories for more salads and vegetables. Athletes in either group can perform poorly because of dietary imbalances.

Josh, for example, pushed a lot of protein into his menu. A college hockey player, he routinely recovered after practice with a big protein bar (30 grams protein) plus a protein shake (20 grams protein). Little did he know that 20 to 25 grams of postexercise protein maximally stimulates muscular growth, and only very large athletes or those on a very low-calorie reducing diet might use up to 40 grams of protein at one time. (ACSM 2016; Moore et al. 2009). For an athlete who is eating plenty of calories, more protein does not translate into bigger muscles.

Paulo, a vegetarian marathon runner who ate pasta with tomato sauce seven nights a week, downplayed his need for protein. "Most Americans get way too much protein; I'm sure I get plenty, too." He consumed few protein-rich foods of any type—plant or animal products. He was humbled when he learned that his food intake was deficient not only in protein but also in iron (for red blood cells), zinc (for healing), calcium (for bones), and several other nutrients that accompany protein-rich foods. No wonder he became anemic, suffered lingering cold and flu, and performed poorly despite consistent training.

Hal, a self-described poor student, lived on oatmeal, ramen, and granola bars for the majority of his meals. On Sundays, he'd have a "real meal" when he went home to visit his family, thinking a once-a-week slab of roast beef could carry him through the week. Wrong. He has a daily need for protein.

DEFINING PROTEIN NEEDS

In scrutinizing the protein needs of athletes, exercise scientists have found that athletes need slightly more protein than other people do to repair the small amounts of muscle damage that occur with training, to provide energy (in very small amounts) for exercise, and to support the building of new muscle tissue. The exact protein requirements of sports-active people varies based on individual needs. People in the following groups have the highest protein needs:

- Endurance athletes and others participating in intense exercise. About 5 percent of energy can come from protein during endurance exercise, particularly if muscle glycogen stores are depleted and blood glucose is low.
- Dieters consuming too few calories. When calorie intake is low, protein is converted into glucose and burned for energy instead of being used to build and repair muscles.
- Growing teenage athletes. Protein is essential for both growth and muscle development.
- Untrained people starting an exercise program. People in this category need extra protein to build muscles.
- People over 50 years old. Protein needs actually increase with age, so senior athletes should be sure to include adequate protein-rich foods at each meal.

In general, pinpointing exact protein requirements is a moot point because most hungry athletes tend to eat more protein than they require just through standard meals. That is, a hungry 150-pound (68 kg) recreational athlete can easily consume after a workout the recommended 0.15 gram of recovery protein per pound (0.3 g/kg) of body weight. That's only about 20 grams of protein, the amount in 12 ounces (360 ml) of Fairlife (protein-rich, lactose-free) chocolate milk. Note that you want to consume protein evenly throughout the day, with a target of 0.15 gram of protein per pound (0.3 g/kg) every three to five hours (ACSM 2016). If you are severely restricting your calorie intake, bump that up a bit (Helms et al. 2014).

Protein needs should be based on grams of protein per pound (or kilogram) of body weight, and not by percent of calories. Table 7.1 provides safe and adequate recommendations for daily protein intake for a range of people. These recommendations include a margin of safety and are not minimal amounts. If you have excessive body fat, base your protein needs closer to your ideal body weight.

TABLE 7.1 Protein Recommendations

While protein requirements have traditionally been set in terms of daily needs, the current view for athletes is to focus on even distribution of protein throughout the day. Depending on your body size, you may need 15 to 25 grams of protein (more precisely, 0.15 gram of protein per pound [0.3 g/kg]) every three to five hours, with a particular focus on refueling after workouts with adequate protein. If you are severely restricting your food intake, you need even more protein than that (ACSM 2016). The following information offers an overview of daily protein needs.

Type of individual	Grams of protein per lb body weight per day	Grams of protein per kg body weight per day
Sedentary adult	0.4	0.8
Recreational exerciser, adult	0.5-0.7	1.1-1.6
Endurance athlete, adult	0.6-0.7	1.3-1.6
Growing teenage athlete	0.7-0.9	1.6-2.0
Adult building muscle mass	0.7-0.8	1.6-1.8
Athlete restricting calories	0.8-0.9	1.8-2.0
Athlete severely restricting calories to make weight	1.0-1.4	2.1-3.0
PROTEIN REQUIREMENTS VS. AMOUNT CONSUMED		
Estimated upper requirement for adults	0.9	2.0
Average protein intake for male endurance athletes	0.5-0.9	1.1-2.0
Average protein intake for female endurance athletes	0.5-0.8	1.1-1.8

Data compiled from ACSM 2016; Helms E. 2014; and Institute of Medicine Food and Nutrition Board, 2002, *Dietary reference intakes for energy, carbohydrate, fiber, fatty acids, cholesterol, protein and amino acids*, Washington, DC: National Academies Press.

Estimating Protein Intake

To learn whether you are meeting your protein needs in your current diet, follow two easy steps. First, using table 7.1, identify which category you belong to. For example, if you are a 35-year-old 140-pound (64 kg) bike racer, you would fit the category of an "endurance athlete, adult" and would need 85 to 100 grams of protein per day:

$$140 \text{ lb} \times 0.6 \text{ g/lb} = 84 \text{ g protein}$$
$$140 \text{ lb} \times 0.7 \text{ g/lb} = 98 \text{ g protein}$$

Second, divide the daily protein need into four to six meals or snacks. Using the previous example, this comes to 20 to 25 grams of protein every four hours. Or, if you prefer three meals and three snacks, target 20 to 25 grams of protein at every meal and 10 grams of protein with each snack.

Tally your protein intake by using either the information on the labels of the foods you ate (see table 7.2 for a list of the protein content in common foods), or use a food tracker or one of the websites in the Dietary Analysis and Nutrition Assessment section in appendix A to analyze your diet and assess your protein intake.

TABLE 7.2 Protein in Common Foods

Protein source	Serving size	Protein (g)
ANIMAL SOURCES		
Egg white	From 1 large egg	3
Egg	1 large egg	6
Yogurt, Yoplait vanilla	6 oz (180 g) tub	6
Cheddar cheese	1 oz (30 g)	7
Milk, 1%	8 oz (240 ml)	8
Milk, instant dry	1/2 cup milk powder	10
Yogurt, Greek Chobani	5.3 oz tub	13
Cottage cheese	1/2 cup (115 g)	15
Haddock	4 oz (120 g) cooked	23
Tuna	5 oz can (150 g)	25
Hamburger	4 oz (120 g) broiled	30
Pork loin	4 oz (120 g) roasted	30
Chicken breast	4 oz (120 g) roasted	35

Protein source	Serving size	Protein (g)
PLANT SOURCES		
Almonds, dried	12 nuts	3
Sunflower seeds	2 tbsp	4
Gardenburger (original)	2.5 oz (75 g) patty	5
Quinoa	3/4 cup cooked, 1/4 cup dry	6
Refried beans	1/2 cup	6
Kidney beans	1/2 cup	8
Peanut butter	2 tbsp	9
Hummus	1/2 cup	10
Lentil soup	10.5 oz (315 g)	11
Tofu, extra firm	3.5 oz (105 g)	11
Baked beans	1 cup	12
Boca Burger	2.5 oz (75 g) patty	12
COMMERCIAL PRODUCTS		
Clif Builder's bar	2.4 oz (70 g)	20
PowerBar ProteinPlus	2.4 (70 g) 4 oz.	20

Data from USDA National Nutrient Database for Standard Reference (2011).

Note that you need to eat a generous portion (more calories) of beans and other forms of plant protein to equal the protein in animal foods. Most fruits and vegetables contain only small amounts of protein, which may contribute a total of 5 to 10 grams of protein per day, depending on how much you eat. Butter, margarine, oil, sugar, soda, alcohol, and coffee contain no protein, and most desserts contain very little.

Table 7.3 shows what a day's worth of ample protein might look like for an active 150-pound (68 kg) adult. Of course, you'll need to eat other foods to round out your calorie and nutrition requirements, and those foods will offer a little more protein, as well.

For optimal muscle building, evenly distribute your protein throughout the day, including some before bed so you have a continual supply of amino acids throughout the night (Phillips and van Loon 2011). This is in contrast to a standard pattern of consuming very little protein at breakfast (oatmeal) and lunch (energy bar and banana), and then a huge steak for dinner.

TABLE 7.3 Protein for a Day

How much protein-rich food should a 150-pound athlete eat to meet his or her protein needs? As you can see from this chart, an athlete can easily consume adequate protein without supplements.

Meal	Primary source of protein	Protein (g)
Breakfast	3 eggs 1/4 cup milk in coffee	20
Lunch	1 (5 oz) can tuna	25
Afternoon	1 tub (5.3 oz) Greek yogurt 24 almonds	20
Dinner	4 oz. (120 g) chicken	25
Bed time	2/3 cup cottage cheese	20

Protein Without Cooking

Whether you are looking for a companion to carbohydrate for your recovery meal, a satiating snack, or protein to meet your daily need, here are a few cooking-free food suggestions if you tend to grab meals and snacks on the run.

Almonds, pistachios, or other nuts

Cheese stick or individual portions of (low-fat) cheeses

Chicken, rotisserie

Cottage cheese

Deli turkey or lean roast beef

Edamame

Eggs, hard-boiled

Hummus

Jerky, turkey or beef

Latte made with low-fat milk

Milk chugs (16 ounces)

Peanut butter

Soy nuts, roasted

Tuna, can or pouch

Veggie patty

Yogurt, Greek or regular

Protein Powders, Shakes, and Bars

Powerful advertisements in sports magazines and on the Internet can easily convince you that protein supplements are essential for optimal muscle development. Athletes who come to me for protein advice often lug gym bags bulging with assorted powders and bars. They wonder whether these supplements are better than the protein in standard food, whether they are worth the price, and whether they are better than whole foods (see table 7.4). Research does not support the claims that protein supplements yield super-strong bulging muscles. In a study of untrained young men who added 20 grams of whey protein to their standard diet, both before and after a 12-week strength training program, muscle growth was the same compared to the group that did not supplement protein (Erskine et al. 2012). The body needs only 20 to 25 grams of protein in one dose to stimulate muscle growth.

In certain instances, protein supplements can be a handy addition to a sports diet. For example, protein bars can be convenient for traveling athletes, busy athletes on the run, and vegetarians. Protein powders are an easy way to turn a fruit smoothie or a bowl of oatmeal into a balanced breakfast. Suzy, a vegetarian fitness exerciser, chose protein supplements because they eliminated guesswork; the label told her exactly how much protein she would consume. In today's grab-and-go fast-food society, protein supplements are a mindless way to get seemingly healthy (low-fat) protein. In the case of missed meals, any protein is better than no protein, so keeping a protein bar handy for emergency food is a wise choice. My advice is to use them to supplement wise eating, not to replace it.

TABLE 7.4 Comparison of Protein Powders, Bars, and Protein-Rich Foods

Protein source	Cost*	Protein (g)	Cost per gram protein
Tuna, 5 oz (150 g) can white	$2.39	24	10¢
Clif Builder's bar	$1.89	20	9.5¢
Vega plant-based protein powder, 18.6 oz (520g) container	$30.89	360	8.5¢
Tuna, 5 oz (150 g) can chunk light	$1.29	20	6.5¢
Nonfat milk,1 qt (1 L)	$1.69	32	5.0¢
Nonfat milk, 1/2 gal (2 L)	$2.59	64	4.0¢
Nonfat milk, 1 gal (4 L)	$3.99	128	3.1¢

*Prices in grocery store in Massachusetts, 2018

That said, protein supplements can be helpful in a few medical situations, such as for malnourished patients with AIDS or cancer. Protein supplements can benefit people with anorexia who have cut out animal products as a way to eliminate calories from their diets.

My main concerns about protein supplements (apart from their cost) are they are highly processed and fail to offer the complete package of health-protective nutrients found in a balanced diet. Because supplements are not regulated as rigorously as food and drugs are, you may not be getting the amount of protein listed on the Nutrition Facts label. Protein supplements may also contain questionable ingredients. According to Consumer Reports (2018), many brands contained significant amounts of lead and arsenic, two health-erosive heavy metals. (Buyer beware!) Plus, if you are filling up on too much protein, you can easily be displacing the carbohydrates needed to refuel your muscles.

What is the difference between whey and casein?

Whey (which is 20 percent of the protein found in milk) is digested and quickly absorbed into the bloodstream faster than other forms of protein such as casein. Casein makes up the other 80 percent of milk's protein and is slowly absorbed. Whey is a rich source of the branched-chain amino acids (BCAAs) leucine, as well as isoleucine, and valine. BCAAs are taken up directly by the muscles instead of being first metabolized by the liver. Hence, whey is fast acting and a good source of raw materials for protecting muscles from breaking down during exercise and for building muscles after exercise. Casein supplies a longer-lasting and sustained source of amino acids, and it's also important in the muscle-building process (Tipton et al. 2004). Bedtime casein (think cottage cheese) can enhance the availability of amino acids throughout the night.

Dairy milk offers both rapid and extended protein activity in the body. Dairy milk and powdered milk (but not almond or other plant milks, apart from soy milk) are good alternatives to expensive protein supplements and are easy to use in smoothies. They offer protein the way nature intended, as well as possible bioactive, growth-promoting compounds that are yet to be discovered. And remember, whey powders often lack the carbohydrate needed to refuel muscles. Hence, chocolate milk (with carbohydrate plus protein) can be the better recovery choice than just a low-carb whey protein shake after a workout.

Too Much Protein

Some athletes these days are eating excessive amounts of protein, including fans of the paleo and other low-carb diets. While a high-protein intake is unlikely to cause kidney problems (the kidneys excrete by-products of protein metabolism) (Phillips, Chevalier, and Leidy 2016), too much protein can create other problems with health and performance. Jasper, an aspiring bodybuilder, chowed down on chicken and beef, yet avoided pasta and potatoes, much to the detriment of his athletic aspirations. He tired easily and asked me whether this high-protein diet might be hurting his performance. Here's what I told him:

- If you fill your stomach with too much protein, you won't be fueling your muscles with carbohydrate.
- A diet high in protein can easily be high in saturated fat (e.g., juicy steaks, spareribs, pepperoni pizza). To date, the American Heart Association recommends you reduce your intake of the saturated fat found in animal protein. A diet high in processed animal protein (salami, pepperoni, sausage) may also increase your risk of certain cancers.
- Your body can use only 20 to 25 grams of protein at one time to build muscle (Phillips and van Loon 2011). That means that if you eat 8 ounces (240 g) of chicken breast (about 70 grams of protein) for dinner, you will burn (or store as fat) less than half of that protein—a waste of money! Plus, if you haven't eaten much protein at breakfast or lunch, thinking that your high-protein dinner will compensate for your lack of protein earlier in the day, think again.
- Protein breaks down into urea, a waste product eliminated in the urine. Anyone who eats excess protein should drink extra fluids. Frequent trips to the bathroom may be an inconvenience during training and competition.
- A diet based on animal protein takes its toll on both your wallet and the environment. You can save money (and the environment) by eating smaller portions of beef, lamb, and other forms of animal protein. Use that money to buy more sources of plant protein (beans, lentils, tofu) and more fruits, vegetables, grains, and potatoes.

I encouraged Jasper to reduce his meat portions at dinner to one-third of his plate and to fill two-thirds with sweet potatoes, green vegetables, and whole-grain bread. Within two days, he noticed an improvement in his energy level. He then changed his breakfast from a four-egg omelet with ham and cheese to two hard-boiled eggs with cereal and a banana, and lunch became a burrito rather than burgers. His diet gradually became a winner. "I'm amazed," he now says, "at the power of food. Eating carbohydrate-based meals that fuel my muscles definitely enhances my sports performance!"

Healthy and Convenient Meat Choices

"I rarely eat meat except when I go home to visit my family," commented Christina, a college student who lived off campus and was responsible for her own food. "I like meat, but it's expensive and seems to spoil before I get around to cooking it for dinner." She ate a lot of ramen for quick and easy dinners, and consequently wondered whether she consumed too little protein.

If you, like Christina, believe you eat too little protein and therefore too little of the accompanying nutrients iron and zinc, and if you are agreeable to eating animal protein, choosing a small amount of lean red meat two to four times per week can enhance the nutrient density of your sports diet, particularly if you are prone to anemia. Here are tips to keep in mind for health-promoting, low-fat meat eating:

- Take advantage of the deli. For precooked meats, buy rotisserie chicken or slices of lean roast beef, ham, and turkey in the deli section at the grocery store.
- Buy extra-lean cuts of beef, pork, and lamb to reduce your intake of saturated fat. Forgo cuts with a marbled appearance, and trim the fat off steaks and chops before cooking them.
- Get rid of more fat. After browning ground beef or ground turkey, drain it in a colander and rinse it with hot water to remove the fat before adding it to spaghetti sauce.
- At a cafeteria, request the hamburger be served on the plate with the roll on the side. Sandwich the burger between a few napkins, then squish out the grease. Place the degreased burger on the roll and enjoy a lower-fat meal.
- Integrate meat into a meal as an accompaniment. Add a little extra-lean hamburger to spaghetti sauce, stir-fry a small piece of steak with lots of veggies, or serve a pile of rice along with one lean pork chop.

PROTEIN AND THE VEGETARIAN

Many active people do not eat animal protein. Some just eat no red meat; others eat no red meat, chicken, fish, eggs, or dairy foods. They may find animal protein hard to digest or believe it is bad for their health, unethical to eat, or erosive to the environment. (Cattle are a source of greenhouse gas that contributes to global warming.) Meatless Mondays (and other days, too) are a good idea for the planet! And a balanced vegetarian diet is indeed a good investment in good health. A plant-based diet tends to have more fiber, less saturated fat, and more phytochemicals—active compounds that bolster the immune system, reduce inflammation, and are health protective.

The trick to eating a balanced vegetarian diet is to make the effort to replace meat with plant proteins. That is, if you eliminate the meatballs from your pasta dinner, add an alternative source of plant-based protein. Do not simply fuel up only on pasta and neglect your protein needs. You can get adequate protein to support your sports program by including kidney beans, chickpeas, hummus, nut butter, tofu, nuts, veggie burgers, edamame, and other forms of plant protein in each meal.

Peter, a 150-pound (68 kg) runner, is an example of a vegan athlete with a marginal protein intake. Each day he consumed only about 0.4 gram of protein per pound of body weight (0.85 g/kg), a bit less than the recommended intake for athletes. I suggested ways he could easily boost his protein intake (table 7.5).

All these changes were easy to make. Yes, he could have added vegan protein shakes and bars to boost his protein intake, but real food offers a more complete nutrition package that includes all of the health-enhancing compounds, some of which we may not even know about.

Tofu (soybean curd) and other soy products, such as soy burgers and soy milk, are smart additions to a meat-free diet. They contain a source of high-quality protein that is similar in value to animal protein. Note that a Boca Burger (soy protein) has far less protein than a hamburger, however (refer to table 7.2). Despite popular belief among male athletes, the plant estrogens in soy do not have a feminizing effect, do not reduce testosterone levels, and do not impair fertility (Messina 2010). All athletes can enjoy soy foods in moderation, as with any food, as a health-promoting part of a balanced sports diet.

For lacto-vegetarians (who consume dairy foods), milk and (Greek) yogurt are simple ways to add extra high-quality protein to meals and snacks. Although they have been given a bad rap because they are high in saturated fat, recent studies question whether a connection exits between dairy fat and heart disease and stroke regardless of the milk fat levels (de Oliveira Otto et al. 2018). This controversial topic is worthy of continued research, so until the American Heart Association gives the green light for full-fat dairy foods, a wise plan is to choose mostly reduced-fat dairy foods and balance full-fat choices into an overall healthy eating pattern. That said, blue cheese and other "moldy cheeses" may be a positive addition to the diet regardless of their saturated fat: They support gut bacteria that promote good health (Petyaev and Bashmakov 2012).

Milk, other dairy foods, eggs, and all animal sources of protein contain all the essential amino acids and are often referred to as complete proteins. The protein in soy foods such as tofu, tempeh, edamame, and soy milk are

TABLE 7.5 How to Boost Your Intake of Plant Proteins

	Low-protein vegetarian meal	Protein (g)	Higher-protein vegetarian meal	Protein (g)
Breakfast	Oatmeal, 1 cup dry, cooked in water	10	Oatmeal, 1 cup dry, cooked in 12 oz. soy milk with peanut butter	20
	Ezekiel bread, toasted, 2 slices	8	2 tbsp nut butter (mixed into oatmeal	9
Breakfast total		18		29
Lunch	Salad greens, dressing	—	Salad greens, dressing	—
	Beets, 1/2 cup	1	Hummus, 1/4 cup (2 oz)	4
	Sweet potato, 1 cup	3	Quinoa, 1 cup	8
	Sunflower seeds, 1/4 cup	14	Sunflower seeds, 1/4 cup	14
Lunch total		18		26
Dinner	Tofu, extra firm, 1/4 cake	10	Tofu, 1/2 cake	20
	Rice, 1 cup	4	Rice, 2/3 cup	3
	Broccoli, 2 medium stalks	8	Broccoli, 2 medium stalks	8
Dinner total		22		31
Total for the day		58		86

also complete proteins. The protein in rice, beans, pasta, lentils, nuts, fruits, vegetables, and other plant foods are incomplete because they contain low levels of some of the essential amino acids. Therefore, vegetarians must eat a variety of foods to get a variety of amino acids that combine with incomplete proteins to make them complete. Vegetarians who drink milk can easily do this by adding soy milk or dairy products to each meal, for example, combining (soy) milk with oatmeal or sprinkling grated low-fat (soy) cheese on beans. Note that rice and almond milks are not nutritionally equal to soy milk, but rather are very poor protein sources (see chapter 1).

Vegans (strict vegetarians who eat no dairy, eggs, or animal protein) need to consistently eat a variety of foods to optimize their intake of a variety of amino acids over the course of the day. The following combinations work particularly well together; they complement each other by boosting the limiting amino acid:

- Grains plus beans or legumes, such as rice and beans, bread and split-pea soup, tofu and brown rice, corn bread and chili with kidney beans
- Legumes plus seeds, such as chickpeas and tahini (as in hummus), tofu and sesame seeds
- Added soy products (or dairy, if nonvegan), such as cereal and (soy) milk, baked potato and Greek or soy yogurt, hummus wrap with low-fat (soy) cheese

By following these guidelines, vegetarian athletes can consume an adequate amount of complete protein every day. They may, however, lack iron and zinc, minerals found primarily in meats and other animal products. Vegans also need to be sure they get adequate riboflavin, calcium, and vitamin B_{12}, either through a supplement or from carefully selected food sources.

FACT OR FICTION

Athletes who choose to eat a vegan diet will hurt their ability to perform well.

The facts: Vegans, who eat only plant foods, can certainly meet their protein needs by eating a variety of plant foods. Most grains contain all nine essential amino acids, just in lower amounts than an equivalent serving of animal foods. Hence, vegans need to consume generous portions of plant protein (grains, beans, legumes, nuts, soy) to compensate for both the lower density of the protein and the fact that plant proteins are less bioavailable (because of their fiber content).

The wisest way for any type of vegetarian to optimize protein intake is to consume adequate calories because a calorie deficit easily leads to muscle loss. Dieting vegans who want to lose fat (not muscle) need to focus their limited food intake on protein-rich plant foods, and less on protein-poor fruits and fats. Luckily, the beans, lentils, and edamame that offer protein also offer carbohydrate for muscle fuel.

Female Vegetarians and Amenorrhea

Jessica, a weight-conscious vegetarian gymnast, used to live on melon for breakfast, a salad for lunch, and steamed vegetables with brown rice for dinner. Once or twice a week, she'd sprinkle a few garbanzo beans on a salad or add soy cheese to the vegetables. She thought her vegetarian diet was great, when in fact it was deficient in several nutrients. At one point she suffered a stress fracture that healed very slowly. She had spindly arms and legs with tiny muscles (despite her exercise program), and her menstrual period was absent, a sign of an unhealthy body.

Like Jessica, some athletic women, in their obsession to lose weight, consume a very low-calorie and low-protein "vegetarian" diet. This drastic restriction of food intake can lead to amenorrhea (loss of regular menstrual cycles) and protein deficiency. Research suggests that amenorrheic athletes have a two to four times higher risk of stress fractures than do regularly menstruating athletes (Mountjoy et al. 2014; Nattiv 2000). Eating a balanced diet containing adequate calories can enhance the resumption of menses, provide adequate protein for building and protecting muscles and bones, and enhance overall health. (See chapter 12 for more information on amenorrhea.)

Iron and Zinc Requirements

Iron is a necessary component of hemoglobin, the protein that transports oxygen from the lungs to the working muscles. If you are iron deficient, you are likely to fatigue easily upon exertion. Other symptoms include dizziness, headaches, spoon-shaped fingernails and toenails, and cravings for licorice or ice. Talk to your doctor if you chew an abnormal amount of ice cubes! The recommended iron intake for men is 8 milligrams; for women it is 18 milligrams until menopause, after which it is 8 milligrams. This target iron intake is set high because only a small percentage is absorbed. See table 7.6 for the iron content of some foods. The best iron sources are animal products (including dark fish); the body absorbs far less iron from plant foods.

Following are athletes with the highest risk of developing iron-deficiency anemia:

- Female athletes who lose iron through menstrual bleeding
- Vegetarians who do not eat red meat (one of the best dietary sources of iron) or choose *all-natural* as opposed to *iron-enriched* breakfast cereals

TABLE 7.6 Iron and Zinc in Food

Foods	Iron (mg)	Zinc (mg)
ANIMAL SOURCES*		
Alaskan king crab, 4 oz (120 g)	1	9
Beef, 4 oz (120 g) top round	4	5
Chicken thigh, 4 oz (120 g)	1.5	2
Egg, 1 large	1	0.5
Oysters, 6 medium raw	4	50
Pork loin, 4 oz (120 g)	1	3
Tuna, 3 oz (90 g) light canned	1.5	1
Turkey, 4 oz (120 g) breast	2	2
FRUIT AND JUICE		
Prune juice, 8 oz (240 ml)	3	0.5
Raisins, 1/3 cup	1	0.1
VEGETABLES AND LEGUMES**		
Broccoli, 1/2 cup	0.5	0.3
Peas, 1/2 cup	1.5	0.5
Refried beans, 1 cup	4	1.5
Spinach, 1/2 cup cooked	3	0.7
SOY SOURCES		
Edamame, 1/2 cup	2	1
Gardenburger, original	1	0.8
Tofu, 3 oz (90 g), firm	2	1
GRAINS		
Bread, 1 slice enriched	1	0.5
Brown rice, 1 cup cooked	1	1.2
Raisin Bran, Kellogg's, 1 cup	4.5	2
Cereal, Total, 3/4 cup	18	15
Cream of Wheat, 1 cup cooked	12	0.4
Pasta, 1 cup cooked, enriched	1	1
Wheat germ, 1/4 cup	2	3.5
OTHER		
Molasses, 1 tbsp blackstrap	3.5	0.2

*Animal sources of iron and zinc are absorbed best (except for iron from eggs).

**Vegetable sources of iron and zinc are poorly absorbed.

Data from USDA National Nutrient Database for Standard Reference (2011).

- Marathon runners (and other athletes in running sports) who may damage red blood cells by pounding their feet on the ground during training
- Endurance athletes who may lose iron through heavy sweat losses
- Teenage athletes, particularly girls, who are growing quickly and may consume inadequate iron to meet expanded requirements

Even marginal iron deficiency (found in about 12 percent of women in the United States) can hurt athletic performance. Hence, you want to eat iron-rich foods each day. Apart from taking a multivitamin and mineral pill with iron, you can boost your iron intake in several easy ways:

- If you are not opposed to consuming animal protein, eat lean cuts of beef, lamb, pork, and the dark meat of skinless chicken or turkey three or four times per week (two lunches and two dinners).
- Combine poorly absorbed vegetable sources of iron (nonheme iron, 10 percent absorption rate) with animal sources (heme iron, 40 percent absorption rate). For example, eat broccoli with beef, spinach with chicken, chili with lean hamburger, and lentil soup with turkey.
- If you are vegetarian, select breads and cereals with the words *iron enriched* or *fortified* on the label. This added iron supplements the small amount that naturally occurs in grains. Eat these foods with a source of vitamin C (e.g., orange juice with cereal, tomato on a sandwich), which may enhance iron absorption. *Note:* Cereals that are *all natural* or *organic* are not fortified with iron or zinc. By mixing them with enriched cereals, you can boost the iron content of your breakfast.
- Cook in cast-iron skillets. These vessels offer more nutritional value than do stainless-steel cookware. The iron content of spaghetti sauce simmered in a cast-iron skillet for three hours may increase from 3 to 88 milligrams for each 1/2 cup (120 ml) of sauce.
- Don't drink coffee or tea with every meal, particularly if you are prone to being anemic. Substances in these beverages can interfere with iron absorption. Drinking them an hour before a meal is better than drinking them afterward.

If you are feeling unusually fatigued during your workouts, you should determine whether your suboptimal performance is caused by iron deficiency. One of my clients went on a reducing diet to try to improve her performance, but iron deficiency—not excess body fat—was slowing her down. Get your blood tested for not only hemoglobin and hematocrit (the standard tests for anemia) but also serum ferritin. Ferritin measures the iron stores in your body; you want a level of at least 20 nanograms per deciliter (ng/dL), preferably 60 or higher. (The normal range is 12 to 300 ng/dL for men and 12 to 150 ng/dL for women.) If the stores are low, you may be preanemic; this can hurt performance (DellaValle and Haas 2011). If you are diagnosed with iron-deficiency anemia, you will need to take iron supplements, typically in the form of ferrous sulfate, ferrous gluconate, or ferrous bisglycinate (which might be easier to tolerate). Your doctor may prescribe 25 to 65 milligrams of elemental iron once a day if your ferritin is between 20 and 35 ng/dL, or 65 to 100 milligrams, if your serum ferritin is less than 20 ng/dL. You may need about four months of supplementation to resolve the problem, but you will feel better in two to three weeks.

However, you should not take iron supplements unless recommended by your physician because too much iron has been linked to heart disease. About 1 in 250 people has a genetic condition that makes him or her susceptible to iron overload. Men and postmenopausal women are most susceptible because they have relatively low iron requirements. The best way to identify iron overload is by having a blood test for serum ferritin to measure the amount of iron stored in your body. An above-normal level signals danger.

In addition to iron, your body needs zinc. This mineral is part of more than 100 enzymes that help your body function properly. For example, zinc helps remove carbon dioxide from your muscles when you exercise. Zinc also enhances the healing process. Because the zinc from animal protein is absorbed better than zinc from plants, vegetarian athletes are at risk of eating a zinc-deficient diet.

The recommended intake for zinc is 8 milligrams for women and 11 milligrams for men (refer to table 7.6 for foods that provide zinc). Like the target for iron, this target is also set high and may be hard to meet. Athletes who sweat heavily and incur zinc losses through sweat should try to hit the target intake.

NUTRIENT TIMING

If you want to build muscle, when is the best time to eat protein: before, during or after you lift weights? It might not actually matter because resistance exercise stimulates a muscle-building effect that is most robust within the first four hours but lasts for one to two days. You need not carry a protein shake around the gym or wake up in the middle of the night to eat cottage cheese! More important is to pace your protein intake evenly throughout the daytime.

As you can see in table 7.7, maximal anabolic (muscle-building) effects are seen with 12 to 40 grams of protein per meal (with small bodies needing

TABLE 7.7 Protein Pacing

If you want a more precise estimate of your protein needs, target about 0.75 gram of protein per pound (1.7 g/kg) of body weight per day, or better yet, 0.1 to 0.2 gram of protein per pound (0.2 to 0.4 g/kg) per meal. Here are some targets to help you pace your protein evenly throughout the day:

Weight	Protein (g) per day	Protein (g) per meal	Meal example
125 lb (57 kg)	95	12-25	2 to 4 eggs
150 lb (68 kg)	115	15-30	1/2 to 1 cup cottage cheese
175 lb (80 kg)	130	18-35	Bean or chicken burrito
200 lb (91 kg)	150	20-40	3 to 6 oz chicken

less and larger bodies needing more). More than that offers little or no further benefit.

However, these recommendations do change with age. If you are more than 50 years old and want to optimize your musculature, don't skimp! Target a slightly larger portion of high-quality protein (milk, egg, fish, soy) per meal. That said, resistance exercise is far more potent for increasing strength and muscle gains than is adding extra protein. Most conditioned athletes might see a gain of only about 2 pounds (1 kg) of muscle in 13 weeks. That's not very much compared to what they really want to see.

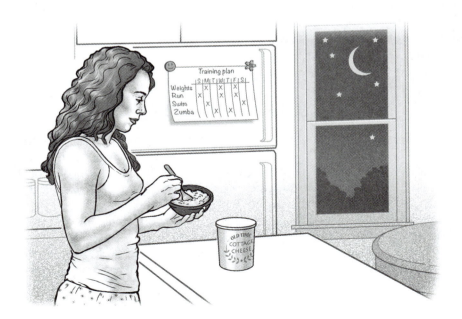

The following are common questions that athletes ask about when and what to eat.

What should I eat before lifting weights?

By eating protein along with carbohydrate in your preexercise snack, you'll start to digest the protein into amino acids, which are used by the muscles during and after exercise. Preexercise protein can also reduce the muscle breakdown that happens during exercise (van Loon 2013). Whether or not this translates into bigger muscles has yet to be determined, but it certainly won't hurt.

What should I eat after lifting weights?

After a hard gym workout, your muscles are primed for breaking down: Their glycogen (carbohydrate) stores are reduced, levels of cortisol and other hormones that break down muscle are high, the muscle damage that occurred during exercise causes inflammation, and the amino acid glutamine that provides fuel for the immune system is diminished. If you just guzzle water after your workout and dash to work, you'll miss the 45-minute postexercise window of opportunity to *optimally* nourish, repair, and build muscles. You can switch out of the muscle breakdown mode by eating a carbohydrate–protein combination as soon as tolerable after you exercise. If you are not feeling hungry then, eat as soon as you can tolerate fluid or fuel. If possible, back your training into a meal, so you soon enjoy breakfast, lunch, or dinner. If not, popular recovery choices are chocolate milk (or any flavored milk), a fruit smoothie (made with milk, Greek yogurt, banana, and berries), and half or all of a peanut butter and jelly sandwich with a glass of milk. Rapid refueling is particularly important if you do two workouts in a day.

Fret not if you miss that 45-minute postexercise *refueling window of opportunity*. Recovery continues for the next day or two, just at a slower rate. So be sure to consume 20 to 25 grams of protein about every four hours (or somewhere between three to five hours). A high-protein bedtime snack might be a good idea as well; although more research is needed to confirm this suggestion (Burke and Hawley 2018; Joy et al. 2018).

Note that people of all ages and athletic abilities have been building muscles for centuries with unfocused eating patterns. Also keep in mind that your muscles have a maximum size that is influenced by genetics. Not everyone can build bulging biceps. For more information on how to add size, develop your physique, and get stronger, read chapter 15, which is where I address how to gain weight healthfully.

If you are an avid learner about all things protein in sports nutrition, see appendix A for more protein information.

CHAPTER 8

FLUIDS: REPLACING SWEAT LOSSES TO MAINTAIN PERFORMANCE

During hard exercise, your muscles can generate 20 times more heat than when you are at rest. You dissipate that heat by sweating. As the sweat evaporates, it cools the skin. This in turn cools the blood, which cools the inner body. If you did not sweat, you could cook yourself to death. A body temperature higher than 106 degrees Fahrenheit (41 degrees Celsius) damages the cells. At 107.6 degrees Fahrenheit (42 degrees Celsius), cell protein coagulates (as egg whites do when they cook), and the cell dies. This is one serious reason why you shouldn't push yourself beyond your limits in very hot weather. You can try to keep yourself cool by drinking a preexercise slushy. During exercise, drink cold fluids (if possible), hold onto a cold water bottle (keep them filled in your freezer), and drape a wet kerchief around your neck or wear a wet hat.

Some people sweat a lot. For example, James had to put a towel under the exercise bike to mop the sweat that dripped from his body. Although it was a source of embarrassment, I reminded James that sweating is good. It's the body's way of dissipating heat and maintaining a constant internal temperature (98.6 degrees Fahrenheit, or 37 degrees Celsius).

James, like many men, produced more sweat than he needed to cool himself. He'd sweat large drops of water, which dripped off his skin rather than evaporated, resulting in a reduced cooling effect. In comparison, women tend to sweat more efficiently than men. But both men and women need to be equally diligent about replacing the fluid lost in sweat.

James wondered how much he needed to drink to replace his sweat loss. I suggested that he learn his sweat rate by weighing himself nude before and after an hour of exercise. For every pound (16 oz, or 0.5 kg) he lost, he needed to drink about 80 to 100 percent of that loss (13 to 16 oz, or 400 to 480 ml) while exercising to stay in optimal fluid balance; this would require training his gut to handle this volume. I also suggested that he figure out how many gulps of water equated to 16 ounces (480 ml).

By knowing his sweat rate (4 lb [almost 2 kg], or 64 oz, per hour), he was able to practice "programmed drinking" during exercise to minimize sweat losses. James started to drink 16 ounces (16 gulps; half of a 32 oz, or 1 qt [1 L] water bottle) every 15 minutes; this matched his thirst and more than doubled what he had previously consumed. His programmed drinking required that he have the right quantity of enjoyable fluids (chilled, palatable) readily available and even setting a wristwatch alarm to remind him to drink on schedule. He felt so much better after his workout that the extra effort was worthwhile.

Thirst, as defined by a conscious awareness of the desire for water and other fluids, usually controls water intake. The sensation of thirst is triggered when body fluid concentrations are abnormally high. When you sweat, you lose significant amounts of water from your blood. The remaining blood becomes more concentrated and has, for example, an abnormally high sodium level. This triggers the thirst mechanism and increases your desire to drink. To quench your thirst, you need to replace the water losses and bring your blood back to its normal concentration.

Unfortunately for athletes, this thirst mechanism can be an unreliable signal to drink. Thirst can be blunted by exercise or overridden by the mind. Hence, you should plan to drink before you are thirsty. By the time your brain signals thirst, you may have lost 1 percent of your body weight, which is the equivalent of 1.5 pounds (3 cups, or 24 oz [720 ml]) of sweat for a 150-pound (68 kg) person. This 1 percent loss corresponds with the need for your heart to beat an additional three to five times per minute (Casa et al. 2000). A 2 percent loss fits the definition of dehydrated. A 3 percent loss can significantly impair aerobic performance. Keep in mind that you will voluntarily replace only two-thirds of the water you lose in sweat. To be safe, drink enough to quench your thirst—but stop drinking if your stomach is sloshing. Enough is enough!

Young children, in particular, have a poorly developed thirst mechanism. At the end of a hot day, children often become very irritable, which may be partially caused by dehydration. If you are going to spend the day with children at a place where fluids are not readily available, such as the beach or a baseball game, bring a cooler stocked with lemonade, juice, and ice water, and schedule frequent fluid breaks to increase everyone's enjoyment of the whole day.

Senior citizens also tend to be less sensitive to thirst sensations than are younger adults. Research with active, healthy men aged 67 to 75 showed that they were less thirsty and voluntarily drank less water when water deprived for 24 hours compared with similarly deprived younger men aged

20 to 31 (Phillips et al. 1984). In another study, older hikers became progressively dehydrated during 10 days of strenuous hill walking. The younger hikers remained adequately hydrated (Ainslie et al. 2002). Athletic seniors who participate in sports should monitor their fluid intake.

FLUID PHYSIOLOGY 101

To help you understand the importance of balancing fluids correctly in your sports diet, here are some of the key points from the National Athletic Trainers' Association Position Statement on fluid replacement for the physically active (McDermott et al. 2017)

Fluid and Electrolyte Requirements

Fluid needs vary greatly from person to person, so it's hard to make a one-size-fits-all recommendation. Sweat rates commonly range between 1 and 4 pounds (0.5 and 2 qt, or L) per hour, depending on your sport, body size, intensity of exercise, and clothing; the weather conditions (hot or cold); whether you are heat acclimatized; and how well trained you are. Sweat rates for a 110-pound (50 kg) slow runner might be 1 pound

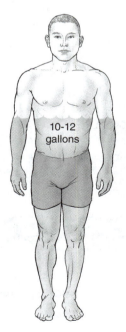

10-12 gallons

150 lb man

Water in saliva and gastric secretions helps digest food.

Water in sweat dissipates heat through the skin. During exercise water absorbs heat from your muscles, dissipates it through sweat, and regulates body temperature.

Water in blood transports glucose, oxygen, and fats to working muscles and carries away metabolic by-products such as carbon dioxide and lactic acid.

Water in urine eliminates metabolic waste products. The darker the urine, the more concentrated the wastes.

Water throughout the body lubricates joints and cushions organs and tissues.

(16 oz, or 480 ml) of sweat per hour, whereas a 200-pound (91 kg) fast runner might lose about 4 pounds (2 qt, or L) per hour. Even swimmers sweat—almost a pound (0.5 kg) per hour during hard training. Football players wearing full equipment in the summer heat might lose more than 16 pounds (2 gal, or 8 L) of sweat in a day.

On a daily basis, the simplest way to tell whether you are adequately replacing the fluid lost in sweat is to check the color and quantity of your urine. For specific colors, search "urine color chart" on the Internet. If your urine is very dark and scanty, it is concentrated with metabolic wastes, and you need to drink more fluids or eat more foods with a high water content such as prepared oatmeal, yogurt, and fruit. (Most people get 20 to 30 percent of their fluids from foods; some people actually eat all their daily water requirement.) When your morning urine is pale yellow, your body has returned to water balance. Your urine may be dark if you are taking vitamin supplements; in that case, volume is a better indicator than color.

In addition to monitoring urine and weight loss, you should also pay attention to how you feel. If you feel chronically fatigued, headachy, or lethargic, you may be chronically dehydrated. This is most likely to happen during long hot spells in the summertime. Dehydration can be cumulative.

Sweat contains more than just water; it has electrically charged particles (electrolytes, more commonly called minerals) that help keep water in the right balance inside and outside of your cells. The amount of electrolytes you lose via your sweat depends on how much you sweat, your genetics, your diet, and how well you are acclimatized. Table 8.1 shows the electrolyte loss that can occur with sweating—and how the losses can be replaced with food.

Muscle cramps might sometimes be associated with dehydration and electrolyte deficits, but the current hypothesis points to muscle fatigue as the key trigger (Casa, DeMartini, and Bergeron 2015) Yet, if you sweat profusely, are left caked with salt, and experience cramps, take extra care to drink plenty of sodium-containing fluids before and during exercise. If

TABLE 8.1 Electrolyte Loss in Sweat

Electrolyte	Average amount lost in 2 lb (1 L, 1 qt) of sweat	Food comparison
Sodium	1,000 mg (range 200-1,600)	1 small packet salt = 590 mg sodium 1 qt (1 L) Gatorade = 440 mg sodium
Potassium	200 mg (range 120-600)	1 medium banana = 450 mg potassium
Calcium	20 mg (range 6-40)	8 oz (230 g) yogurt = 300 mg calcium
Magnesium	10 mg (range 2-18)	2 tbsp peanut butter = 50 mg magnesium

your diet has a high salt content, you can likely replace sodium losses after exercise with standard postexercise meals. Consuming extra salt on your food if you have sweated heavily can be a smart way to enhance recovery, retain fluid, and stimulate thirst. See chapter 10 for more information about muscle cramps and sodium replacement.

Dehydration and Performance

Dehydration stresses the body: Your body temperature rises, your heart beats faster, you burn more glycogen, your brain has trouble concentrating, and exercise feels harder. Some athletes are more tolerant of dehydration than are others, but for the most part, the more dehydrated you are, the greater the strain you will experience.

Whereas fitness exercisers (who work out for 30 to 60 minutes at a moderate pace three or four times a week) can easily maintain water balance by eating and drinking normally, athletes who exercise hard day after day can become chronically dehydrated if they fail to fully rehydrate daily. Football players in full uniform might lose far more fluids than they would think to consume. Having sweat-loss data eliminates the guesswork.

Most athletes who lose more than 2 percent of their body weight through sweat, lose both their mental edge and their physical ability to perform well, especially in hot weather. Yet during cold weather, you are less likely to experience reduced performance even at 3 percent dehydration. That is, a runner feels less impact of dehydration on her performance during a cold winter run than she does during the same run in the summer heat.

FACT OR FICTION

The best way to prevent dehydration is to drink when you feel thirsty.

The facts: During days of repeated hard exercise, the best way to determine whether you are drinking enough to replace sweat losses and maintain normal water balance is to weigh yourself nude each day in the morning after emptying your bladder and bowels. Your weight should remain stable, assuming the following:

- You are not restricting calories to lose fat weight.
- You have not eaten abnormally high amounts of sodium the night before, such as a water-retaining Chinese dinner.
- You are not experiencing 2 to 4 pounds (1 to 2 kg) of premenstrual bloat.

Dehydration of 3 to 5 percent negatively affects muscle strength and short intense bursts of anaerobic performance, such as weightlifting. A sweat loss of 9 to 12 percent of body weight can lead to death. Warning signs of heat illness are muscle cramps, nausea, vomiting, headache, dizziness, confusion, disorientation, weakness, reduced performance, an inability to concentrate, and irrational behavior.

Fluids Before Exercise

The goal of drinking before you exercise is to start exercising when your body is in water balance, not in deficit from the previous exercise session. You might need 8 to 12 hours to rehydrate. The goal is to drink 2 to 4 milliliters per pound (5 to 10 ml/kg) of body weight at least four hours before the exercise task (ACSM 2016). For a 150-pound (68 kg) athlete, this equates to 300 to 600 milliliters, or 10 to 20 ounces, of fluid (1 ounce is about 30 ml). By hydrating several hours preexercise, you have time to eliminate the excess before starting the exercise event.

If you drink a beverage containing sodium (110 to 275 ml of sodium per 8 oz, or 240 ml) or eat a few salty snacks or sodium-containing meals, the

FACT OR FICTION

Caffeine has a dehydrating effect.

The facts: While caffeine might hasten the urge to urinate when you are sedentary, it does not induce diuresis during exercise. Caffeine in amounts normally consumed does not contribute to excessive water loss and is OK for athletes, even in hot weather (McDermott et al. 2017). The military became intensely interested in the physiological effects of caffeine on hydration among soldiers enduring extreme heat. They researched the effects of moderate (approximately 12 ounces of coffee; 200 mg caffeine) and high (approximately 24 ounces of coffee; 400 mg caffeine) doses of caffeine on hydration in soldiers who habitually consumed only one 6-ounce (180 ml) cup of brewed coffee (100 mg of caffeine per day). They found no detrimental effects of caffeine. By day's end, the 24-hour urine losses were similar (Armstrong et al. 2005). In another study testing endurance in hot weather (100 degrees Fahrenheit, or 37.7 degrees Celsius), the subjects who consumed about 225 milligrams of caffeine—the equivalent of a 12-ounce (360 ml) mug of coffee—exercised for 11 minutes longer (86 versus 75 minutes) compared with the group that consumed no caffeine (Roti et al. 2006).

sodium will stimulate your thirst so that you drink more; the sodium also helps retain the fluid so it doesn't go in one end and out the other. If you sweat heavily, consuming 300 to 700 milligrams of sodium in the two to three hours before exercise can help maintain your sodium balance. (See table 10.4 for the sodium content of popular sports foods.) There's no need to try to hyperhydrate. As I mentioned earlier, the body can absorb just so much fluid—and you will end up needing to urinate during the event. Overhydrating can also dilute your blood sodium; if you then continue to aggressively drink fluids during exercise, you can increase your risk of becoming waterlogged and developing hyponatremia, a potentially fatal condition related to diluted blood, causing an abnormally low sodium level.

Fluids During Exercise

The goal of drinking during exercise is to prevent excessive dehydration, as defined as a loss of more than 2 percent of body weight as a result of a water deficit. If you are exercising hard enough to risk becoming dehydrated, you should drink periodically during exercise. If you will be exercising for more than two or three hours, you should know your sweat rate to prevent the performance decline associated with small cumulative mismatches between how much fluid you need and how much fluid you are losing via sweat. Because few athletes actually make the effort to learn their sweat rates, a starting point is to drink as desired, according to thirst.

What should you drink during exercise? The recommended fluid replacer contains a little sodium to stimulate thirst and enhance carbohydrate absorption, and a little carbohydrate (sugar) to provide energy. You can consume these nutrients through standard foods such as pretzels and bagels as well as commercial sports foods (see chapter 11), which can be more convenient for runners, triathletes, and other endurance athletes.

When you are exercising hard for more than an hour (or doing less-intense, longer exercise), consuming 120 to 240 calories of carbohydrate (30 to 60 g) per hour along with water can improve your performance. If you'll be out for more than two and a half hours, bump that intake up to 60 to 90 grams of carbohydrate per hour (ACSM 2016). Carbohydrate helps maintain normal blood glucose levels so you are able to enjoy sustained energy. Sports drinks are an easy way to get carbohydrate plus water. For example, 16 ounces (480 ml) of Gatorade offers 25 grams of carbohydrate and 100 calories; 16 ounces of Powerade offers 35 grams of carbohydrate and 140 calories. Practice drinking large volumes of fluid during training to help you adapt to the fluid load and prevent stomach sloshing and discomfort during competition.

What to Look for in a Sports Beverage

Many niche sports beverages are fighting for shelf space wherever fluids are sold. With so many options to choose from, you might wonder what to look for in a sports drink. Here's a brief summary:

The Basics

- **Good taste.** If you like the flavor, you'll drink more and be less likely to become dehydrated.
- **Carbohydrate.** Look for beverages with 50 to 70 calories of carbohydrate (12 to 18 g of carbohydrate per 8 oz, or 240 ml). Too much carbohydrate slows absorption; too little leaves you lagging in energy. For long, hard, intense exercise, such as bike racing and marathon running, carbohydrate from a variety of sources (glucose, fructose, and sucrose—or dried fruit, energy bar, and Gummi Bears) is better absorbed and offers an energy advantage.
- **Sodium.** Important for maintaining fluid balance, sodium stimulates thirst and enhances fluid retention. If you experience significant sweat losses, the sodium found in sports drinks helps replace some (but not all) of the sodium lost in sweat. The drink should contain 110 to 170 milligrams of sodium per 8 ounces (20 to 30 milliequivalents [mEq] of sodium per L) (ACSM 2007).

Add-Ins of Questionable Value

- **Vitamins.** The vitamins in sports drinks are not incorporated quickly enough during exercise to be of any benefit.
- **Ginseng, guarana, and other herbs.** There are no solid data to support any claimed benefits of these substances, and the amounts in beverages are probably too small to make a difference.
- **Caffeine.** Because of individual responses, caffeine might enhance endurance or cause side effects such as anxiety, jitters, and irritability.
- **Protein.** The addition of protein may or may not enhance performance (McDermott et al. 2017). The benefit noticed after exercise might be reduced muscle soreness. You can get this same benefit by eating protein before exercise (let's say, a snack of cereal with milk).

- **Potassium, calcium, magnesium, and other minerals.** In most cases, the amount of these minerals that is lost in sweat is too small to create problems. The recommended 20 to 50 milligrams of potassium per 8 ounces (2 to 5 mEq of potassium per L) can be easily replenished with fruits, vegetables, and wholesome foods, as can the other minerals.

What You May Not Want

- **Carbonation.** Bubbles can make you bloated and fill you up sooner.
- **Plastic bottles.** They litter the environment if not recycled and are also potentially a source of hormone-disrupting BPA (as noted by a 7 inside a triangle on the bottom of the bottle). How about having just one BPA-free bottle (stainless steel, aluminum) that you refill daily?

Fluids After Exercise

After sweaty exercise, your goal is to fully replace all lost fluids and electrolytes. How aggressively you rehydrate depends on how quickly you need to recover before your next exercise session and how big a fluid–electrolyte deficit you incurred. Most active people can recover with normal meals (that contain a little sodium) and plain water. If you are significantly dehydrated and need to exercise again within 12 hours, then you need to be more aggressive with your rehydration program and sprinkle extra salt on your food if you had high sodium losses through sweat.

Drinking 50 percent more fluid than you lost in sweat will enhance rapid and complete recovery from dehydration. (The extra fluid accounts for what gets lost via urine.) Sipping fluids over time maximizes fluid retention and is preferable to drinking large amounts in one sitting. If you become dehydrated during an unusually long and strenuous bout of exercise, you should drink frequently for the next day or two. Your body may need 24 to 48 hours to replace the fluid you lost in sweat.

If you become more than 7 percent dehydrated (via sweat losses, diarrhea, or vomiting), you will likely end up requiring intravenous fluid replacement under a doctor's care. In most cases, there is no advantage to taking fluids by IV, unless for medical necessity. Your best bet is to stay out of the medical tent in the first place by knowing your sweat rate and drinking accordingly.

HYPONATREMIA AND SODIUM LOSS

There's no need to try to superhydrate before you exercise; your body can absorb just so much fluid. The kidneys regulate water balance by adjusting urine output—from a minimum of about a tablespoon to a maximum of about 1 quart (1 L) per hour. If you overdrink, you then may need to (inconveniently) urinate during exercise. A wise tactic is to drink two or more hours before exercise; this allows time for your kidneys to process and eliminate the excess. Then drink again 5 to 15 minutes preexercise.

For the most part, frequent trips to the bathroom simply inconvenience people who drink too much water. But in some cases, drinking too much water can actually be lethal if it dilutes body fluids and creates a sodium imbalance. A condition known as hyponatremia occurs when blood sodium levels become abnormally low. In general, hyponatremia that occurs in events that last four hours is caused by overdrinking water before, during, and even after the event. Hyponatremia that occurs in endurance events that last more than four hours in the heat is often related to extreme sodium loss without adequate replacement as well as overhydration. During exercise and heat stress, the kidneys make less urine. Therefore, if athletes overhydrate during exercise, their bodies may make too little urine to excrete the excess volume.

Athletes likely to experience a sodium imbalance caused by extreme sodium loss are slow marathoners, triathletes, ultrarunners, and unfit weekend warriors who have a higher sweat loss (and therefore a sodium loss) than their fit counterparts. These athletes may diligently consume high amounts of preexercise water plus consistently drink water during the event. As a result, they accumulate too much water by consuming it faster than their bodies can make urine, and they end up with a relative excess of water compared with sodium. The plain water dilutes their electrolyte balance and makes matters worse.

Most athletes get too much salt in their daily diets. Even with extended exercise, you can easily replace sodium losses with salty foods. Also, remember that the more you train in the heat, the less sodium you lose because your body learns to conserve sodium as well as other electrolytes (table 8.2).

TABLE 8.2 Electrolyte Content of Sweat in Unfit and Fit Subjects

Electrolyte	Unfit, unacclimatized	Fit, unacclimatized	Fit, acclimatized
Sodium	3.5 g/L	2.6 g/L	1.8 g/L
Potassium	0.2 g/L	0.15 g/L	0.1 g/L
Magnesium	0.1 g/L	0.1 g/L	0.1 g/L
Chloride	1.4 g/L	1.1 g/L	0.9 g/L

Adapted, by permission, from T. Noakes, 2003, *Lore of Running*, 4th ed. (Champaign, IL: Human Kinetics), 214.

The symptoms of hyponatremia include feeling tired, bloated, nauseated, and headachy. Any of these symptoms may become increasingly severe. A person with hyponatremia may also experience swollen hands and feet, undue fatigue, confusion and disorientation (due to progressive swelling of water in the brain), a decline in coordination, and wheezy breathing (due to water in the lungs). Blood sodium levels that drop too low can lead to seizures, coma, and death. To prevent hyponatremia if you will be exercising for more than four hours in the heat, observe the following guidelines:

- Add sodium before hot-weather events.
- Eat salted foods and fluids (soup, pretzels, salted oatmeal) 90 minutes before you exercise. This dose of sodium results in water retention in your body. This extra fluid not only can help you exercise longer but also may make the exercise seem easier and more enjoyable (Sims et al. 2007).
- Consume an endurance sports drink with higher sodium amounts than the standard sports drink during exercise in the heat that lasts for more than four hours.
- Consume salty foods during the endurance event, as tolerated (broth, pickles, pretzels, salted gels).
- Stop drinking water during exercise if your stomach is "sloshing," as may happen if you drink more than a quart (32 oz, or 1 L) of water per hour for extended periods.

FACT OR FICTION

Sports drinks are the best way to replace sodium losses from sweat.

The facts: Sports drinks generally contain too little sodium to balance sweat loss. The better choices are endurance sports drinks and salty snacks (e.g., pretzels, olives, pickles, V8 juice), salt sprinkled on foods, and brothy soups. Your target should be 250 to 500 milligrams of sodium per hour, the amount in 20 to 40 ounces (0.6 to 1.2 L) of Gatorade, for example. That's a lot of sports drink! Note that some salt tablets, such as Endurolytes, offer only 40 milligrams of sodium per tablet. One long-distance cyclist enjoyed boosting his sodium intake by eating little boiled potatoes rolled in olive oil and sprinkled with salt. He'd prepare them the night before a ride, store them in a plastic baggie, and munch on them at rest stops.

RETHINK YOUR DRINK

Many sweaty athletes wonder what to drink to quench their thirst; they feel confused by the abundant choices of fluids. There's plain ol' water, sports drinks, soft drinks (sugar sweetened or diet), 100 percent fruit juices, juice drinks, milk (chocolate, skim, low fat, or whole), beer, wine . . . the list goes on. As a sports dietitian, I get lots of questions about what's the best (or worst) to drink, so here's my advice about a variety of liquids with calories:

• **Orange juice (and other 100 percent fruit juices).** Many athletes ask whether they should stop drinking orange juice because they're worried it is loaded with (fattening) carbohydrate and sugar. My answer is no. To start, carbohydrate is not fattening, and it is an important fuel for your muscles (see chapter 6). Please do not knock orange juice—or other 100 percent fruit juice—out of your breakfast (and then, gulp, replace it with an extra-large coffee with sugar and double cream). Certainly, eating a whole orange is preferable to drinking its juice, but for eat-and-runners who won't take the time to peel the orange, OJ is better than no-J. Orange juice offers a strong dose of vitamin C, potassium, folate, and other health-protective nutrients that accompany the natural sugar. The trick is to balance the calories from orange juice—and any other juice or food—into your daily calorie budget.

Red, purple, and blue juices offer a potent dose of antioxidants that can reduce muscle soreness, protect against heart disease, and offer other health benefits. These include tart cherry juice, purple grape juice, blueberry juice, and cranberry juice cocktail (this is not 100 percent juice because cranberries are just too tart to enjoy). You need not spend extra money on acai or other tropical fruits from the Amazon rainforest—locally grown products are just as good!

• **Soft drinks.** After a hard workout, some tired athletes reach for a Coke or Pepsi, yearning for cola's combination of sugar, caffeine, and water to refuel, rehydrate, and revive themselves. Although juice would offer far more vitamins and minerals, dietary guidelines indicate that 10 percent of calories can appropriately come from refined sugar. Hence, you can enjoy, if desired, 200 to 300 calories of daily sugar—a can or two of soft drink. There is little doubt, however, that Coke and Pepsi—either regular or diet—do nothing to improve your health and are bad for your teeth. They are acidic and, with chronic exposure, can erode tooth enamel and leech calcium from your teeth. This can lead to dental decay (Borjian et al. 2010). Rinse your mouth with plain water after consuming such beverages, but don't brush within an hour, because that can actually worsen the damage caused by the acids. The same goes for sports drinks, particularly for endurance athletes such as elite triathletes who continuously sip sports drinks for extended periods of time (Bryant et al. 2011).

Many athletes wonder about a possible link between soft drinks and weight gain. Some studies suggest that people who drink sugary beverages tend to be heavier than those who abstain. This might be because fluid calories fail to "register" (i.e., they may not curb one's appetite), so soda drinkers consume more calories per day. Other studies report that soda might trigger the desire to eat more food. Hence, if soda drinking culminates in consuming more calories than you burn off, the result is indeed weight gain (Drewnowski and Bellisle 2007; Vertanian, Schwartz, and Brownell 2007).

As an athlete, you can enjoy a daily soda without fat gain if you keep the soda calories within your daily calorie budget, choosing wholesome foods for the rest of your sports diet. And if you are concerned about soft drinks being fattening, also pay attention to how much sports drink you consume. Many thirsty athletes overlook the fact that chugging a quart of sports drink during and after a workout (or during lunch, for that matter) contributes 200 to 300 sugar calories—and these calories do count.

• **Water.** Remember plain old tap water? Maybe not! Today we can choose from not only bottled spring waters but also designer waters that are flavored, vitamin fortified, and enhanced with herbs and supposed energizers. Many bottled waters come from municipal water supplies—not from the mountain streams pictured on the label—which validates the high quality of our standard municipal tap water. In the United States, municipal water is strictly regulated by the Environmental Protection Agency (EPA), and most municipal water also contains fluoride, a mineral added to reduce dental cavities. In comparison, bottled water is (loosely) regulated by the Food and Drug Administration (FDA)—but only if it is shipped across state lines or is imported. If you don't trust the safety of your local tap water, you might want to invest in a water filter and a refillable water bottle. Otherwise, you likely will buy water in plastic containers. More than a million tons of plastic are used every year to make water bottles, most of which end up as litter or in landfills, which is not environmentally friendly.

Vitamin water has wide appeal to many health-conscious people who equate vitamins with energy. (This is a misconception. Energy comes from carbohydrate.) Some of these beverages are, indeed, high in energy—there are 120 calories in a 20-ounce (600 ml) bottle of Glacéau vitaminwater. That's enough to contribute to undesired weight gain. Vitamin waters will not improve your health; many contain too few vitamins (because of aftertaste) to make much of a health difference. If they are highly fortified, they still lack the phytochemicals and other health enhancers found in real

FACT OR FICTION

The artificial sweeteners in diet soda cause cancer.

The facts: According to the National Cancer Institute (www.cancer.gov), this rumor is false. Studies show no clear relationship between artificial sweeteners and cancer. The choice of whether to drink regular soft drinks or diet soft drinks is a personal one. I'd vote for all-natural water, myself. Regular soda is filled with nutritionally empty sugar calories.

---

food. You'd be better off drinking the original vitamin water—orange juice or any other 100 percent juices—or adding a splash of juice to seltzer water for a flavor boost.

Sparkling water, or fizzy water, is a little more exciting than plain water, particularly if you are trying to wean yourself off of carbonated soft drinks. It is made by pumping carbon dioxide into water. The problem is, the carbon dioxide turns into carbonic acid, which can erode tooth enamel. The solution, don't sip on it all day and don't brush your teeth for at least 30 minutes after drinking it.

• **Coconut water.** Marketed as "100 percent pure" and "all natural," coconut water has only two ingredients: coconut water (the watery liquid inside a green coconut) and added vitamin C. Coconut water is naturally rich in potassium and has a high price tag (about $3 for a 17 oz, or 500 ml, carton). Table 8.3 shows how it compares to other popular postexercise drinks.

Because serious athletes have a higher need for sodium than potassium during sweaty exercise (and they will simply flush excess vitamin C down the toilet), I suggest that they choose a higher-sodium sports drink during endurance workouts and spend their money on orange juice, chocolate milk and other nutrient-rich foods afterward. That is, unless they happen to prefer the taste of coconut water.

• **Energy drinks.** Energy comes from calories, and energy drinks such as Red Bull and Rockstar tend to be rich in calories from sugar. For example, an 8.3-ounce (250 ml) can of Red Bull has 110 calories, and a 16-ounce (480 ml) can of Rockstar has 240 calories. If you are looking for an energy boost, the better bet is to fuel your body with appropriate meals and snacks. No amount of energy drink will compensate for a suboptimal sports diet.

Energy drinks also contain caffeine, a known ergogenic (energy enhancing) aid (see chapter 11 and appendix A.). Red Bull has 80 milligrams of

TABLE 8.3 Comparison of Postexercise Drinks

Fluid	Serving size	Calories	Sodium (mg)	Potassium (mg)	Vitamin C
Coconut water (2 ingredients)	17 oz (500 ml)	90	60	1,030	350% DV (fortified)
Gatorade (12 ingredients)	20 oz (600 ml)	125	275	75	0
Orange juice (1 ingredient)	16 oz (480 ml)	220	0	900	200% DV
Nesquik chocolate milk (10 ingredients)	14 oz bottle (400 ml)	250	230	640	0

caffeine, similar to the 100 milligrams in an eight-ounce (240 ml) cup of coffee but far more than the 20 milligrams in a packet of caffeinated Gu. The jury is still out on whether the other ingredients, such as taurine, guarana, ginseng, and yerba mate, add a boost. A study of college football players that compared a taurine-containing energy drink (AdvoCare Spark) with and without caffeine suggested the caffeine is the primary "magic ingredient" (Gwacham and Wagner 2012). Yet, too many emergency room visits are related to overdoses of caffeine-laced energy drinks that result in rapid heartbeat, muscle tremors, and seizures.

Like soft drinks, energy drinks are erosive, and can cause lasting damage to teeth. Another concern about energy drinks is that many athletes and sports fans use them as mixers with alcohol. The caffeine masks the effects of the alcohol, so consumers may not realize how intoxicated they are. This increases the likelihood of drunk driving (Ferreira et al. 2006; Marczinski and Fillmore 2006).

• **Green tea.** Many athletes I talk with want to know whether green tea is health protective and whether it enhances fat loss. Green tea is made from fresh tea leaves and does have a higher concentration than black and oolong teas of compounds that may protect against heart disease and cancer, particularly cancer of the breast, stomach, and skin. Many of the green tea studies have been done on animals or in research labs. To date, the FDA says there is not enough scientific evidence from studies with human subjects to prove that green tea is a miracle cure for all ailments. You need to look at the whole diet; you can certainly incorporate green tea into an overall heart-healthy, cancer-protective diet without harm and with potential complementary benefits.

We do know that tea drinkers tend to be healthier overall than coffee drinkers, and there appears to be no downside to drinking tea (unless you are caffeine sensitive). But use your common sense. I have a client who

Liquid Calories

Be aware of how quickly liquid calories can add up, especially when they come in large portions. Guzzling a quart (32 oz, or 1 L) of any calorie-containing beverage—even a sports drink after a workout—can hinder weight management. Table 8.4 shows the calorie counts for a number of popular beverages. Also take another look at table 3.3, Gulp! It's a Calorie Cafe!

TABLE 8.4 Liquid Calories

Beverage	Calories
Water, any size	0
Diet soda, any size	0
Coffee and tea, black, any size	0
Vita Coco coconut water, 11oz (330 ml)	60
Milk, nonfat, 8 oz (240 ml)	80
Coffee with 2 creamers, 2 sugars	80
Soy milk, vanilla, 8 oz (240 ml)	100
Gatorade, 16 oz (480 ml)	100
Beer, light, 12 oz (360 ml)	110
Orange juice, 8 oz (240 ml)	110
Milk, 2%, 8 oz (240 ml)	120
Glacéau vitaminwater, 20 oz (600 ml)	120
Wine, red, 5 oz (150 ml)	125
Regular soda, 12 oz (360 ml)	150
Beer, regular, 12 oz (360 ml)	150
Snapple iced tea 16 oz (480 ml)	150
Nesquik chocolate milk, 14 oz (480 ml)	250
Minute Maid lemonade, 20 oz (600 ml)	260
Naked Juice smoothie, 15 oz (450 ml)	320
Starbucks strawberry banana smoothie, 24 oz (700 ml)	340
Starbucks double chocolate chip vanilla Frappuccino, 16 oz (480 ml)	420
Jamba Juice peanut butter chocolate smoothie, 24 oz (700 ml)	550

Nutrient information from food labels, company websites, and USDA National Nutrient Database for Standard Reference.

started drinking Starbucks Matcha Green Tea Latte with steamed 2 percent milk (240 calories in 16 oz, or 480 ml, and 130 calories from sugar). This was a questionable way to invest in good health and likely wiped out the possible health benefits of the green tea—and certainly did not help with weight management!

ALCOHOL AND ATHLETES

Alcohol and athletes seem to go hand in hand. Adult athletes gather at the pub after a team workout, celebrate victories with champagne, and quench their thirsts with cold beers. You might think that the detrimental effects of alcohol on performance would make athletes less likely to drink it, but that is not the case. Even serious recreational runners drink more than their sedentary counterparts do.

When asked whether beer is good for runners, running legend Jim Fixx's answer was "Sure, if it's the *other* guy drinking it." If you stay sober, you can take advantage of other athletes' poor judgment. But if you are determined to drink alcohol as a part of your sports diet, keep in mind the following facts:

- Alcohol is a depressant. It slows your reaction time; impairs eye–hand coordination, accuracy, and balance; and, apart from killing pain, offers no edge for athletes. You can't be sharp, quick, and drunk. And you might be more likely to end up in the medical tent. Exercise physiologist Doug Casa of the University of Connecticut reported preevent alcohol consumption was the common denominator among the 20 heat-stricken runners at a summer road race. Don't drink excessive alcohol before an event—especially in the summer heat!

- Late-night drinking that contributes to getting too little sleep can wreck the next day's training session. Drinks that contain congeners (chemicals produced during the fermentation process that add flavor and aroma—red wine, cognac, whiskey) are more likely to cause hangovers than other alcoholic beverages are. The best hangover remedy is to avoid drinking excessively in the first place. That said, a modest amount of alcohol, consumed along with a balanced meal, is unlikely to have a negative impact.

- Alcohol is a poor source of carbohydrate. A 12-ounce (360 ml) can of beer has only 14 grams of carbohydrate, as compared with 40 grams in a can of soft drink. You can get loaded with beer, but your muscles will not get carbohydrate loaded—unless you consume pretzels, thick-crust pizza, or other carbohydrate-rich foods along with the beer. Adding alcohol to the recovery diet slows muscle repair, protein synthesis, and adaptation processes. Heavy alcohol intake does not make the list of best recovery practices for athletes.

- Alcohol is a diuretic. One unit (10 g) of alcohol stimulates the formation of 100 ml of excess urine. Whiskey and other spirits with a high alcohol content cause more water loss than they contribute. In comparison, the alcohol content of beer is lower—and beer has a lot of water—so dehydrated athletes can rehydrate with a beer or two, if desired, and if no important workout is scheduled for the near future (Maughan et al. 2016). That said, drinking water along with the beer and adding salt (pretzels) can improve the rehydration process.

- Alcohol is absorbed directly from the stomach into the bloodstream; it enters the bloodstream within five minutes of drinking it. After a hard workout, alcohol on an empty stomach can quickly contribute to a drunken stupor, while hampering muscular adaptations to training. You are better off enjoying the natural high from exercise than being brought down by a few postexercise beers.

- Your liver breaks down alcohol at a fixed rate—about 4 ounces (120 ml) of wine or one can of beer (360 ml) per hour. Exercise does not hasten that process; nor does coffee.

- Hot tubs, alcohol, and athletes are a bad combination. The hotter your body becomes, the drunker you may feel. Alcohol impairs your ability to control your body temperature, and the high temperature of the hot tub heightens the response of your body to alcohol.

- Winter sports and alcohol are a dangerous combination. Don't drink while skiing. If you succumb to alcohol, at least alternate with soft drinks or juices for carbohydrate and fluids.

- The calories in alcohol are easily fattening. People who drink moderately often consume alcohol calories on top of their regular caloric intake because alcohol can stimulate the appetite. These excess calories promote body fat accumulation, commonly in the trunk area—the well-known beer belly. If you are trying to maintain a lean machine, abstaining is preferable to imbibing. That six-pack of beer equates to 900 calories—the equivalent of four slices of cheese pizza!

- If you are destined to drink, drink moderately and have at least one glass of water for every alcoholic drink you consume. The definition of moderate drinking is two drinks per day for men and one for women. Having 18 drinks or more per week can cut life expectancy by four to five years (Wood et al. 2018)

- Don't start drinking if you can't easily stop. Be conscious of your ability to keep alcohol consumption within socially and medically acceptable bounds.
- If you believe you need to drink to fit in and be popular, think again. A survey of 117 student-athletes in Texas found that 22 percent abstained from drinking alcohol, 68 percent described themselves as light to moderate drinkers, and 59 percent did not binge drink (Wagner, Keathley, and Bass 2007).

Alcohol: Want to Take a Break?

Athletes tend to drink more alcohol than nonathletes. Often my clients comment they want to take a break from drinking alcohol. While they don't see themselves as alcoholics, they know they feel better the next morning and can manage their weight better when they don't drink. But drinking less can be easier said than done.

If you face this struggle, first assess the role drinking plays in your life: Is it a stress reliever? A means to socialize? A way to mark the end of your workday? Can you find another way to meet those needs? Try these alternatives:

- Socialize with a mocktail.
- Unwind with a cup of tea.
- Destress with five minutes of high-intensity exercycling.
- Reward yourself with self-care (e.g., massage, calming stroll around block).
- Trade your alcohol calories for a food reward such as a larger potato at dinner or apple crisp for dessert. (People often crave carbs when they stop drinking.)

Make a list of all the reasons you don't want to drink and read it daily—particularly at vulnerable times. You can also strive to break the routine of, let's say, immediately having a drink when you come home. Maybe you can first check e-mails, take a shower, walk the dog. Do something different than the activities you associate with drinking. For further information, see appendix A.

If you think before you drink, you can talk yourself into moderation. That is preferable to dealing with a hangover. Or if you know you will be drinking, at least eat a hearty meal and drink extra water to buffer the impending flood of alcohol. Drink slowly, don't mix liquors, and please have a designated driver.

If you fail to heed this advice, you will likely be dealing with the symptoms of a hangover: headache, light-headedness, irritability, anxiety, sensitivity to light and noise, trouble sleeping, difficulty concentrating, nausea, and vomiting. These symptoms generally dissipate over 12 (or more) hours, but you may be looking for a way to hasten the process.

Anecdotal remedies for a hangover include drinking sodium-containing (nonalcoholic) fluids. The sodium helps retain the fluid in your body. Try chicken soup, sports drink (with or without added Alka-Seltzer), Pedialyte, or more water or sports drink every time you wake up to urinate during the night. Do not take acetaminophen (Tylenol); this combination can be damaging to the liver.

PART II

THE SCIENCE OF EATING AND EXERCISE

CHAPTER 9

FUELING BEFORE EXERCISE

I am forever amazed at how little people eat and drink before they exercise. For example, while on a two-hour 30-mile (48 km) group bike ride, I have observed people who "ride to eat" rather than "eat to ride." One woman complained about how hungry and tired she'd get one hour into a ride—and then added she preferred to hold off to eat until the postride breakfast. She thought she was tired because she hadn't been training hard enough (not because she had run out of fuel). Other riders complained about how parched they were by the end of the ride.

My message to those cyclists and to all athletes and everyday exercisers is this: Just as you put fuel in your car before you take it for a drive, you need to put fuel in your body before you exercise. Your ability to perform well depends on proper fueling, not just training.

Preexercise fuel has five main functions:

1. It helps prevent hypoglycemia (low blood sugar) and its symptoms of light-headedness, needless fatigue, blurred vision, and indecisiveness—all of which can interfere with your performance.
2. It helps settle your stomach, absorb some of the gastric juices, and ward off hunger.
3. It fuels your muscles and feeds your brain.
4. It gives you the peace of mind that comes with knowing your body is well fueled.
5. It helps you exercise harder so you can burn more calories, which might help you lose undesired body fat, if that is your prime motive for exercise.

GO BY YOUR GUT

Preexercise foods that settle comfortably can enhance stamina, endurance, strength, and enjoyment. But many people are afraid that preexercise food will result in an upset stomach, diarrhea, and undesired pit stops. Of course, eating too much of the wrong kinds of foods can cause intestinal problems. But you want to be curious and experiment with small amounts of a variety of options to learn what works—and what doesn't—and train the gut so that adequate fueling can support your exercise goals.

Each person has unique food preferences and aversions, so no one food or magic meal will ensure top performance for everyone. Frank, a competitive runner, avoids any food within four hours of training or competing. Otherwise, he needs to find bathrooms along the route. Kristin, a loyal exerciser at a health club, thrives best on overnight oats (see recipe in chapter 18) an hour before her morning routine. "It absorbs the stomach juices and settles my stomach," she said. Sarah, a gymnast and eighth-grade student, snacks on a banana before practice sessions but on nothing before a competition. She gets so nervous that she can't keep anything down. "I make sure I eat extra the day before a competition," she said.

Choices of what to eat before exercising vary from person to person and from sport to sport—there is no single right or wrong choice. My experience has shown that each athlete needs to learn through trial and error during training and competition what works best for his or her body and what doesn't work. From day 1 of your training program, you need to train not only your heart, lungs, and muscles but also your intestinal tract.

To train your intestinal tract to tolerate preexercise fuel, start with a cracker or a sip of a sports drink; gradually add more until you can enjoy 200 to 300 calories within the hour before you work out. Keep in mind the following predisposing factors that might trigger gastrointestinal (GI) problems:

- **Type of sport.** Cyclists, swimmers, cross-country skiers, and others who exercise in a relatively stable position report fewer GI problems than do athletes in running sports that jostle the intestines.

- **Training status.** Untrained people who are starting an exercise program report more GI problems than do well-trained athletes who have built up a tolerance to exercise. If you are a novice who is experiencing GI distress, gradually increase your training volume and intensity so that your body can adjust to the changes.

- **Age.** GI problems occur more frequently in younger athletes than in veterans. The younger athletes may be less trained and possibly have less nutrition knowledge and experience with precompetition eating. Veterans, on the other hand, have had the opportunity to learn from years of nutrition mistakes.

- **Gender.** Women report more GI problems than men do, particularly at the time of their menstrual periods. The hormonal shifts that occur during menstruation can contribute to looser bowel movements.

- **Emotional and mental stress.** Athletes who are tense are more likely to report that food in the stomach lingers longer and settles like a lead balloon.

- **Exercise intensity.** During easy and even moderately hard exercise, the body can both digest food and comfortably exercise. But during intense exercise, the shift of blood flow from the stomach to the working muscles may be responsible for GI complaints.

- **Precompetition food intake.** Eating too much high-protein and high-fat food (such as bacon and fried eggs or a burger and french fries) shortly before exercise can cause GI problems. Tried-and-true low-fat, carbohydrate-rich favorites (such as oatmeal or bananas) that are part of your day-to-day training diet are a safer bet.

- **Fiber.** High-fiber diets intensify GI complaints. If you are eating large amounts of fruits, vegetables, beans, legumes, and whole grains, try cutting back for a week to see whether you feel better.

- **Caffeine.** Some athletes try to enhance their performance by drinking a larger-than-usual mug of coffee but end up with an upset stomach, diarrhea, and substandard performance.

- **Level of hydration.** Dehydration enhances the risk of intestinal problems. During training, start exercising in a well-hydrated state and be sure to practice drinking different fluids on a regular schedule (about 8 oz, or 240 ml, every 15 to 20 minutes of strenuous exercise) to learn how your body reacts to water, sports drinks, diluted juice, and any fluids that you will be drinking during competition.

- **Hormonal changes.** The digestive process is under hormonal control, and exercise stimulates changes in these hormones. For example, postmarathon levels of GI hormones tend to be two to five times higher than resting levels. These hormonal changes can result in food traveling faster through the digestive system and explain why some people experience GI problems regardless of what they eat.

- **Undiagnosed celiac disease.** The same people who routinely have "sensitive stomachs" and bowel issues find that exercise exaggerates the problem. Marta, a 17-year-old high school runner, kept getting sidelined with fecal urgency during cross country races. She came to me for help with figuring out the GI problem. When I asked about her medical history, she mentioned that she had an underactive thyroid, three broken bones in the past four years, and recurrent anemia. Her father had colon cancer, his mother had severe osteoporosis, and her aunt had diabetes. All of these medical issues raised a red flag for celiac disease.

I suggested that Marta meet with a GI doctor. Sure enough, celiac disease was the problem. Once she went on a gluten-free diet (no wheat, barley, or rye), the intestinal distress started to abate over the next few weeks. Given that 1 percent of Americans have celiac disease, and only about 10 percent of those are diagnosed (and others are misdiagnosed as having irritable bowel syndrome), you might want to talk with a medical professional if you can relate to Marta's story. (See chapter 6 and appendix A for more information on celiac disease.)

- **Gels and concentrated sugar solutions.** Highly concentrated sugar solutions consumed during exercise may cause stomach distress. Don't confuse the high-carbohydrate recovery drinks (about 200 calories per 8 oz, or per 240 ml) with low-carbohydrate fluid replacers.

- **Irritable bowel syndrome.** An estimated 10 to 20 percent of Americans experience irritable bowel syndrome. That number includes a lot of athletic people who may be sidelined by their symptoms during exercise. Yet, in general, exercise can improve symptoms (Johannesson et al. 2011). Sometimes irritable bowels can be calmed by a low-FODMAP diet, which is described in the following section.

- **Sugar-free foods with sorbitol.** If you get gassy and feel bloated after chewing sugar-free gum or eating sugar-free candies that are sweetened with sorbitol, you might have trouble digesting certain kinds of carbohydrate (sugar alcohols). A dietitian who specializes in FODMAP diets can help you.

What's a FODMAP?

FODMAP stands for fermentable oligo-, di-, and monosaccharides and polyols. Fermentable means *gas producing*; the oligo-, di-, monosaccharides, and polyols are different kinds of carbohydrate. For example, the disaccharide lactose (milk sugar) is difficult for some people to digest. Other kinds of carbohydrate, such as those in apples, onion, or mushrooms, can also create intestinal distress in people who lack certain digestive enzymes. Many people who claim to feel better when they avoid gluten are actually reacting to a carbohydrate in wheat called a *fructan*. They have no need to be on a diet for celiac disease if the problem is not gluten, which is a protein.

Joccelyn, a 45-year-old consultant and marathon runner, came to me feeling discouraged about her inability to complete long runs without having to take frequent bathroom breaks. Fecal urgency had become increasingly problematic over the previous five years. When she started choosing more low-FODMAP foods—particularly on the day or two before long runs and races—the issue was resolved. She was able to reach her goal of qualifying for the Boston Marathon after all!

If you experience digestive issues, you want to become a food detective and keep food logs to pinpoint potential culprits, or at least narrow down the problem. For several days, eliminate a suspected problem food such as milk, broccoli, corn, onions, garlic, kidney beans, or sugar-free gum. Does the problem go away when that food is out of your system? Does the problem return when you reintroduce the suspected food into your diet? A registered dietitian can help you with this process. For more information on FODPMAPS, see the resources in appendix A.

Are You Training Your Gut?

Endurance athletes and those in running sports commonly live with fear of transit troubles, but they fail to train their gut. As one marathoner reported, "I was so afraid of getting diarrhea during long training runs that I did not eat or drink anything beforehand. I really struggled after 14 miles." A high school soccer player admitted, "I'm so afraid I'll throw up if I run with food in my stomach." He ate only a light lunch at 11:00 a.m. and then practiced on fumes at 3:30. No wonder he had a disappointing season.

An estimated 30 to 50 percent of endurance athletes (including up to 90 percent of distance runners) have experienced gastrointestinal issues during and after hard exercise. Issues with bloat, gas, nausea, stomach cramps and pain, side stitch, diarrhea, vomiting, and urge to defecate arise during long bouts of exercise because blood flow to the gut is reduced for an extended time. When combined with dehydration, elevated body temperature, and high levels of stress hormones, normal intestinal function can abruptly end (Jeukendrup 2017).

If you are an athlete with a finicky GI tract, restricting your diet before and during exercise will not solve the problem. Instead, you want to learn how to train your gut to accommodate performance-enhancing carbs and water. That way, you can train better—hence compete better—without stressing about undesired pit stops.

Thankfully, the gut is trainable. Competitive eaters have proven this point. Look up Nathan's Hot Dog Eating Competition on the Internet and watch the video of a champ who stuffed 72 hotdogs into his stomach in 10 minutes. Clearly, he had to train his gut to be able to complete that task. Competitive eating is unlikely your goal, but you may want to be competitive in your sport. That means you need to fuel wisely in order to perform optimally. While some "keto athletes" choose to train their bodies to rely on abundant stores of body fat for fuel (hence reducing their need for consuming fuel during extended exercise), training the gut is a far easier alternative for most of us.

BURNING FAT INSTEAD OF CARBOHYDRATE

Athletes burn fat for fuel when they exercise in a fasted state, with no preexercise fuel. While some believe this will help them lose body fat, that is not the case. To lose body fat, you need to create an energy deficit by the end of the day regardless of whether you burn carbohydrate or fat during exercise. You'll be able to exercise harder, burn more calories, and

Tips for Competitive Athletes

To determine the right precompetition snack or meal for your body, experiment with the following guidelines:

- Always eat familiar foods before a competition. Don't try anything new! Schedule a few workouts of similar intensity to and at the same time of day as an upcoming competition, and experiment with different foods to determine which (and how much) will be best on race day.

- If you know that you'll be jittery and unable to tolerate food before an event, make a special effort to eat well the day before. Have an extra-large bedtime snack instead of breakfast.

- If you have a finicky stomach, experiment with liquid meals (smoothie, Boost) to see whether they offer you an advantage.

- When traveling to an event, pack a supply of tried-and-true foods in case of an emergency. If you should encounter delays, such as being stuck in traffic or on an airplane, you'll still be able to fuel your body adequately. Suggestions for a traveling athlete's emergency food kit include protein bars, dried fruit, trail mix, nuts, soy nuts, and sandwiches with peanut butter and honey or jam.

- If you have a "magic food," be sure to take it with you. Even if it's a standard item such as a Clif Bar, pack it so that you will be certain to have it on hand.

- Drink extra fluid the day before so that your urine is very pale. On the day of the event, drink 2 to 4 milliliters per pound (5-10 ml/kg) of body weight in the two to four hours before the event. This helps you hydrate optimally plus allows sufficient time to void the excess (ACSM 2016). For a 150-pound (68 kg) athlete, that's 300 to 600 milliliters (10 to 20 oz)—a mug of coffee and a glass of water!

potentially lose more body fat if you eat a preexercise snack (Paoli et al. 2012). See chapter 16 for more information on appropriate methods for losing weight.

Caitlyn, a competitive marathon runner, experimented with a high-fat, very low-carbohydrate ketogenic diet, hoping it would give her endless energy as she tapped into her body's abundant fat stores. She didn't know that burning fat requires more oxygen than burning carbohydrate (glycogen). Hence, she was less efficient and less powerful when she wanted to make a high-intensity surge up a hill or a sprint to pass a competitor.

Instead of "going all-out keto" and severely restricting carbohydrate, some highly competitive athletes "train low." They limit their intake of grains, fruits, and vegetables around specific low-intensity training sessions, so they train with low carbohydrate stores a few times a week to gain a metabolic advantage but still train well-fueled most of the time to support high-intensity workouts. To train depleted, these elite athletes might work out hard in the evening, limit their carb intake afterward (eat just chicken and a spinach salad with lots of dressing for dinner), and then train again the next morning with depleted glycogen stores. Training in a carb-depleted state in that second workout triggers beneficial metabolic adaptations that might help improve sports performance in subelite athletes (Burke and Hawley 2018). Stay tuned for more research. Note that training low is not fun, but it does boost mental toughness! I recommend keeping the enjoyment in exercise for most of my clients.

EAT THE RIGHT FOODS AT THE RIGHT TIME

The trick to completing your workout with energy to spare is to fuel up with the right foods at the right time before the event. Figure 9.1 shows the steps of digestion. For workouts less than 60 to 90 minutes, the preexercise snack should be predominantly carbohydrate because it empties quickly from the stomach (as compared to protein and fat) and becomes readily available to be used by the muscles. But before extended exercise such as a long run or bike ride, adding peanut butter to that bagel will contribute sustained energy. Here are suggestions for different types of events at different times of the day:

Time: 8:00 a.m. event, such as a road race, swim meet, or intense spin (stationary cycling) class

Meals: Eat a carbohydrate-based dinner, and drink extra water the day before. On the morning of the event, at about 6:00 or 6:30, have a light 200- to 400-calorie meal (depending on your tolerance) such as toast and a banana or a granola bar, a latte, and extra water. Eat familiar foods. If you want a larger meal, consider eating between 5:00 and 6:00 a.m.

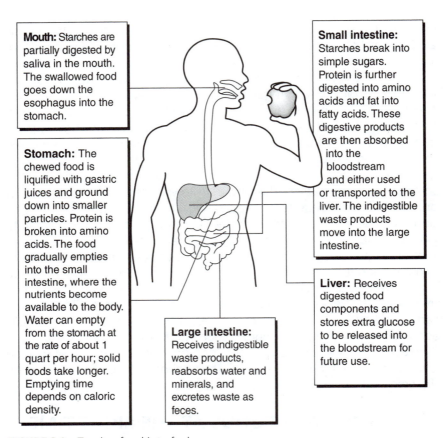

Mouth: Starches are partially digested by saliva in the mouth. The swallowed food goes down the esophagus into the stomach.

Stomach: The chewed food is liquified with gastric juices and ground down into smaller particles. Protein is broken into amino acids. The food gradually empties into the small intestine, where the nutrients become available to the body. Water can empty from the stomach at the rate of about 1 quart per hour; solid foods take longer. Emptying time depends on caloric density.

Small intestine: Starches break into simple sugars. Protein is further digested into amino acids and fat into fatty acids. These digestive products are then absorbed into the bloodstream and either used or transported to the liver. The indigestible waste products move into the large intestine.

Liver: Receives digested food components and stores extra glucose to be released into the bloodstream for future use.

Large intestine: Receives indigestible waste products, reabsorbs water and minerals, and excretes waste as feces.

FIGURE 9.1 Turning food into fuel.

If your body cannot handle breakfast before early-morning hard exercise, eat your breakfast before going to bed the night before. A bowl of cereal, bagel with peanut butter, or packets of oatmeal can help boost liver glycogen stores and prevent low blood sugar the next morning.

Time: 10:00 a.m. event, such as a bike race or soccer game

Meals: Eat a carbohydrate-based dinner such as a chicken stir-fry with extra rice, and drink extra water the day before. On the morning of the event, eat a familiar breakfast by 7:00 or 8:00 a.m. to allow two to three hours for the food to digest. This meal will prevent the fatigue that results from low blood sugar. Popular choices are oatmeal with nuts and raisins, an english muffin with peanut butter and a banana, and yogurt with Grape-Nuts and berries. You might even want a snack right beforehand, such as applesauce or a gel.

Time: 11:00 a.m. event, such as a lightweight crew race, wrestling match, or other weight-class sport that requires a weigh-in one to two hours beforehand

Meals: Athletes who have crash dieted and dehydrated themselves to reach a specific weight for their sport have only a few hours after weigh-in to prepare for the competition. They need to replace water, carbohydrate, and sodium. An ideal target for a 150-pound (68 kg) depleted athlete would be 700 calories (primarily from carbohydrate), 2,200 milligrams of sodium, and 2 quarts (2 L) of water (Slater et al. 2007). The intake will vary greatly depending on the athlete's tolerance for food. Too many wrestlers end up vomiting on the mat after having pigged out after the weigh-in. The following are appropriate food choices:

- Chicken noodle soup, bread, and lots of water
- Salted boiled potatoes, broth, salted crackers, and water
- Ginger ale or cola, a bagel sandwich with ham and mustard, and water
- Gatorade Endurance plus pretzels

Time: 2:00 p.m. event, such as a football or lacrosse game

Meals: An afternoon game allows time for you to have either a hearty carbohydrate-based breakfast such as French toast and a light lunch or a substantial brunch by 10:00, allowing four hours to digest. As always, eat a carbohydrate-based dinner the night before, and drink extra fluids the day before and up to noon. Popular brunch choices include French toast, pancakes, cereal, scrambled eggs, poached eggs on toast, Canadian bacon, bagels, fresh fruit salad, 100 percent fruit juice, fruit yogurt, and fruit smoothies. Eat a light snack within the hour beforehand if you feel hungry and can tolerate, let's say, animal crackers or pretzels.

Time: 8:00 p.m. event, such as a basketball game

Meals: You can thoroughly digest a hefty carbohydrate-based breakfast and lunch by evening. Plan for an early dinner, as tolerated, by 5:00 p.m., and you might even want a pregame snack at 7:00 p.m. Drink extra fluids all day. Two popular dinner choices are pasta with tomato sauce and meatballs, and chicken with a large serving of rice or potato, plus rolls, fruit salad, and low-fat frozen yogurt.

Time: All-day event, such as a hard hike, 100-mile (160 km) bike ride, or a day of cross-country skiing

Meals: Two days before the event, cut back on your exercise. Take a rest day the day before to allow time for your muscles to replace depleted glycogen stores. Eat carbohydrate-rich meals at breakfast, lunch, and dinner (see chapter 6 for information about preparing for an endurance event). Drink extra fluids. On the day of the event, eat a tried-and-true breakfast depending on your tolerance. Oatmeal and bagels with peanut butter are favorites.

While exercising, plan to eat carbohydrate-based foods (banana bread, energy bars, dried fruit, sweet potato in a pouch [baby food], sports drinks, gels) every 60 to 90 minutes to maintain normal blood sugar levels. If you stop at lunchtime, eat a comfortable-sized meal, but in general try to distribute your calories evenly throughout the day. Include foods with protein and fat such as hummus, nuts, nut butters, and cheese. They offer sustained energy because dietary fat takes a few hours to be digested into fuel. Drink fluids before you get thirsty; you should need to urinate at least three times throughout the day.

Fueling Three to Four Hours Before a Workout

In general, most athletes prefer to allow a full meal three to four hours to digest before exercising. A meal at this time has plenty of time to empty from the stomach, particularly if the athletes don't stuff themselves with high-fat foods (cheeseburgers and fries) that take longer to digest than a carbohydrate-based pasta-type meal. Kyle, a collegiate runner, slept through breakfast, but had a big brunch at 11:00 a.m., knowing it would help fuel his 4:00 p.m. team practice. (He also snacked on graham crackers with a little peanut butter and a banana at 3:00 p.m., a smaller amount of food to offer fuel as well as abate hunger.) Table 9.1 shows suggested amounts of food to consume before exercising.

TABLE 9.1 Suggested Targets for Preexercise Fueling

Because each person differs in tolerance to preexercise food, these numbers are just suggestions. Experiment during training to determine how much food works best for your body. The amount of food tolerated varies according to sport and intensity of exercise. That is, cyclists often eat more than runners.

Preexercise time	Grams of carbohydrate based on body weight	Calories for a 150-pound (68 kg) athlete
4 hours	2 g/lb (4 g/kg)	1,200
2 hours	1 g/lb (2 g/kg)	600
5-60 minutes	0.5 g/lb (1 g/kg)	300

For a 150-pound (68 kg) triathlete who will be starting a 50-mile bike ride at 10:00 a.m., 600 calories of breakfast carbohydrates at 8:00 a.m. translate as follows:

- A bowl of granola with a large banana and milk
- Three or four pancakes with maple syrup
- Three packets of oatmeal with a snack box of raisins

This is more than many athletes tend to eat!

Please don't go crazy counting carbohydrate grams; this is just a guide. Adding a little fat or protein (such as eggs or peanut butter) can help keep you feeling fed longer, as well as protect your muscles from breaking down, but carbohydrate is the most important factor here for fueling. Too much protein or fat (a big cheese omelet with bacon and hash browns) could sit heavily in your stomach, making for an unpleasant workout. Also add a sprinkle of salt in hot weather. Consuming 300 to 700 milligrams of sodium two to three hours preexercise can help prevent sodium depletion. You can easily get that much from food (see chapter 10).

Sherman and colleagues (1989) conducted a study that demonstrates the importance of eating a hearty meal four hours before you exercise. In their study, cyclists ate either nothing or 1,200 calories of carbohydrate (about 2 g of carbohydrate per lb, or 4 g/kg, of body weight) four hours before an exercise test to exhaustion. When they ate the 1,200-calorie meal (That's a lot of pasta and juice!), they were able to bike 15 percent harder during the last 45 minutes, as compared to when they ate nothing. Given that road races and many competitive events are won or lost by fractions of a second, being 15 percent stronger offers a huge advantage. The carbohydrate the cyclists ate before they exercised supplied extra fuel for the end of the workout, when their glycogen stores were low.

Although this study looked at cyclists, who tend to report fewer gastrointestinal complaints than do athletes in running sports that jostle the stomach, the benefits are worth noting. If you've always done afternoon exercise on an empty stomach, you may discover that you can exercise harder and longer by enjoying a heartier breakfast and lunch, as well as a preexercise snack within the hour before you work out. Even if you are dieting, you should follow this pattern; you need to fuel during the active part of your day. You can lose weight at night, when you're sleeping! (See chapter 16.)

Fueling an Hour or Less Before a Workout

Morning exercisers who work out before breakfast, in particular, need to be sure they have fueled themselves adequately. If you roll out of bed and eat nothing before you jump into the swimming pool, participate in a CrossFit class, or go for a run, you may be running on fumes. If you've eaten nothing since a 6:00 p.m. dinner the night before, your blood sugar will definitely need a boost. But if you had a large bedtime snack the night before, you'll be less in need of early-morning food.

Experiment to figure out whether you will perform better if you eat something before your early-morning exercise. During the night, you deplete your liver glycogen, the source of carbohydrate that maintains normal blood sugar levels. When you start a workout with low blood sugar, your brain fails to get adequate fuel and the result is needless fatigue because your brain controls your muscles. Plus, you'll enjoy the workout more. Exercising on empty is hard work.

How much people should eat before a morning workout varies from person to person, ranging from a few crackers to a slice of toast, a swig of juice, or a bowl of cereal. The rule of thumb is to consume about two calories of carbohydrate per pound (4 cal/kg) of body weight 5 to 60 minutes before exercising (ACSM 2016). Whether fueling for a morning run or an after-work CrossFit session, 300 preexercise calories of carbohydrate for a 150-pound (68 kg) athlete translates into the following:

- Two packets of instant oatmeal (flavored)
- A bagel with jam
- A baggie of "munchies" made with dried fruit, cereal, and pretzels
- An energy bar and 16 ounces (480 ml) of a sports drink

Because tolerances vary so much, defining the best amount of preexercise food is difficult. Some competitive athletes get up two hours early just to eat and then go back to bed and allow time for the food to settle. Others have an energy bar, a banana, or some other easy-to-digest food as they dash out the door. Then there are those who habitually exercise on empty. If that's you, an abstainer, here is a noteworthy study that might convince you to experiment with eating at least 100 calories of a morning snack before you work out.

Researchers asked a group of athletes to bike moderately hard in the morning for as long as they could. When they ate breakfast (400 calories of carbohydrate), they biked for 136 minutes, as compared with only 109 minutes when they had no breakfast, just water (Schabort et al. 1999). Clearly, these athletes were able to train better with some fuel in their tanks. Preexercise morning fuel will likely work for you, too (table 9.2). I encourage you to experiment and observe the benefits. Catherine, an early-morning swimmer, learned that she simply didn't want to eat at 5:00 a.m., so she enjoyed her breakfast the night before: a 9:00 p.m. bowl of cereal before she went to bed. This works well for her, as well as for many other morning exercisers.

TABLE 9.2 Guidelines for Preexercise Carbohydrate Intake

If you are a numbers geek, here is more precise information to help guide your food choices (ACSM 2016). But rather than spend hours counting grams of carbohydrate (a daunting task), grasp the concept that this could easily be more carbohydrate than you currently consume. Could you perform better if you were better fueled? Be sure to experiment during training to learn the amount of carbohydrate that works best for your body. Refer to table 6.6 for more information about the carbohydrate content of common foods.

Carbohydrate needs based on exercise	Carbohydrate: recommended intake	Grams of carb for a 150-lb (68 kg) athlete	Translating grams of carb into calories	Food example
One hour before exercise	0.5 g carb/lb (1 g/kg) body weight	75	300	2 packets flavored oatmeal
Two hours before exercise	1.0 g carb/lb (2 g/kg) body weight	150	600	2 Starbucks bagels with jam
Three hours before exercise	1.5 g carb/lb (3 g/kg) body weight	225	900	4 large pancakes + syrup + orange juice
Four hours before exercise	2 g carb/lb (4 g/kg) body weight	300	1,200	6 large pancakes + syrup + orange juice
Exercise 60-90 min/day, such as a solid gym workout or a soccer practice or game	3-5.5 g/lb body weight (7-12 g/kg body weight)	450-825 g carb/day or 110-205 g carb at each of 4 meals per day	1,800-3,300 cal from carb per day = 450-825 cal from carb at each of 4 meals per day	2 bagels from Starbucks offer 110 g carb (440 calories from carb)
Carbohydrate loading, to prepare for a competitive endurance event longer than 90 minutes	4.5-5.5 g carb/lb/day (10-12 g carb/kg/day) for 1.5 to 2 days	675-825 g carb/day for 1.5 to 2 days	2,700-3,300 cal from carb	Two 1-lb (455 g) boxes of uncooked pasta offer 640 g carb (2,560 calories from carb)
Speedy refueling	~0.5 g carb/lb/hour (~1 g/kg/h) for the first 4 hours then resume regular meals	75 g carb/hour for 4 hours	300 cal of carb/hour	2 packets of flavored instant oatmeal + 8 oz. orange juice offers 75 g carb (300 cal)

FACT OR FICTION

The food you eat in the hour before you exercise sits in your stomach and is not useful.

The facts: You can grab a small snack just five minutes before exercise and the food will get put to good use—as long as you are exercising at a pace that you can maintain for more than half an hour. That is, you might not want to eat much five minutes before a hard track workout, but you could likely enjoy a banana before you put on your jogging shoes. Research suggests that eating an energy bar 15 minutes before moderate exercise offers the same energy boost as eating one 60 minutes before exercising (Kerr et al. 2008).

Sugar Crashes

In general, people who are in good physical condition can regulate their blood glucose with far less insulin than sedentary people can, and they do not experience "sugar crashes" (rebound hypoglycemia). But some people are far more sensitive than others are to drops in blood glucose. For a few people, eating a high-sugar food 15 to 45 minutes before exercise can have a negative effect. A concentrated dose of sugar (either natural sugar in fruit juice or refined sugar in sport drinks and jelly beans) rapidly boosts your blood sugar but simultaneously triggers the pancreas to secrete a large amount of insulin. Insulin transports excess sugar out of the blood and into the muscles. Exercise, like insulin, similarly enhances this transport. Thus, your blood sugar can drop to an abnormally low level once you start to exercise.

To be on the safe side, if you are hungry and craving sweets before your afternoon workout, eat the sweets within 10 minutes of exercise. If you are sugar sensitive, choose a carbohydrate that includes fiber or protein, such as a pear, dried apricots, or chocolate milk. This plan will minimize the risk of a hypoglycemic reaction because the insulin will not have greatly increased in that short period. Alternatively, consume a gel, honey, gummy candy, or another form of carbohydrate while you warm up or at the start of the exercise, and every 20 to 30 minutes during exercise.

Most of my clients who complain about "sugar shakes" have simply undereaten before exercising. Kathy, a teacher who went directly to the gym after a busy school day, experienced low-blood-sugar "crashes" simply because she'd skimped on calories all day. She was trying hard to lose weight and ate only small portions at breakfast and lunch. Within 15 minutes of beginning her exercise class, she felt light headed, shaky, uncoordinated, and unmotivated to continue. To resolve the problem, I suggested that she do the following:

- Eat a bigger breakfast and lunch (and smaller dinner).
- Enjoy a preexercise snack of applesauce and graham crackers.

By doing these two things, she discovered that she had energy to enjoy her workout, was less hungry when she arrived home, and was able to eat fewer calories at night. She learned to lose weight when she was sleeping and not when exercising. (See chapter 16.)

Preexercise Caffeine

Caffeine is a popular preexercise energizer and is known to help many athletes train harder and longer when taken in moderate amounts. Caffeine stimulates the brain and contributes to mental alertness and greater concentration. Many good studies address the use of caffeine for both endurance exercise, such as long runs and bike rides, and short-term, higher-intensity exercise, such as soccer. The vast majority of the studies conclude that caffeine taken an hour before exercise does indeed enhance performance (by about 11 percent) and makes the effort seem easier (by about 6 percent).

A target dose of caffeine is 1.5 to 3 milligrams per pound (3-6 mg/kg) (Maughan et al. 2018). For a 150-pound (68 kg) athlete, this is 225 to 450 milligrams of caffeine. Table 9.3 lists the caffeine amounts in common perk-me-ups.

TABLE 9.3 Caffeine Content of Common Beverages and Other Products

Sources of caffeine	Average caffeine content (mg)
COFFEE, 16 OZ (480 ML) MUG	
Starbucks brewed, grande	330
Brewed, drip method, Maxwell House	135-215
Dunkin'	180
Decaffeinated, Dunkin' or Starbucks	15-23
OTHER BEVERAGES	
Starbucks espresso (Doppio) (6.5 oz, or 195 ml)	150
Starbucks Refreshers, 12 oz	45-55
Espresso, generic, 1 oz (30 ml) shot	40 (30-90)
Hot cocoa, 12 oz (360 ml)	12

(continued)

TABLE 9.3 (continued)

Sources of caffeine	Average caffeine content (mg)
TEA	
Tea, brewed, 16 oz (480 ml)	60-160
Starbucks Tazo Chai Tea Latte, 16 oz (480 ml)	95
Snapple Lemon Tea, 16 oz (480 ml)	62
Lipton Pure Leaf Iced Tea, 16 oz (480ml)	60
Arizona Iced Tea, green, 16 oz (480 ml)	15
SOFT DRINK, 12 OZ (360 ML) CAN*	
Mountain Dew, regular or diet	54
Pepsi One	54
Pepsi	38
Diet Pepsi	35
Coca-Cola, classic or diet	35
Barq's Root Beer	23
Mug Root Beer	0
7-Up	0
ENERGY DRINKS	
5-Hour Energy, 2 oz (60 ml)	200
Red Bull, 8.3 oz (250 ml)	80
Rockstar Energy Drink, 8 oz (240 ml)	80
Monster Energy Drink, 8 oz (240 ml)	80
CAFFEINATED SPORTS SUPPLEMENTS	
Jolt Gum, 1 piece	45
Gu, vanilla, 1 oz (30 g)	20
DRUGS	
NoDoz, maximum strength, 1 tablet	200
Excedrin, 1 tablet	130
Dexatrim, 1 tablet	80
Anacin, 1 tablet	64

*Small children who drink a can of cola can receive the equivalent in caffeine to an adult who drinks a cup of coffee.

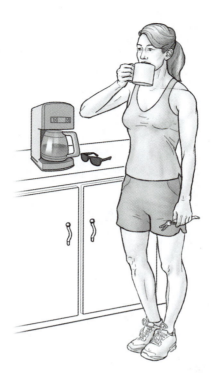

Although a cup or two of coffee before exercise may be a helpful ener-gizer, more may be of little value. Well-trained cyclists performed equally well with about 350 milligrams of caffeine as they did with 850 milligrams (Pasman et al. 1995). So if you're tempted to jazz yourself up with a second mugful, think again. You may find that the second mug will do you in with the caffeine jitters.

Because each person responds differently to caffeine, in part due to genetic differences, do not assume that you will perform better with a caffeine boost. You might just end up nauseated, coping with a "coffee stomach," or feeling agitated at a time when you are already nervous and anxious. And be forewarned: Although a morning cup of coffee can assist with a desirable bowel movement, a precompetition mugful might lead to transit troubles. Experiment during training to determine whether a caffeinated beverage or plain water is the better bet.

If you are sleep deprived and seek coffee for its stimulant effect, think again before buying that large cup of brew for a morning eye-opener. Perhaps, instead, you should be resting and not dragging yourself through a workout. Be sure no trouble is brewing in your desire for caffeine!

CHAPTER 10

FUELING DURING AND AFTER EXERCISE

Just as what you eat before you exercise greatly affects your energy levels, so does what you eat during and after extensive and intensive exercise. Students who do sustained hard training after school from 3:30 to 5:30 p.m., businesspeople who de-stress with a tiring workout from 5:30 to 7:00 p.m., marathoners who train for hours, and others who exercise hard for more than 60 to 90 minutes need to think about fueling not only before but also during exercise. Unfortunately, many of these folks are in such a rush to start their workouts that they fail to bring with them the foods and fluids that will enhance their exercise efforts. They forget that endurance performance depends on fueling, not just training!

This chapter will help you enjoy high energy and enhanced stamina during challenging exercise sessions that last longer than an hour. Standard healthy eating practices should take care of shorter sessions. But when you're pushing the limits, you'll want to pay proper attention to what you eat and drink before (see chapter 9), during, and after your hard workouts. Research on well-trained cyclists suggests that those who followed specific scientific fueling plans performed 6 percent better than those following self-chosen plans (Hottenrott et al. 2012). Six percent—that's a lot! Keep reading to learn how you can develop your own scientific plan.

FUELING DURING EXTENSIVE EXERCISE

Your goals during sustained hard exercise that lasts more than 60 minutes are to 1) prevent dehydration by drinking enough fluid to balance your sweat losses and 2) maintain a normal blood sugar level by consuming adequate carbohydrate. Optimal intake of fluids and fuel can significantly increase your stamina. During high-intensity exercise (basketball, soccer), you'll likely want to stick with gels and sports drinks—no need to chew! (Just be sure to drink enough water with the gels.) But with lower-intensity exercise (long runs and bike rides), you can consume and digest standard foods while you are working out. Table 10.1 shows several plans for fueling.

Research involving cyclists suggests that Sport Beans, sports drinks, and gels all offer similar performance benefits (Campbell et al. 2007). Your body also doesn't care whether you ingest solid or liquid carbohydrate; both are equally effective (Mason, McConell, and Hargreaves 1993). Even sugar can be a positive snack during exercise (see chapter 6). The key is to eat enough carbohydrate: 60 to 90 grams (240 to 360 calories) is more than many endurance athletes would ever consider ingesting. (Refer to table 6.6, Carbohydrate Content of Common Foods, to learn what 60 to 90 grams looks like.) Could you also adapt your body to burning more fat by going

TABLE 10.1   Suggestions for Fueling During Exercise

Exercise type	Carbohydrate intake during exercise	Examples
<45 minutes, such as a workout at the health club	Nothing needed other than a preexercise snack.	Water, if thirsty
Sports with half-times, such as soccer, football, basketball	Easily digested carbohydrate as tolerated during and right before returning to play (to reduce risk of rebound hypoglycemia).	Watermelon, grapes, apple sauce, sports drinks, gel, maple syrup, animal crackers
1 to 2.5 hours, such as triathlon training, half-marathon, or swim team practice	30-60 g (120-240 calories) of carbohydrate/hour, after the first hour. (The preexercise snack fuels the first hour.)	Sports drink, gels, banana, dried pineapple, dried apple rings, fruit puree in squeeze pouches, gummy candy, pretzels
>2.5 hours, low to moderate intensity, such as walking a marathon, an all-day bike ride, or hiking	According to appetite, but at least 60 to 90 g (240 to 360 calories) if not more.	Banana bread, trail mix, dried fruit, hummus wrap, peanut butter and jam sandwich, any food that settles well
>2.5 hours, moderate to high nonstop intensity, such as running a marathon, an adventure race, or a triathlon	60-90 g carbohydrate/hour (240 to 360 calories of carbohydrate/hour) from a variety of foods. (Higher intakes are associated with better performance.) If digestive issues, swish and spit out sports drink.	Sports drinks, gels, sports candies, energy bars, simple cookies and candies, and standard foods, as tolerated, for carbohydrate, protein, and flavor change, nut butter and honey wrap, chocolate milk, jerky, cheese stick

on a ketogenic diet? Perhaps, but that's a lot of effort for questionable added performance benefit. (See chapter 6.)

Your best bet is to mix up your foods and fluids so you consume a variety of types of carbohydrate from commercial and natural foods. Instead of just sports drinks, choose a sports drink and dried apple rings or (part of) an energy bar plus extra water. Because different sugars use different transporters, you can absorb more carbohydrate and have more fuel to support your endurance exercise if you choose a variety of foods that offer a variety of forms of carbohydrate (Jentjens et al. 2006). You need to experiment during training to determine which foods and fluids work best for you and how much is appropriate.

During a moderate to hard endurance workout, carbohydrate supplies about 50 percent of your energy. As you deplete carbohydrate from muscle glycogen stores, you increasingly rely on blood sugar for energy. By consuming carbohydrate during exercise, such as the sugar in sports drinks, you give your muscles and your brain an added source of fuel. Because much of performance depends on mental stamina, you want to maintain a normal blood sugar level to keep your brain fed so you can think clearly, concentrate well, and remain focused.

Is more carbohydrate better? Not if the source of carbohydrate just sits in your stomach. Keep in mind that too much sugar or food taken at once can slow the rate of digestion. Be more conservative with your carbohydrate intake during intense exercise in hot weather, when rapid fluid replacement is perhaps more important than carbohydrate replacement. In cold weather, however, when the risk of becoming dehydrated is lower, more carbohydrate can provide much-needed energy.

Because consuming 120 to 250 calories or more per hour (after the first hour) may be far more than you are used to consuming during exercise, you need to practice eating during training to figure out which foods and fluids work and which do not.

Alex, a novice marathoner, tucked Gummi Bears, dried mango, and caffeinated gels in a waist pack that he wore on his long runs. He also hid along his running loop a bag containing pretzel nuggets and bottles filled with water and the brand of the sports drink that would be available during his planned marathon. Between the snacks and the fluids, he was able to maintain adequate energy during his three-hour training runs and simultaneously learn what he liked to eat during exercise. On marathon day, he assigned friends to specific checkpoints along the route. Their job was to keep him well supplied with a variety of carbohydrate and caffeine sources. He never hit the wall, and he was pleased with his time.

Allie, another marathoner, would generally get a "crummy tummy" after two hours of running. She couldn't tolerate fluids, but she learned that swishing with a sports drink made her feel better. Mouth swishing sends a message to the brain that energy is forthcoming. Swishing can enhance performance by 2 to 3 percent if the athlete is running on empty (Rollo and Williams 2011).

Whatever the situation, endurance athletes such as marathon runners, ultradistance cyclists, and Ironman triathletes need to make a nutrition plan far in advance of the event and experiment during training to learn their preferences. The same goes for team sports; half-time nutrition can offer the winning edge. Sports drinks, bananas, watermelon, and pretzels can be a welcomed energizer, as can a gel or sugar-fix right before going on the field.

By developing a list of several tried-and-true foods that taste good even when you are hot and tired, you need not worry about what to eat (and what not to eat) during the competitive event. If you are concerned about intestinal problems, see chapter 9.

Ideally, you should know more or less how much fluid to drink and how many calories to ingest. Here's how to estimate your needs:

- Determine your target fluid intake by weighing yourself naked before and after a workout in different temperatures to determine your sweat loss per hour.

- Estimate your calorie targets by working with a sports nutritionist, exercise physiologist, or the calorie information on heart rate monitors, Fitbits and other wearable sports technology, and exercise equipment. The information on calculating calories in chapter 16 can also be helpful.

Like Alex, you should also figure out how to make these foods and fluids available during your training and competitions. If you have a support crew, instruct them to feed you on a defined schedule to prevent hypoglycemia and dehydration.

Fueling Midworkout

Jameel, a fitness buff, noticed that he ran out of energy after running on the treadmill for 45 to 60 minutes and then trying to lift weights. "I think my lifting would be better if I refueled a bit after the run," he said. I agreed! I suggested 150- to 300-calorie postrun snacks that would boost his energy so he could then lift harder and better enjoy the second half of his workout. The cafe in the health club offered these options:

- Chocolate milk (low fat or skim), flavored yogurt
- Fruit juice, fruit smoothie

- Banana, melon chunks, dried pineapple, raisins
- Pretzels, Fig Newtons, belVita breakfast biscuits, energy bars

A quick-to-digest sugary midworkout snack can also be incorporated into an overall wholesome diet given that 10 percent of daily calories can appropriately come from sugar. This includes (defizzed) Coke and Pepsi, sweetened iced tea (for a caffeine boost), sports drinks, gels, gummy candy, any kind of sugary candy, and marshmallows. Sugary midworkout snacks offer a quick fix and are unlikely to cause a "sugar crash" (Lambert 2018), but they do not contribute to good health. If you go that route, simply choose primarily nutritious calories at other times throughout the day.

Fueling During Tournaments and Back-to-Back Events

If you are a competitive swimmer or wrestler or a tennis, soccer, or basketball player, you may frequently face the nutrition challenge presented by back-to-back events and tournaments that require top performance for hours on end, sometimes for days in a row. If you pay careful attention to what you eat, you'll be able to win with good nutrition. I've talked to many swimmers who gave no thought to their nutrition plan for an all-day swim meet. They cheated themselves of the ability to perform well in the late-afternoon events.

When you will be at a daylong event, be sure to bring along proven foods. Following are just a few suggestions to help you stock your gym bag or cooler (preferably using reusable food storage containers, to minimize packaging waste).

Fruit

Dried fruits such as dried cherries, pineapple, and mango

Applesauce

Canned fruit, such as peaches, pears, or pineapple

Bananas, oranges, and dates

Protein

Almonds or any nuts

Peanut butter

Tuna

Hummus*

Jerky

Hard-boiled eggs*

Cheese sticks*

Cheddar cheese,*

Yogurt,* Greek or regular

*Refrigeration is recommended, but these foods can withstand short periods without being refrigerated. The safest bet is to invest in a small cooler.

Grains

Granola, granola bars

Oatmeal Squares or your favorite brand of dry cereal

Pretzels, preferably whole grain

Pita chips, preferably whole grain

Snacks and Treats

Energy bars, such as Clif, Kashi, Lara, and Rx

Animal crackers

Oatmeal raisin cookies

Dark chocolate

Fluids

Water, plain or sparkling

Sports drink

100 percent juice

Chocolate (dairy or soy) milk

When engaging in daylong tournaments and events, as I mentioned before, your goals are to maintain proper hydration and normal blood sugar levels. Plan your strategies for refueling as soon as possible after the first event to prepare for the next. Know the portions of foods and beverages that will hit your calorie and fluid targets and have these proven sports foods in your gym bag or a cooler.

Following good nutrition practices can certainly give a team the winning edge. But persuading athletes to dedicate themselves to eating a proper sports diet can be a challenge. One college coach felt frustrated by his team's ritual of preevent high-fat pepperoni pizza parties (often accompanied by alcohol) that filled players' stomachs but left their muscles under fueled and the players dehydrated. No wonder the team was having a bad season. The coach took a strong stance. He hired a sports nutritionist to educate the players about the performance benefits of proper preevent carbohydrate and fluid intake. He instructed all coaches and athletic trainers to enforce appropriate between-game eating.

With the support of several parents, players were provided bagels, bananas, juices, pretzels, yogurt, chocolate milk, and other high-carbohydrate sports snacks and drinks on tournament days. When traveling to a game, the coach preselected an appropriate restaurant that could handle the whole team, and he prearranged an economical buffet of minestrone soup, spaghetti with tomato sauce, turkey meatballs, green beans, fresh whole-grain rolls, low-fat (chocolate) milk, cider, and apple crisp with frozen yogurt. He instructed each player to pack his gym bag with his own favorite sports foods (e.g., sports drinks, fig bars, trail mix, oranges, energy bars) to eat before, during, and between practice sessions and games.

The players noticed that proper fueling helped them perform better, and they respected the value of this winning nutrition program. Sure enough, they did start to have greater stamina and strength and better moods. Although they didn't always win, they no longer got clobbered in the final minutes, and they felt better about their overall effort.

If you are among the many athletes who give no thought to a sports nutrition plan during daylong tournaments and repeated events, think again. The right sports diet can indeed enhance your performance. If you and your teammates are performing well despite poor food choices, just think how much better you could be! See chapter 13 for additional information about how to manage team nutrition.

CRAMPING YOUR STYLE?

If you have ever experienced the excruciating pain of a severe muscle cramp, you may fearfully wonder whether it will strike again. Unfortunately, no one totally understands what causes muscle cramps, but if you've suffered one, you are at risk for having more. A field study of 433 Ironman triathletes suggests that those who cramped had exercised harder than usual, had a family history of cramping, and had had previous tendon or ligament injuries (Shang, Collins, and Schwellnus 2011). Because cramps commonly occur when muscles are fatigued, the problem may be related to a nerve malfunction that creates an imbalance between muscle excitation and inhibition, which prevents the muscle from relaxing (Schwellnus et al. 2004). Shocking the system with a pungent taste, such as Hotshot or pickle juice, can disrupt the cramp.

Although cramps are likely related to overexertion, other predisposing factors may include fluid loss, inadequate conditioning, and electrolyte imbalance. The solution often can be found with massage and stretching. Other times, nutrition may be involved. Although the following nutrition tips are not guaranteed to resolve this malady, I recommend that people who are predisposed to getting cramps rule out these possible contributing causes:

- **Lack of water.** Cramps commonly coincide with dehydration. To prevent dehydration-induced cramps, drink enough fluids before, during, and after you exercise. Always drink enough fluids daily that your urine is clear, pale yellow, and copious. During a long exercise session, a target for a sweaty 150-pound (68 kg) athlete might be about 8 ounces (240 ml) of fluid every 15 to 20 minutes. See chapter 8 for more information on fluid recommendations.

- **Lack of sodium.** Athletes who exercise hard for more than four hours in the heat, such as tennis players, triathletes, and ultrarunners, may be putting themselves at risk of developing a sodium imbalance that could contribute to cramps if they consume only water during the event and no foods or beverages that contain sodium. Endurance sports drinks and salted pretzels might be wise snack choices during extended sweaty exercise. Aaron, a tennis player, would bring pickles to tournaments, swearing they helped spare him from cramping. That said, a survey of ultrarunners found no difference in salt intake during the 100-mile (161 km) event or blood sodium levels afterward among the runners who cramped and those who did not. (Hoffman and Stuempfle 2015). Maybe sodium intake does not prevent muscle cramps, after all?

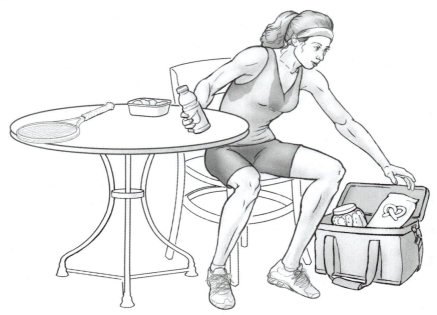

- **Lack of calcium.** Calcium plays an essential role in muscle contractions. Some active people report that their problem with cramping disappears when they boost their calcium intake. For example, one ballet dancer found that once she reintroduced yogurt and skim milk into her diet, her cramping disappeared. A mountaineer resolved his muscle cramps by taking antacid tablets containing calcium, such as Tums, when hiking. But some exercise scientists argue that a calcium imbalance seems an unlikely cause of muscle cramps because when dietary deficiencies occur, calcium is released from the bones to provide what is needed for proper muscle contraction. Nevertheless, to rule out any possible link between a calcium-poor diet and muscle cramps, athletes who experience cramps should consume dairy products or other calcium sources (calcium-fortified orange juice or soy milk) at least twice each day.

- **Lack of magnesium.** Just as muscles need calcium to contract, they also need magnesium to relax. Magnesium can help reduce leg cramps that occur in the middle of the night (Roffe et al. 2002). Whether magnesium also helps with exercise-related cramps is unclear. Many people do not meet the RDA for magnesium: 320 milligrams per day for women and 420 milligrams per day for men. The richest sources of magnesium are green leafy vegetables, whole grains, nuts, beans, and legumes. One cup of spinach has 155 milligrams of magnesium; a half cup of All-Bran, 110 milligrams; a cup of brown rice, 85 milligrams; and one whole-wheat pita, 45 milligrams. I hear marathoners claim that antacids like Rolaids are helpful. One tablet contains 45 milligrams of magnesium and 220 milligrams of calcium.

- **Lack of potassium.** An electrolyte imbalance, such as a lack of potassium, may play a role in muscle cramps. However, a potassium deficiency is unlikely to occur as a result of sweat losses because the body contains much more potassium than even a marathoner might lose during a hot, sweaty race. Nevertheless, you can rule out this issue by eating potassium-rich foods such as bananas and oranges daily. (Refer to table 10.3.)

Although these tips for preventing muscle cramps are only suggestions and not proven solutions, you might want to experiment with them if you repeatedly experience muscle cramps. Adding extra fluids, low-fat dairy products, potassium-rich fruits and vegetables, and a sprinkling of salt certainly won't harm you, and it may resolve this worrisome problem. Fueling well before and during to delay muscle fatigue might reduce cramping (and will enhance overall performance). You might want to try a "nervous-system shocker" such as Hotshot that claims to disrupt cramps. I also recommend that you consult with a physical therapist, athletic trainer, or coach regarding proper stretching and training techniques. And if you are taking statins to lower cholesterol, talk with your doctor. The medication may be contributing to the problem.

RECOVERING FROM EXTENSIVE EXERCISE

When you deal with the rigors of a tough training schedule, remember that what you eat after a hard workout or competition affects your recovery. Right after exercise, the muscles easily assimilate protein (amino acids) from the blood and use it to build muscle. The muscles are also most efficient at absorbing carbohydrate from the blood to replenish depleted glycogen stores. So don't be like Kevin, a competitive triathlete who dashed from workout to work to another workout, claiming he had no time to eat a recovery meal. I told him to think again, and reminded him, "You haven't finished your training until you have refueled. If you can make time to train, you can also make time to refuel. Refueling is part of your training program."

Kevin added that he wasn't hungry and had a hard time tolerating postexercise food. I suggested he just sip on low-fat chocolate milk and nibble on pretzels within half an hour after a workout. He didn't need to consume a lot of food; as few as 100 calories can make a big difference (Flakoll et al. 2004). That snack turned on his appetite, and within an hour and a half, he was ready for a full meal.

Refueling with carbohydrate plus protein is beneficial in two ways:

1. Carbohydrate stimulates the release of insulin, a hormone that helps build muscles as well as transports carbohydrate into the muscles to replenish depleted glycogen stores.

2. Carbohydrate combined with a little protein (10 to 20 g) creates an even better response, and it reduces cortisol, a hormone that breaks down muscle. You'll more rapidly convert from a state of breaking down muscle to repairing and rebuilding muscle, thus speeding your recovery and improving your next bout of exercise.

For the serious athlete, food eaten after exercise should be selected as carefully as food eaten before exercise. By wisely choosing your foods and fluids right after you finish exercising and also throughout the day, you prepare your body the best you possibly can for the next workout. And if you can do a good job of fueling *during* your endurance workouts, you'll have less depletion from which to recover.

The key to effective recovery is to consume three times more carbohydrate (which refuels depleted glycogen stores) than protein (which rebuilds and repairs damaged muscles). That means, don't reach for just a protein shake for your recovery meal; also grab a banana and some pretzels. Or

FACT OR FICTION

You need to eat immediately after exercise to take advantage of the recovery window of opportunity.

The facts: Although depleted muscles are indeed primed to refuel most rapidly during the first 4 hours after a hard workout, the muscles continue to take up carbohydrate over the next 24 to 48 hours, but at a slower pace. If you are a recreational exerciser who works out three or four times per week, you have plenty of time to refuel your muscle glycogen stores between workouts without immediate refueling.

If you are a competitive athlete who will be doing intense training again within 24 hours, you should target 0.5 gram per pound of body weight (1 g/kg) per hour during the first 4 hours postexercise (Burke, van Loon, and Hawley 2017). For a 150-pound (68 kg) athlete, that's about 300 calories of carbohydrate per hour that you need to have readily available. Hence, if you are a soccer player at a training camp with morning and afternoon practices or an Ironman triathlete who trains twice a day, plan ahead to have high-carb recovery foods at your fingertips for easy grazing.

whip up a fruit smoothie made with Greek yogurt, berries, and banana! Or enjoy chocolate milk. You can also back your training into a mealtime and enjoy a meal such as pasta with meatballs or chicken with sweet potato. This saves calories for weight-conscious athletes who need to recover rapidly but do not want additional "recovery calories."

Recovery Fluids

After you finish a hard workout, your top dietary priority should be to replace the fluids you lost by sweating so that your body can get back into water balance. As discussed in chapter 8, if your exercise puts you at risk of becoming underhydrated, you should know your sweat rate. The goal is to drink on a schedule and lose no more than 2 percent of your body weight (e.g., 3 lb for a 150 lb, or 1.4 kg for a 68 kg, person). Ideally, you should minimize dehydration during the event—but that can be hard to do during intense exercise.

Lenny, a large, muscular man who spent two hours at the gym doing an hour of cardio and an hour of strength training was shocked to discover that he'd lost about 8 pounds (3.6 kg) during the morning sessions—5 percent of his body weight and the equivalent of a gallon (4 L) of sweat!

TABLE 10.2 Comparing Milk and Sports Drinks

Beverage (8 oz, or 240 ml)	Sodium (mg)	Potassium (mg)	Protein (g)	Carbohydrate (g)
Low-fat milk	100	400	8	12
Powerade	55	45	—	19
Chocolate milk	150	425	8	26
Water	—	—	—	—

(One pound [0.5 kg] of sweat loss represents 16 oz, or about 500 ml, of fluid.) Weighing himself made him aware of the importance of drinking more. He started bringing a gallon of water to the gym. He'd drink 1 quart (1 L) every half hour and make sure that he finished the whole gallon by the end of the workout. These steps to prevent dehydration helped him recover far more quickly—and he felt much better the rest of the day.

After a hard workout, many athletes reach for a sports drink such as Gatorade or Powerade to quench their thirst and replace sweat losses. Little do they realize that low-fat and skim milk can be effective rehydrators (Karp et al. 2006)! Yup, skim milk has electrolytes (as do all natural foods) that enhance fluid retention and restore normal fluid balance (Shirriffs, Watson, and Maughan 2007). Use sports drink *during* exercise; they are not needed afterward! Table 10.2 shows how plain and chocolate milk compare to Powerade.

The bottom line: After a hard workout, recovery foods such as chocolate milk, a bagel with peanut butter, or pasta with meat sauce offer far more electrolytes than you'll get in a sports drink.

Recovery Foods

If you will be exercising hard again in four to six hours, you should plan to eat as soon as tolerable after your first workout. The key is to plan ahead so you can easily consume a combination of carbohydrate sources to refuel depleted muscle glycogen stores and protein to repair and build muscles. Although engineered sports foods may advertise a 3-to-1 or 4-to-1 ratio of carbohydrate to protein, you need not get obsessed about the exact ratio. The idea is to eat primarily carbohydrate with 10 to 20 grams of protein as the accompaniment, depending on your body size (more precisely 0.15 g protein/lb or 0.3 g/kg of body weight). That offers plenty of protein to optimize muscle synthesis. Most hungry athletes naturally do this (if not initially, then within an hour or so) as they repeatedly seek wholesome snacks and meals—unless they are swayed by high-protein, low-carbohydrate fad diets.

If you enjoy tracking your food and want a more specific recommendation, target about 0.5 gram of carbohydrate (1 g/kg) and 0.1 to 0.15 gram of protein per pound (0.25 to 0.3 g/kg) of body weight every hour for four to six hours (ACSM 2016). Let's assume that you weigh 150 pounds (68 kg). The equation would look like this:

150 lb × 0.5 g carbohydrate
= 75 g carbohydrate = 300 cal carbohydrate

150 lb × 0.1-0.15 g protein
= 15-22 g protein, more easily 20 g protein = 80 cal protein

Following are carbohydrate–protein combinations that fit this formula:

- Three scrambled eggs and a bowl of oatmeal with maple syrup
- 16 ounces (480 ml) chocolate milk and energy bar
- Peanut butter and honey sandwich and yogurt
- Fruit smoothie (1 cup sweetened Greek yogurt with banana and berries)
- Turkey sub and grape juice

You can eat more than the calculated amount, but extra carbohydrate and protein will not hasten the recovery process. Choose foods that taste good, settle well, and help you feel better. By tracking your food intake, you can learn how close you come to meeting these recommendations. Athletes who train 10 hours a week should consume about 2.5 to 3 grams of carbohydrate per pound of body weight (5 to 7 g/kg) per day; those who train 20 hours a week need 3 to 5.5 grams of carbohydrate per pound (7 to 12 g/kg), depending on the length and intensity of the workout. (See chapter 6 and table 6.4.)

If exercise diminishes your appetite, you might find liquids more appealing than solid foods. Liquids and solid foods refuel your muscles equally well. Start off with chicken broth, ginger ale, or a fruit smoothie. But, if you are ravenous, there's little wrong with a bowl of beans and rice or a ham and cheese sub sandwich with 100 percent fruit juice.

Some exhausted athletes seek protein—hamburgers and steaks. After hours of sugary sports drinks and gels, their bodies want protein. If that's your case, enjoy the lean steak—along with a potato and rolls.

Recovery Electrolytes

When you sweat, you lose not only water but also minerals (electrolytes) such as potassium and sodium that help your body function normally. A pound (16 oz, or about 500 ml) of sweat contains 80 to 100 milligrams of potassium and 400 to 700 milligrams of sodium. Assuming that the harder you exercise, the hungrier you'll get and the more you'll eat, you'll consume more than enough electrolytes from standard postexercise foods (tables 10.3 and 10.4). You won't need salt tablets or special potassium supplements. For example, a marathoner who guzzles a liter of orange juice after completing the event replaces three times the potassium she might have lost. Munching on a bag of pretzels or sprinkling salt on a recovery meal will more than replace sodium losses.

Active people who exercise for more than four hours and athletes who sweat excessively should be sure to consume extra salt. But for the ordinary exerciser, salt depletion is unlikely, even though this electrolyte is lost the most. The concentration of sodium in your blood actually increases during exercise because you lose proportionately more water than sodium. Hence, your first need is to replace the fluid. You can replace sodium by eating salty items such as olives, pickles, crackers, or soup. And please notice (by reading food labels) that popular recovery foods such as yogurt, bagels, and spaghetti sauce have more sodium than you may realize (refer to table 10.4).

If you are tempted to replace sodium losses with commercially prepared fluid-replacement beverages such as Gatorade or Powerade, note that most of these special sports drinks are sodium poor. Commercial fluid-replacement drinks are designed to be taken *during* intense exercise. They are very dilute, which helps them empty quickly from the stomach. They are

TABLE 10.3 Potassium in Popular Recovery Foods

Food	Potassium (mg)
Potato, 1 large, baked, 10 oz (300 g)	1,650
Yogurt, low fat, 8 oz (230 g)	530
Orange juice, 8 oz (240 ml)	445
Banana, 1 medium	420
Pineapple juice, 8 oz (240 ml)	325
Raisins, 1/4 cup (40 g)	310
Beer, 12 oz (360 ml) can	90
Cran-apple juice, 8 oz (240 ml)	50
Gatorade, 8 oz (240 ml)	30
Cola, 12 oz (360 ml) can	10
Potential loss in a 2-hour workout	**300**

Data from USDA National Nutrient Database for Standard Reference.

TABLE 10.4 Sodium in Popular Recovery Foods

Food	Sodium (mg)
Chicken noodle soup, 1 can Campbell's	2,235
The Right Stuff, 1 pouch (0.7 ounce)	1,780
Macaroni and cheese, 1 box Kraft (7.25 oz, or 225 g)	1,710
Ramen noodles, Maruchan, 1 packet	1,660
Spaghetti sauce, 1 cup Prego	960
Salt, 1 small packet	590
Pretzels, 1 oz (30 g) Rold Gold thins	490
Cottage cheese, 1/2 cup	400
Bagel, 1	370
Gatorade Endurance, 8 oz (240 ml)	200
Bread, 1 slice	170
Potato chips, 15 Lay's	170
Gatorade, 12 oz (360 ml)	160
Saltine crackers, 5 (0.5 oz, or 15 g)	150
Cheerios, 1 cup multigrain	120
Wheat Thins, 8 (0.5 oz, or 15 g)	115
SaltStick Fastchews, 1	50
Coke, 12 oz (360 ml) can	45
Endurolytes, 1	40
Beer, 12 oz (360 ml) can	10-15
Potential loss in 2-hour workout	**1,000-2,000**

Note: Nutrient information from food labels.

not the best recovery foods in terms of electrolyte content, carbohydrate, and overall nutritional value unless you drink large volumes or choose the endurance formulation, such as Gatorade Endurance.

Recovery Vitamins

Many people believe that extra vitamins are needed after exhaustive exercise. To date, no research supports this belief. Vitamins are not used up during exercise; they are recycled.

Some people believe that vitamins can help repair the oxidative damage that occurs during exercise and is thought to hinder muscle repair and enhance cancer risk. Hence, they take antioxidant vitamins (C, E, beta-carotene). Large doses of these vitamins, however, can create an imbalance that hinders recovery. Your better bet is to consume colorful fruits and vegetables that offer the right balance of antioxidants. See chapter 11 for more information on vitamin supplements.

TAKING TIME TO RECOVER

Although proper nutrition can optimize recovery, even active people who eat well can become chronically fatigued for a variety of reasons, including excessive training, inadequate rest, or too little sleep. If you have a strenuous and prolonged training schedule in addition to other commitments and responsibilities, you may find yourself with too little time for proper eating, sleeping, and self-care.

Overtraining symptoms can vary. Physical symptoms include loss of appetite, weight loss (without trying), insomnia, frequent colds or respiratory infections, and muscle or joint pains that seem to have no cause. Mental symptoms included irritability and anxiety, either of which may be accompanied by depression. Unusually poor performance in training or competition and lack of improvement even when you're maintaining diligent training can also indicate overtraining. If you are experiencing two or more of these symptoms, be aware that your training could be doing more harm than good.

Rather than overtrain to the point of chronic fatigue, you should take steps to prevent it. Eat a proper sports diet that provides adequate carbohydrate and protein, allow recovery time between bouts of intense exercise, and plan your schedule so that you get enough sleep at night. Try to minimize stress in your life and curtail disruptive activities that might drain your physical and mental energy reserves.

Rest days with little or no exercise are an important part of every training program. Yet, some people feel guilty when they don't train every day. They fear becoming unfit, fat, and lazy if they miss a day of training. That scenario is unlikely. These compulsive exercisers overlook the important physiological fact that rest is essential for top performance. Rest enhances the recovery process, reduces the risk of injury, and is an investment in future performance. To replace depleted glycogen stores completely, the muscles may need up to two days of rest with no exercise and a high-carbohydrate diet. True athletes recognize that bad things happen when they train and good things happen when they rest. They plan days with no exercise! Compulsive exercisers, in comparison, push themselves relentlessly and often pay the price in poorer performance and overuse injuries.

The same athletes who avoid rest after an event also tend to overtrain while preparing for an event. Many sub-elite athletes train for two or three hours per day, thinking that such a regimen will help them improve. However, that sort of training program may hurt, not enhance, performance. Research has shown that swimmers performed just as well after one 90-minute training session per day as they did with two 90-minute sessions (Costill et al. 1991). *Quality* training is better than *quantity* training. Do not underestimate the power of rest.

CHAPTER 11

SUPPLEMENTS, PERFORMANCE ENHANCERS, AND ENGINEERED SPORTS FOODS

Once upon a time, athletes enjoyed well-balanced diets filled with natural sports foods—bananas, orange slices, yogurt, pasta, spinach, and chicken. Today, many athletes fuel themselves from a shopping basket piled with highly processed protein powders, bars, shakes, and supplements. They graze throughout the day, with little mention of enjoyable meals shared with family, friends, and teammates.

There's no denying that the sports food and supplement industry is booming. Competitors are fighting for a niche, and advertisements for their products lead us to believe that engineered nutrition is a better way to optimize health and performance. Doubtful. A review of the research mentioned in sports supplement advertisements and websites indicates that only 3 of 74 studies were judged to be high quality with low risk of bias (Heneghan et al. 2012).

Although there is a time and a place for engineered nutrition, commercial products should be used knowledgeably, at the right times, and for the right reasons. Commercial products advertise promises of enhanced performance and nutritional excellence, but please don't miss this important point: Natural foods contain components that interact in highly complex ways to synergistically benefit your overall health. Dietary supplements, in comparison, commonly contain isolated components with no synergistic effect but rather a high likelihood of being tainted with unapproved substances.

Eating food that is as close to its natural form as possible is by far the best bet for improving health, preventing disease, optimizing healing, and thus enhancing performance. Vegetables, fruits, whole grains, nuts, beans, legumes, lean meats, and low-fat dairy foods are all rich in a combination of the important vitamins, minerals, fiber, protein, fat, carbohydrate, antioxidants, and phytochemicals that athletes need daily to stay in the game. The purpose of this chapter is to help you wade through the plethora of confusing information so you understand the appropriate situations for choosing engineered sports foods, vitamin supplements, and commercial energy enhancers.

VITAMIN AND MINERAL SUPPLEMENTS

What are vitamins and minerals? Vitamins are metabolic catalysts that regulate biochemical reactions within the body; they are found in the plants you eat and are created by the plants themselves. The peak of nutrient value occurs at peak ripeness; hence, buying freshly picked local produce can offer slight nutritional benefits. Minerals are natural substances that plants must absorb from the soil. If the soil is void of the needed minerals, the plant fails to thrive or yields small fruits or vegetables that have a poor appearance.

Your body cannot manufacture vitamins (except for vitamin D, which is actually a hormone) or minerals, which is why you must obtain them through your diet. By eating a variety of wholesome foods, you can consume the proper balance of vitamins and minerals needed for optimal health and performance. To date, 14 vitamins and 15 minerals have been discovered, each with a specific function. Here are a few examples:

- Calcium maintains the rigid structure of bones.
- Sodium helps control water balance.
- Iron transports oxygen to the muscles.
- Thiamin helps convert glucose into energy.
- Vitamin D controls the way your body uses calcium.
- Vitamin A is part of an eye pigment that helps you see in dim light.

Many of my clients take vitamin supplements. They assume that active people need extra vitamins and supplements to pave the way to better health and performance. This is not the case. You can get the recommended amount of most nutrients (except possibly iron) by eating 1,500 calories of a variety of wholesome foods. This amount not only prevents nutritional deficiencies but also invests in good health. You are unlikely to live any longer if you take vitamin supplements (Macpherson, Pipingas, and Pase 2012).

Although you do need adequate vitamins and minerals to function optimally, no scientific evidence to date proves that extra vitamins and minerals offer a competitive edge. Despite claims to the contrary, vitamin supplements do not enhance performance, increase strength or endurance, provide energy, or build muscle in healthy, active people. Nor does exercise significantly increase your vitamin and mineral needs.

According to the International Olympic Committee (Maughan et al. 2018), the best way to get all the needed vitamins, minerals, and protein is to eat a variety of foods from all the food groups. Although supplements may be appropriate in certain situations, athletes should plan to maximize performance by eating quality foods. Taking a general multivitamin is unlikely to be harmful, but high doses of vitamin C, vitamin E, beta-carotene, selenium, and manganese might negatively suppress the body's immune system.

Keep in mind that the more you exercise, the more you eat. Compared with inactive people with smaller appetites, most athletes consume more calories and therefore more vitamins and minerals. Deficiencies are more likely to occur in sedentary people who eat very little, such as elderly people, than in active people who eat hefty portions.

Vitamin and mineral deficiencies do not develop overnight but over the course of months or years, as in the case of a person with anorexia or someone who eats an inadequate vegetarian diet. Your body actually stores some vitamins in stockpiles (A, D, E, and K—the fat-soluble vitamins) and others in smaller amounts (B and C—the water-soluble vitamins). Most healthy people have enough vitamin C stored in the liver to last about six weeks. One day of suboptimal eating will not result in a nutritionally depleted body.

Paul, a triathlete, had heard that exercise increases harmful free radicals (particles that can cause oxidative damage and cancer). He was told to take supplements of cancer-protective antioxidants, including vitamins C and E, beta-carotene, and selenium. Little did he realize that high doses of antioxidants can sometimes turn into pro-oxidants and blunt the training response (Maughan et al. 2018). A good reason to get antioxidants from food is that food contains them in the right amounts (as well as other nutrients the body needs).

By eating a variety of wholesome fruits, vegetables, whole grains, beans, legumes, nuts, lean meats, and low-fat dairy foods, you will consume the vitamins and minerals you need. As a bonus, many of today's foods (including energy bars and breakfast cereals) are highly fortified, so many active people actually consume far more vitamins and minerals than they realize, further negating the need to take supplemental pills. For the most part, the people who take vitamins are health conscious, eat well, and do not need supplements. Table 11.1 shows commonly eaten sources of several vitamins and minerals.

TABLE 11.1 Common Sources of Vitamins and Minerals

Vitamins or minerals	Fruits	Vegetables	Grains	Protein-rich foods	Dairy and calcium-rich alternatives
B vitamins	Oranges or orange juice	Green leafy vegetables	Whole-grain and enriched bread, cereals, pasta, rice, noodles	Meats, milk, eggs, nuts, seeds	Milk, yogurt
Vitamin C	Oranges grapefruit, strawberries, melon	Broccoli, peppers, greens, potatoes	Fortified breakfast cereal	—	—
Vitamin D	—	Mushrooms (sun exposed)	Fortified breakfast cereal	Salmon, tuna, eggs	Fortified milk, yogurt, cheese
Calcium	Fortified orange juice	Broccoli, kale, turnip greens	Chia (technically, a seed, not a grain)	Canned salmon with edible bones, calcium-processed tofu	Milk, yogurt, cheese. fortified (soy, rice, and nut) milks
Iron	Raisins, dates, figs, dried apricots, plum (prune) juice	Spinach, Swiss chard, turnip greens, collards, broccoli, brussels sprouts	Enriched bread, cereals, pasta, rice, noodles; quinoa, wheat germ	Beef, pork, chicken thighs, soy nuts, lima and kidney beans, egg yolk	—
Magnesium	Dates, figs, dried apricots, dried plums (prunes)	Spinach, broccoli, green vegetables, cocoa	Whole grains, nuts, wheat bran	Peanut butter, almonds, cashews, dried beans, lentils, edamame	—

FACT OR FICTION

Nutrition supplements are highly regulated to meet tight government standards.

The facts: Vitamin and herbal supplements abide by a set of government regulations different from those for prescription drugs and other medications. The government has very little control over their purity, potency, safety, or effectiveness, and the supplement industry can therefore hype their products with little need to prove their claims. *High potency* and *all-natural* tend to be promotional buzzwords. In 2019, the FDA announced it is implementing changes (for the first time in 25 years) to better regulate this industry so that consumers have access to safe, well-manufactured, and appropriately labeled products. That is good news!

Are Supplements Health Insurance?

Although taking a simple multivitamin is unlikely to hurt your health, does taking vitamin supplements improve your health if you already have a good diet? In a review of carefully controlled research studies on the impact of vitamin supplements on cancer, heart disease, cataracts, and age-related macular degeneration and hypertension, the U.S. National Institutes of Health concluded that "the evidence is insufficient to prove the presence or absence of benefits from use of multi-vitamin or mineral supplements to prevent cancer and chronic disease" (Huang et al. 2006, 1; National Institutes of Health 2007).

The latest results of carefully conducted clinical research suggest that most supplements, including vitamins, are not as effective as hyped. That's because much of the hype stems from observational research studies that do not show cause and effect. That is, people who take vitamin supplements tend to be health conscious in the first place. So when you hear that people who take vitamin E pills have less heart disease, you need to wonder whether those people were compared against (less-health-conscious) people who chose to not take vitamin E, or against randomly chosen people.

The American Cancer Society recommends getting vitamins from a healthy diet, and if you choose to take a supplement, take one with 100 percent of the daily value (DV) but not more. Taking a large dose of a single vitamin might upset nature's balance because vitamins work synergistically.

Antioxidants (vitamins A, E, and C, and beta-carotene) have shown potential harm for athletes and no benefits. For example, a review of multiple studies shows that more than 1,000 milligrams of vitamin C might hinder athletic performance (Braakhuis 2012). The consensus is that daily high-dose antioxidant vitamin supplementation is unlikely to be of real practical benefit (Davison, Gleeson, and Phillips 2007).

Taking a multivitamin and mineral supplement does not compensate for a high-fat, low-fiber, nutrient-poor diet. Nor should it allow you to rationalize eating suboptimally because you are overconfident about your vitamin intake. A vitamin pill at breakfast does not compensate for a potato chip lunch. The information in chapters 1 and 2 can help you make smart food choices that provide the nutrients you need. If you choose to take a vitamin supplement, look first at your daily diet to see whether you are already consuming these vitamins through fortified foods such as breakfast cereals.

Dietary Reference Intakes (DRI)

To help you determine whether you are getting the right balance of nutrients, the U.S. government has established dietary reference intakes (DRI). The recommendations for vitamins and minerals exceed the average nutrition requirements of nearly all people, including athletes. The DRIs are divided into the following subgroupings:

- Recommended dietary allowance (RDA) is the amount per day that should decrease the risk of chronic disease.
- Adequate intake (AI) is used when an RDA cannot be determined for a particular nutrient.
- Tolerable upper intake level (UL) is the highest daily level of a nutrient that is likely to pose no health risks. Above the UL, there is potential for increased risk.

Another measurement of intake you've likely seen is the daily value (DV), which is a compilation of DRIs used for food labels. The DV is intended to provide a perspective on overall dietary needs. Table 11.2 lays out the DRIs for several vitamins and minerals.

TABLE 11.2 Vitamin and Mineral DRIs

| Nutrient | Daily value (on food labels, as of January 2020) | Recommended dietary allowance (RDA) or adequate intake (AI) | | Tolerable upper intake level (UL) |
		Women	Men	Women and men
Biotin		10	10	ND
Calcium (mg/day)	1,300	1,000	1,000	2,500
		1,200 (>age 50)	1,200	

Nutrient	Daily value (on food labels, as of January 2020)	Recommended dietary allowance (RDA) or adequate intake (AI)		Tolerable upper intake level (UL)
		Women	Men	Women and men
Folate (mcg Dietary Folate Equivalents/day)	400	400 600 (if pregnant)	400	1,000
Niacin (mg/day)	20	14	16	35
Riboflavin (mg/day)	1.7	1.1	1.3	ND
Thiamin (mg/day)	1.5	1.1	1.2	ND
Iron (mg/day)	18	18 8 (postmenopause) 27 (pregnant)	8	45*
Vitamin A (IU/day)		2,333	3,000	10,000
Vitamin A** (mcg RAE)	900	700	900	3,000
Vitamin B$_6$ (mg/day)	2	1.3 1.5 (>age 50)	1.3 1.7	100
Vitamin B$_{12}$ (mcg/day)	6	2.4	2.4	ND
Vitamin C (mg/day)	90	75	90	2,000
Vitamin D (IU/day)	20 mcg	600 (<age 50) 600 (ages 50-70) 800 (>age 70)	600 600 800	4,000
Vitamin E (mg alpha-tocopherol/day)	15	15	15	1,000
Vitamin K (mcg/day)	120	90	120	ND
Zinc (mg/day)	15	8	11	40

Note: ND = not determined.

*The upper limit does not apply to people who are taking an iron supplement as a short-term medical treatment for iron-deficiency anemia.

**Starting in 2020, vitamin A will be reported as retinol activity equivalents (RAE) to account for the different types and bioavailability of carotenes (dietary sources of vitamin A) that the body converts into retinol.

Sources: Food and Nutrition Board, Institute of Medicine, 2011, Dietary Reference Intakes (DRIs): Recommended dietary allowances and adequate intakes. [Online]. Available: http://iom.edu/Activities/Nutrition/SummaryDRIs/~/media/Files/Activity%20Files/Nutrition/DRIs/RDA%20and%20AIs_Vitamin%20and%20Elements.pdf [May 21, 2013].

Vitamin A Fact Sheet for Professionals, Office of Dietary Supplements, National Institutes of Health. Available: https://ods.od.nih.gov/factsheets/VitaminA-HealthProfessional

https://blog.watson-inc.com/nutri-knowledge/daily-values-and-unit-changes-on-the-new-nutrition-facts-label

Supplementing in Special Situations

Taking a simple multivitamin and mineral pill can be a good idea for certain people who are at risk of developing nutrition deficiencies. You should indeed consider taking a multivitamin and mineral pill if you fall into any of the following categories:

- **Restricting calories.** Dieters who eat less than 1,200 calories daily may miss some important nutrients.

- **Allergic to certain foods.** People who can't eat certain types of foods, such as fruits or wheat, may need to compensate with alternative vitamin sources to avoid deficiencies in some nutrients.

- **Lactose intolerant.** The inability to digest the milk sugar found in dairy products is a common occurrence among African American and Hispanic people. Avoiding dairy foods can result in a diet deficient in riboflavin, vitamin D, and the mineral calcium.

- **A traveling athlete.** If you will be spending extended periods of time in countries with limited food supplies, or will be doing extensive travel that is likely to dismantle your healthy eating program, you might want to take a multivitamin along for nutritional health insurance.

- **Contemplating pregnancy.** To help prevent certain types of birth defects, women who are thinking about becoming pregnant should be sure to consume a diet rich in folate, and they should take a multivitamin with 400 micrograms of folic acid (the form of folate in supplements).

- **Pregnant.** Expectant mothers require additional vitamins and iron, but they should consult with their physicians before taking supplements. See chapter 12 for more about athletes and pregnancy.

- **Vegan.** People who abstain from eating any animal foods may become deficient in vitamin B_{12}, vitamin D, and riboflavin. Those who eat a poorly balanced vegetarian diet can also become deficient in protein, calcium, iron, and zinc.

- **Elderly.** Poor nutrition is common among frail, elderly people who take in few calories. The fewer the calories, the higher the risk of vitamin and mineral deficiencies.

- **An indoor athlete.** If you spend little time in the sun or consistently use sunscreen when you are outdoors, you might be short on vitamin D, the so-called sunshine vitamin. The sun's ultraviolet rays activate the precursor to vitamin D when the rays shine on the skin. Milk fortified with vitamin D is among the best sources of this vitamin. If you cannot or will not drink milk, taking a calcium pill with vitamin

Vitamin D

Vitamin D helps the body absorb calcium from the intestines; that's why it's important for bone health. Vitamin D may also be involved in immune function, muscle function, recovery from damaging exercise, diabetes, and certain cancers. More research is needed to determine whether vitamin D directly enhances muscle strength and athletic performance (Owens, Allison, and Close 2018).

Indoor athletes (gymnasts, dancers, wrestlers, swimmers, skaters, gym rats) who rarely see the light of day can easily get insufficient vitamin D. Your doctor can order a blood test to determine your vitamin D status and whether or not you should take a supplement. Blood levels less than 30 ng/mL of the form of vitamin D called 25(OH)D are considered deficient; greater than 50 ng/mL are desirable (Owens, Allison, and Close 2018).

Enjoying 15 to 20 minutes of sunshine without sunscreen a few times a week can increase vitamin D levels without increasing the risk of skin cancer. If you live north of Atlanta, Georgia, (more specifically, at a latitude 37 degrees north or south of the equator), vitamin D_3 supplements during the winter months can be a wise choice if your diet contains too little vitamin D (table 11.3) to prevent a decline. At these latitudes, the sun's rays are not strong enough to convert the body's precursor of D into the active form of the vitamin during the winter months.

The current recommended dietary allowance (RDA) for vitamin D is 600 international units (IU). A light-skinned person can make 20,000 to 30,000 IU of vitamin D in 30 minutes of sunbathing with no sunscreen (CSPIa 2006); dark-skinned people make less. Most daily multivitamin pills offer 400 IU; calcium pills offer 200 to 400 IU. When reading the supplement label, note that D_3 (cholecalciferol) is preferable and more potent than D_2 (ergocalciferol).

Whether or not a supplement will offer benefits is yet to be firmly agreed on, Researchers are questioning whether supplements of D (with or without calcium) are proving to be as valuable as touted. Studies show no reduction in bone breaks or hip fractures in older adults without osteoporosis (Kahwati et al. 2018). Yet, the risk of harm is low, so if you rarely see the light of day, plan to increase your intake of vitamin D by consuming the foods in table 11.3, and if a blood test indicates insufficiency, to take a supplement containing 2,000 to 4,000 IU.

(continued)

Vitamin D (continued)

TABLE 11.3 Good Sources of Vitamin D in Foods

Food sources	Vitamin D (IU)
Salmon, pink, 3 oz (90 g) canned	470
Portobello mushroom, 3 oz (90 g) UV-light exposed	375
Shrimp, 4 oz (120 g) raw	175
Tuna, light, 3 oz (90 g)	154
Milk, 8 oz (240 ml)	115-125
Orange juice, fortified, 8 oz (240 ml)	100-130
Soy milk, fortified, 8 oz (240 ml)	80-120
Yogurt, fortified, 6-8 oz (175-230 g)	80
Cereal, fortified (10% DV), 1 oz (30 g)	40
Egg, 1 large	40

National Institutes of Health Office of Dietary Supplements, http://ods.od.nih.gov; USDA National Nutrient Database for Standard Reference, www.ars.usda.gov.

D_3 might be a smart idea, as well as spending 15 minutes of regular activity in the sunshine without sunscreen. Consume mushrooms that have been exposed to ultraviolet light, which causes them to make vitamin D. Look for "UV-treated" or "high in vitamin D" on the label.

Deciding Whether to Supplement

Confused? If you are taking supplements and are not knowledgeable about vitamins or minerals, I recommend that you consult with a registered dietitian (RD), preferably an RD, CSSD (board-certified specialist in sports dietetics). This nutrition professional will be able to evaluate your diet and tell you not only what nutrients you are missing but also how to choose foods that offer what you need. To find a sports RD, use the referral network at the website of the Sports, Cardiovascular and Wellness Nutrition (SCAN) Dietary Practice Group of the Academy of Nutrition and Dietetics, www.SCANdpg.org, and see the Dietitian section in appendix A for other resources.

If you fall into one of the categories of people who can benefit from a supplement, here are guidelines that can help you zero in on the best practices:

- Choose a supplement with the vitamins and minerals close to 100 percent of the daily values (DV). More is not better.
- Don't expect to find 100 percent of the DV for calcium and magnesium listed on a label; these minerals are too bulky to put in one pill.
- Don't buy supplements that contain excessive doses of minerals. A high dose of one mineral can offset the benefits of another. For example, too much zinc can interfere with the absorption of copper. In the Iowa Women's Health study, long-term iron supplementation was associated with an increased risk of death (Mursu et al. 2011).
- Buy and use a supplement before its expiration date. Store it in a cool, dry place.
- Ignore claims about natural vitamins; they tend to be blends of natural and synthetic vitamins and offer no benefits. Vitamin E is more potent in its natural form, but the difference is inconsequential.
- Chelated supplements offer no advantages, and neither do those made without sugar or starch or those with the highest price tag.
- Look for USP on the label. This indicates that the manufacturer followed standards established by the U.S. Pharmacopeia.
- Choose nationally known brands; this may improve the likelihood of actually getting what you believe you are buying.
- To optimize absorption, take a supplement with or after a meal.

Above all, think food first. As I have said before, and will say again, no vitamin pill will compensate for hit-or-miss eating. If you eat wisely and well, you can get the nutrients you need from the foods you enjoy. Your overall dietary pattern is what's health protective, not isolated vitamins. Your best bet is to get your vitamins by eating a variety of foods.

PERFORMANCE-ENHANCING SUPPLEMENTS

Just as whole grains, fruits, vegetables, lean protein, and low-fat dairy foods can provide the vitamins and minerals you need for optimal health, they can also supply the protein you need to build muscles, and the carbohydrate and healthy fat to fuel top performance. Yet, many athletes fail to fuel properly; they look for a quick fix from supplements, pills, and potions.

One of my clients, an aspiring baseball pitcher, skipped breakfast, failed to properly fuel himself before and after exercise, and then gobbled late-night fried rice and egg rolls from a Chinese restaurant. He came to me with abundant questions about supplements, asking about muscle builders, energy boosters, immune system enhancers, and bone and joint protectors. I reminded him that no supplement, no matter how expensive it is, can compensate for a lousy diet. We talked about how many of the popular performance enhancers have been overrated. Some make false claims; others fail to list the "magic" (i.e., illegal) ingredients on the label. (And no government agency has been watching very carefully.)

Some supplements might even be contaminated. If you are a serious athlete who undergoes drug testing, be aware that contaminated nutritional supplements have caused athletes to fail drug tests (Mathews 2018). See the Supplements section in appendix A for a list of websites you can visit for more in-depth information and cutting-edge research.

Supplements with *strong* evidence of improving performance include caffeine, creatine, sodium bicarbonate, beta-alanine, and nitrate (ACSM 2016). Many other supplements offer glimmers of hope, but currently lack the evidence needed to support their claims. With new research and new products appearing weekly, you need to do your own research and draw your own conclusions about products you might read about on the Internet or in muscle magazines. Again, please refer to the Supplements section in appendix A for the latest information.

Whatever you do, remember that no supplement will compensate for a suboptimal sports diet. Be responsible, take mealtimes as seriously as you take your training, and observe the power of good nutrition. And, as exercise physiologist Ron Maughan, PhD, reminds us, some supplements might work for some athletes some of the time, but no supplement works for all athletes all of the time. Very little research on supplements offers definitive evidence, in part because the research is rarely done on elite athletes under real-life conditions. *Real life* includes 1) multiday tournaments, competitions, or events, 2) "stacking" supplements (such as mixing caffeine and nitrates), and 3) determining whether an elite athlete responds the same way to a supplement as does a recreational athlete.

Real life also includes your genetics and unique microbiome (the bacteria in your gut that influence your overall health and well-being). We do not yet know how much a microbiome, which varies 80 to 90 percent between individuals, influences the effectiveness of a sports supplement and contributes to different responses (Maughan et al. 2018).

Muscle Builders

The best muscle builder is resistance exercise that fatigues your muscles. While you may think that the guys at the gym are hulks because of pills and potions, they actually work out very intensely. That hard work lays the true foundation for building muscle mass.

Creatine is a naturally occurring compound found in muscles (meat) and may assist the ability to perform high intensity weight lifting. Creatine is an important source of fuel for sprints and bouts of high-intensity exercise lasting up to 10 seconds. This includes weightlifting; interval or sprint training with repeated short bouts of explosive efforts; and team or racket sports with intermittent work patterns, such as soccer, football, basketball, tennis, and squash. Creatine might reduce the severity of, or enhance the recovery from, mild traumatic brain injury, although more research is needed to verify this hypothesis (Dolan, Gualano, and Rawson 2018). Athletes recovering from broken bones may find that creatine helps rebuild muscle after the cast is removed. The typical diet of meat eaters contains about 2 grams of creatine per day; vegetarians have lower body stores of creatine.

Many athletes who take creatine report increases in lean body mass, perhaps because they are better able to recover during strength training; this allows more weightlifting repetitions. A study of 31 experienced bodybuilders who took a protein–carbohydrate supplement with or without creatine at midmorning, after their afternoon workouts, and before bed (for a total of about 450 calories) suggests that the protein–carbohydrate–creatine group gained more muscle mass and strength than did those who consumed just protein and carbohydrate (Cribb, Williams, and Hayes 2007).

Not all athletes experience enhanced performance with creatine, however. In a study of 11 healthy men, 3 had a strong response, 5 a moderate response, and 3 were classified as nonresponders (Syrotuik and Bell 2004).

In research studies, the subjects commonly "load" by taking 20 grams of creatine (more precisely, 0.15 g creatine monohydrate/lb [0.3 g/kg], in four doses of 5 g each) for five to seven days, and then take a daily maintenance dose of 3 grams per day (Maughan et al. 2018). Taking creatine with a meal is more effective than taking it on an empty stomach. Creatine holds water, so loading the body with creatine results in gaining water weight. This added weight might be counterproductive for weight-conscious athletes, such as sprinters.

Most health professionals agree that only fully developed athletes should take creatine. Young athletes need to learn to improve performance by training hard and developing sports skills. Although creatine is unlikely to cause medical problems, taking it might encourage athletes to develop a desire to look for shortcuts to success.

While creatine has been the front-runner in terms of supplements that enhance muscle growth, leucine and beta-hydroxy beta-methylbutyrate (HMB) have shown promise in promoting muscle health. The essential amino acid leucine acts as a metabolic trigger to stimulate muscle growth. HMB is a by-product of leucine metabolism. In chronically ill, hospitalized patients, HMB helps prevent muscle wasting. In athletes, HMB may reduce

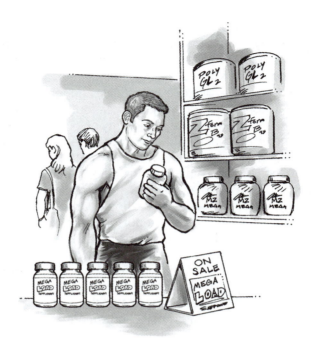

muscle protein breakdown and improve recovery (Wilson et al. 2013). Yet, performance studies suggest that HMB does not enhance muscular growth or strength in young men (Teixeira 2019).

Athletes who consume animal sources of protein get plenty of leucine in their daily diets and have no need to take leucine supplements. Vegan weightlifters, however, have to plan their diets carefully to ensure adequate intakes throughout the day of protein in the form of soy, seeds, nuts, and beans if they want to optimize the response from their programs. Although a 6-ounce (180 g) serving of beef contains about 5 grams of leucine, a cup of edamame (soybeans) offers only 1.6 grams of leucine and a cup of lentils, only 1.3 grams.

Whatever you do, stay away from muscle-building products that contain testosterone, prohormones, "natural steroids," or hormone boosters. You have no idea what is actually in them. The chances are good they contain illegal substances that have not been tested in humans for liver toxicity or harm to the heart (see appendix A, Supplement Safety). Young athletes who take hormones could experience the undesired consequence of stunted growth caused by premature closure of their growth plates (Mathews 2018). That's the opposite of what they want. See chapter 15 for information on how to add bulk healthfully.

If you are an athlete with low testosterone levels, you may be undereating. Just as female athletes experience reduced estrogen when they undereat, men experience low testosterone levels. The solution is to improve your sports diet, not look for a supplement (Mountjoy et al. 2014).

Endurance Enhancers

The best endurance exercise enhancers are carbohydrates consumed as the foundation of each meal and snack, as well as before and during exercise. Food provides the energy you need to exercise longer and harder. Once you have optimized your diet, you can try a few frills such as beetroot juice or beta-alanine to determine the costs and benefits of using such supplements. Highly competitive athletes should plan to experiment with ergogenic aids such as caffeine and beetroot juice during at least four long training sessions that mimic the demands of the competitive event.

Studies suggest that dietary nitrate can improve performance in events that last 12 to 40 minutes by 1 to 3 percent, and with long, slow exercise it can improve time to exhaustion by 4 to 25 percent (Maughan et al. 2018). Strong sources of dietary nitrates are leafy greens (Chinese napa cabbage, spinach, bok choy, arugula) and beets (also called beetroots in the United Kingdom). Dietary nitrate stimulates the production of nitric oxide. Nitric oxide regulates blood flow and oxygen consumption. For the same amount of oxygen uptake, athletes with higher levels of nitric oxide can work harder.

A typical protocol is to consume 300 to 550 milligrams of nitrate (2.5 ounces [75 ml] of concentrated beetroot juice shots, or 7 ounces [200 g] of baked beets or other nitrate-rich sources) two to three hours before an event. That's when nitric oxide peaks; it remains elevated for another six to nine hours before declining toward baseline by 12 hours (Jones, Bailey, and Vanhatalo 2013). The key is to experiment with this during training to be sure your digestive tract can handle this unusual preevent food! Better yet, routinely fuel your body with nitrate-rich fruits and vegetables. This is a positive dietary strategy, particularly for elite-level athletes who seem to have a harder time getting performance gains from a single dose of preevent nitrates (Maughan et al. 2018).

The effects of nitric oxide may be particularly beneficial not only to athletes who train and compete at altitude (such as skiers or mountaineers) because it helps reduce oxygen needs but also helps people with lung disease, impaired circulation, and cardiovascular problems. For example, some people with peripheral artery disease (PAD) who consume beetroot juice can exercise longer before being stopped by pain. For beet lovers with PAD, this is an easy way to improve exercise tolerance and quality of life. Nitrates can also help lower blood pressure, which can reduce the risk for stroke.

Beta-alanine, another performance enhancer, is an amino acid that helps take the "burn" and fatigue out of high-intensity exercise that lasts 30 seconds to 10 minutes. When taken daily for 10 to 12 weeks, beta-alanine can buffer the acid that builds up in muscles. This can contribute to small but meaningful performance benefits of 0.2 to 3 percent—enough to win! Athletes who might benefit from beta-alanine include rowers, swimmers, and sprinters who perform sustained high-intensity exercise for one to seven minutes; sprinters, weightlifters, and other athletes who perform repeated bouts of high-intensity work; soccer, ice hockey, and other athletes who play stop-and-start sports; and marathoners, bike racers, and other athletes who sprint at the end of endurance events. Some athletes who take high doses (more than 800 milligrams) of beta-alanine experience flushing and "beta-tingles"—a tingling sensation in the skin that can range from mild to intolerable; it can be abated by taking sustained-release supplements (Artioli et al. 2010). Beta-alanine can be used in addition to, or instead of, sodium bicarbonate, another buffering agent.

Sodium bicarbonate is known to buffer the lactic acid that accumulates in the blood and can improve performance in high-intensity exercise that lasts 60 to 180 seconds. The known problem with sodium bicarbonate is it creates gastrointestinal distress. The preferred way to take sodium bicarbonate is through capsules (from the pharmacy) and with a small meal to lessen the nausea and diarrhea.

Lastly, caffeine is a known ergogenic aid that increases alertness, decreases reaction time, and makes effort seem easier. Many athletes enjoy a caffeine boost before, during, and after exercise. For more information on caffeine, see chapters 3 and 9 and appendix A.

Immunity Boosters

To fully function as an athlete, you need to stay healthy. That's where a strong immune system is helpful, and you want to support your immune system by eating well every day. Immune system enhancers are found in a variety of foods, including apples, oats, broccoli, tea, spices . . . the list goes on! Taking extra nutrients will not boost your immune response above normal levels, but if you are training rigorously, you can help maintain immune function, for example, by consuming carbohydrate before, during, and after exercise. You can also eat an anti-inflammatory Mediterranean-style diet, which focuses on fruits, vegetables, seafood, and olive oil.

People who have low immunity tend to be people who eat very little and are rapidly losing body weight—a syndrome more commonly seen in frail elderly people and those experiencing a famine than in robust athletes (unless they are in severe calorie deficit). For people with HIV/AIDS, infections, and failing health, "immuno-nutrition" is being intensely researched. But whether the findings will translate to enhanced recovery for athletes is yet to be determined. Until then, optimize your immune system by avoiding overtraining, eating adequate carbohydrate, and sleeping well. The following is a list of a few immunity boosters popular among athletes that certainly will not hurt you.

• **Carbohydrate.** Consuming carbohydrate before, during, and after exercise lowers stress hormones and is the best way for athletes to enhance immune function. Being adequately fueled with a steady stream of carbohydrate defends against the stress response. See chapters 9 and 10 for information about proper fueling tactics.

• **Echinacea.** An herbal remedy, echinacea supposedly prevents or shortens the duration of colds. Well-controlled studies question the effect of echinacea on rates of infection or the severity of cold symptoms (Karsch-Volk, Barrett, and Linde 2015).

• **Glutamine.** Glutamine is an amino acid that is an important source of fuel for immune cells. It is involved in healing wounds, boosting the immune system, fighting infection, and decreasing illness. During physical stress (cancer, surgery), glutamine levels drop. Glutamine supplements have been used with success in very sick patients with HIV/AIDS and cancer, but research into whether glutamine supplements can help healthy athletes when they are intensely training has been weak and inconclusive. Most protein-rich foods are rich in glutamine, including beef, chicken, fish, beans, whey, and dairy.

• **Vitamin C.** An antioxidant, vitamin C is abundant in fruits and vegetables. It is involved in boosting the immune response and reducing the potential cellular damage caused by free radicals. Overtraining and taking part in prolonged exercise can lower your immune response, but don't count on vitamin C to reduce your risk of catching a cold (Hemila and Chalker 2013). If you insist on taking vitamin C, 500 milligrams is more than enough.

• **Vitamin E.** While vitamin E might have an immune-enhancing effect in the frail elderly, no benefit has been seen in healthy athletes. In fact, vitamin E can become a potentially performance-eroding pro-oxidant (Ristow et al. 2009). If you choose to take vitamin E, do so in moderation; 500 IU is more than enough. See chapter 10 for more information.

• **Probiotics.** Probiotic are living microorganisms that can increase the gut's health-enhancing bacteria. For athletes, more research is needed to determine whether taking probiotic supplements might decrease the risk of catching a cold or combat diarrhea related to exercise or travel (Pyne et al. 2015). Until we know how to assess an individual athlete's microbiome, the specific probiotics that might offer the best benefits, how much to supplement, and at what times to do so, your best bet is to regularly consume probiotics in the form of yogurt, kefir, kombucha, and other fermented foods. Also enjoy plenty of whole grains, fruits, and vegetables; their fiber feeds gut microbes, which in turn boosts your immune system.

Bone and Joint Protectors

Runners, basketball players, baseball catchers, and others who put undue stress on their bodies often worry about their aching joints. Can they take anything to invest in bone and joint health? Here are two popular (but unproven) options:

1. **Chondroitin and glucosamine.** Touted to improve joint health and reduce the pain of osteoarthritis, masters athletes often take these two compounds together in hopes of preventing cartilage damage. Chondroitin is believed to give cartilage elasticity by helping it retain water. Glucosamine claims to help maintain and regenerate healthy cartilage in joints. While prescription formulations of a patented crystalline glucosamine sulfate and chondroitin sulfate may help enough to delay total joint replacement surgery (Brevere 2016), the general consensus is that most formulations provide little or no benefit (Liu et al. 2018).

2. **Gelatin (collagen) and vitamin C.** Collagen is the primary structural protein in tendons, ligaments, and cartilage. Gelatin contains amino acids similar to those found in the collagen in those tissues. Will consuming preexercise gelatin along with vitamin C reduce the risk of sprains, strains, rupture, or breaks in those tissues? Some studies suggest it might help strengthen those connective tissues (Shaw et al. 2017). Stay tuned!

COMMERCIAL SPORTS FOODS AND FLUIDS

The sports fuel industry has rapidly grown, starting in the 1970s with the introduction of Gatorade, continuing into the 1980s with the debut of PowerBar, expanding in the 1990s with gels such as Gu, and overwhelming athletes in the 2000s with an array of products. Multitudes of companies have jumped on the bandwagon to create niche fuels for every possible dietary need—gluten free, vegan, kosher, lactose free, fructose free, you name it—and every possible time to eat (before, during, and after exercise).

If you feel confused and overwhelmed by the wide selection of commercial sports fuels to choose from, you are not alone. Athletes and casual exercisers alike inevitably ask me, "What's the best energy bar? Gel? Sports drink?" Some are worried about consuming the best ratio of carbohydrate to protein. The simple answer is that you need to learn which products are best for *your* body by experimenting with them during training. The best choice for one person may be nauseating for another.

In general, commercial sports foods tend to be more about convenience than necessity. They can make fueling easier, take away the guesswork, and offer more benefits than you'd get from drinking plain water. But if you are on a budget, take note: A daily bottle of postexercise sports drink at $1.59 adds up to about $50 a month for sugar water. The homemade sports drink recipe in chapter 25 can save you a bundle of money!

Certainly, there is a time and place for engineered sports fuels, particularly if you are a high-level endurance cyclist, marathoner, triathlete, or adventure athlete who exercises intensely or is limited by a sensitive intestinal tract. But all active people should maintain a foundation of wholesome foods in their day-to-day diets, with engineered choices used just to support their exercise programs. In other words, don't have a sports drink at lunch (instead of orange juice) or eat Jelly Belly Sport Beans (instead of fruit) for an afternoon snack. Be sure you toss a few apple cores and banana peels into the compost bin instead of throwing engineered energy bar wrappers in the trash. (When making your food choices, please consider the negative environmental impact of plastic sports drink bottles, gel packets, and sports food wrappers.)

Many athletes are easily swayed by advertisements to take their sports diet "to the next level" with commercial products. Engineered foods, supplements, and energy boosters seem to offer the magic solution when life is too busy, performance is lagging, meals are hit or miss, and sleep is inadequate. But some of these products offer nutrients in an unnatural balance that will hinder performance. For example, we know that athletes can absorb more carbohydrate when it comes from a variety of sources, not just one source, such as a commercial sports drink might offer (Jentjens et al. 2006; Wallis et al. 2005). We know that fat is important for refueling the intramuscular fat stores that are depleted during endurance exercise (van Loon et al. 2003), but many commercial products offer carbohydrate and protein but no fat. We need more research to prove that natural foods do as good a job as engineered products, if not better. The problem is research comparing the benefits of, let's say, a peanut butter sandwich over sports candy would be very expensive. The peanut butter industry would need to decide whether such a research project would improve its profits.

CHAPTER 12

NUTRITION AND ACTIVE WOMEN

Whether you are a teenage girl wanting to excel in high school sports, a female runner contemplating pregnancy, or a masters runner in menopause, you likely have female-specific nutrition questions. This chapter addresses some of the nutrition-related issues confronted by active women throughout the life cycle.

NUTRITION AND LOSS OF THE MENSTRUAL PERIOD

Women who exercise a lot and eat too little can stop menstruating (a condition known as amenorrhea). Although you may believe that amenorrhea is desirable because you no longer have to deal with the hassles of monthly menstrual periods, amenorrhea can lead to problems that interfere with your health and ability to perform your best, such as the following:

- A four-times-higher incidence of stress fractures that put you on the sidelines (Nattiv 2000)
- Premature osteoporosis that can affect your bone health in the not-too-distant future
- An inability to conceive easily either now or in the future (after you have resumed menses) should you want to start a family

Amenorrhea can happen, for example, when you step up your exercise program without boosting your calorie intake. If this happens, don't ignore it! You may be experiencing what once was called the female athlete triad (disordered eating, amenorrhea, and low bone mineral density) but now is called relative energy deficiency in sports (RED-S) (Mountjoy et al. 2014) because this is not just a female issue. Male athletes also undereat

(Teneforde et al. 2016). RED-S refers to impaired physiological function that includes (but is not limited to) these health issues that range in severity:

- Inadequate energy intake (due to "no time to eat," strict dieting, or an outright eating disorder)
- Irregular or nonexistent menstrual periods (or loss of libido in males)
- Stress fractures and weakened bones (resulting in early osteoporosis)
- Reduced metabolic rate (eating less than peers, without weight loss)
- Decreased glycogen stores (reduced stamina and endurance)
- Decreased muscle strength (loss of power)
- Depression, irritability (reduced quality of life)

Amenorrhea commonly happens in women with eating disorders or disordered eating, but it also occurs in busy students and working women who just don't take the time to eat enough.

To be able to menstruate, your body requires at least 13.5 calories per pound (30 cal/kg) of lean body mass (weight without any body fat). By comparison, the average (nonathletic) woman maintains energy balance at about 20.5 calories per pound (45 cal/kg) of lean body mass (Mountjoy et al. 2014).

An athletic woman who weighs 120 pounds (54 kg) and has 20 percent body fat, for example, has a lean body mass (LBM) of 96 pounds (44 kg) (20% × 120 lb = 24 lb [11 kg] fat, which means that she has 96 lb [44 kg] LBM). She needs to eat at least 1,300 calories (13.5 cal/lb × 96 lb LBM = 1,300 cal) that are not burned off, that are "available energy." If she burns 500 calories in exercise, she needs to consume at least 1,300 + 500 = 1,800 calories for her body to function normally (i.e., menstruate); this is still far too little to fully fuel her muscles and allow her to enjoy optimal performance.

Many amenorrheic athletes have been advised to take the birth control pill to resume menses, and theoretically, this would help prevent bone loss. Current research does not support that theory (Gordon et al. 2017;

FACT OR FICTION

Exercising too much causes amenorrhea.

The facts: Amenorrhea is most commonly caused by eating too little food, not by exercising too much. Most athletic women do have regular menstrual periods. They eat enough calories to support both their exercise programs and their bodies' ability to reproduce.

Mountjoy et al. 2014). Eating enough food to negate an "energy drain" and rebuild muscles is the key to reversing bone loss. Adequate food includes adequate carbohydrate to replace depleted glycogen stores, adequate protein to build muscles that tug on bones and improve bone strength, adequate fat to maintain hormonal balance, and enough fuel to maintain energy balance.

Eating more food, for some women, is easier said than done—particularly if they are struggling with an eating disorder. If the thought of adding more fuel to your sports diet creates panic, you might want to seek help from a registered dietitian (RD) who specializes in sports nutrition. To find someone local, use the referral network at www.scandpg.org. The following tips may also be of help:

• **Practice eating as you did when you were a child.** Focus on eating when you are hungry and stopping when you are content. If you are always hungry and constantly obsessing about food, you are undoubtedly eating too little food. Your body is complaining and requesting more fuel. You likely need 300 to 600 additional calories a day (Mountjoy et al. 2014). Remember: Hunger is simply a request for fuel. The information in chapter 16, plus advice from your doctor and dietitian, can help you determine an appropriate energy intake.

• **Eat on a regular schedule.** Amenorrheic women commonly follow nontraditional, chaotic eating patterns. They may eat little at breakfast and lunch, only to overeat at night, or they restrict themselves on Monday through Thursday and then overeat on the weekends. If your weight is stable, you are somehow consuming the number of calories you need, so you might as well eat them on a regular schedule of wholesome, well-balanced meals, not going longer than three to five hours (or whenever you first feel hunger) without fuel. Again, please seek meal-planning help from a registered dietitian instead of struggling on your own.

• **Eat adequate protein.** Vegetarians, in particular, need to be sure to consume adequate protein to minimize muscle wasting that occurs when a person undereats. Protein needs increase when calorie intake decreases. See chapter 7 for specific protein guidelines.

• **Eat at least 20 percent of your calories from fat.** Some fat is absolutely essential for your health and well-being. Skip the fat-free products! Your body needs fat to build healthy cell membranes and to make hormone-like substances called prostaglandins. You should boost your intake of good fat and carefully balance the saturated ("bad") fat in red meat and other fatty animal proteins. For most active women, eating 40 to 60 grams of fat per day would be a low-fat diet. This plan clearly allows salmon, peanut and other nut butters, avocado, almonds, walnuts, pumpkin seeds, olive oil, and other health-promoting fats, as well as smaller amounts of saturated fat as found in lean beef, low-fat cheese, and other nourishing foods that provide balance to a sports diet. If you just cannot bring yourself to add nut butter to toast or oil to salads, then do the following:

- Sprinkle sunflower seeds or slivered almonds on salads.
- Enjoy trail mix with nuts and raisins for snacks.
- Eat fish rich in omega-3 fat (salmon, tuna) twice a week.
- Use olive or canola oil for cooking.

• **Maintain a calcium-rich diet.** Bones benefit from the strengthening effect of exercise, but exercise does not compensate for lack of calcium, particularly when calorie and vitamin D intake is inadequate. Plus, the bones of athletes with amenorrhea respond less to the bone-building effects of exercise. Your low levels of estrogen reduce the uptake of calcium from the blood and deposition into your bones, and this heightens your risk of stress fractures (Mountjoy et al. 2014).

You should invest in bone (and muscle) health by boosting your energy intake; low energy availability is associated with poor bone health. A wise way to consume more calories is by including a serving of calcium-rich (and protein-rich) dairy or soy milk or yogurt with each meal and snack to reach a total of 1,500 milligrams per day of calcium. (Dietary sources of calcium are preferred to supplements, but any calcium is better than no calcium.) Also take vitamin D if your blood levels are low.

Refrain from almond or plant-based "milks" that lack protein and are more like juice. (See chapter 1 for more information about calcium and dairy alternatives.) Also, if you are eating a diet that includes lots of bran cereal, fruits, and vegetables, you may have an even higher need for calcium because the fiber may interfere with calcium absorption. You have no need for more than 35 grams of fiber per day!

Many amenorrheic women worry about their bone health, and rightfully so. If the amenorrhea is associated with anorexia, you might be losing bone density at the rate of 2.5 percent a year (Miller et al. 2006). Multiply that by several years, and it's no wonder many of my 20- to 30-year-old clients have bones similar to those of 70-year-old women and problems with stress fractures. Teenagers, in particular, need to optimize their bone density because peak bone density is reached by age 19. Teens need to be fully aware they are not only losing bone density, but they are also not gaining bone density as should happen during teenage years. If you don't have dense bones as a teenager, you may never reach your peak bone mass and will have a higher risk of osteoporosis in later life (Weaver 2002). A shocking one-fourth of young women who have anorexia experience early osteoporosis. Some end up in severe pain throughout their lives, others, in wheelchairs.

You can recover much of the bone loss by eating well enough to rebuild muscles and gain weight, but not always all of it (Dominguez et al. 2007). A case study of a 31-year-old distance runner indicates that she was able to bring her bone mineral density back to within normal values by eating better and rebuilding her body, despite a long history of anorexia and amenorrhea (Fredericson and Kent 2005). Not everyone is so lucky.

• **Throw away the bathroom scale.** Rather than strive to achieve a certain number on the scale, let your body settle at its genetic weight. The information in chapters 14 and 16 can help you estimate a weight you can comfortably maintain without constantly dieting. Your physician or dietitian can also offer unbiased professional advice. And if you believe you are overwhelmed by an eating disorder, seek help from a (sports) psychologist.

Although female athletes fear that eating more and exercising less will lead to weight gain that will hurt their performance, this is not the case. Here is just one example: A 19-year-old amenorrheic runner reduced her training by one day per week, increased her daily food intake with one can of a 360-calorie liquid meal supplement, gained 6 powerful pounds (2.7 kg) over about four months (from 106 to 112 lb, or from 48 to 51 kg), and resumed menstruation. She set more personal records than she had during any prior season, broke two school records, and qualified for a national track meet (Dueck et al. 1996). What are you waiting for?

NUTRITION AND PREGNANCY

Many active women have sweet dreams about becoming moms. Others have nightmares about the effect pregnancy will have on their bodies. Competitive athletes, in particular, worry about "getting fat." Remember that pregnancy and obesity are very different! The 25 to 35 pounds (11 to 16 kg) gained during pregnancy can be accounted for by the weight of the baby (8 lb, or 3.6 kg), placenta (2 to 3 lb, or 0.9 to 1.4 kg), amniotic fluid (2 to 3 lb, or 0.9 to 1.4 kg), uterus (2 to 5 lb, or 0.9 to 2.3 kg), breast tissue (2 to 3 lb, or 0.9 to 1.4 kg), blood supply (4 lb, or 1.8 kg), and fat stores for delivery and breastfeeding (5 to 9 lb, or 2.3 to 4 kg). The Institute of Medicine (2009) recommends that women who are underweight at the start of pregnancy gain more weight (28 to 40 lb, or 13 to 18 kg) and higher-weight women gain less (15 to 25 lb, or 6.8 to 11.3 kg).

Nutrition Before Pregnancy

If you are contemplating motherhood, you shouldn't wait until you are pregnant to start eating well. Every day, mothers-to-be should fortify their bodies with the nutrients needed for the current and future well-being of their bodies and those of their unborn children. In particular, a prepregnancy sports diet should be rich in folate (table 12.1), a B vitamin that helps prevent

TABLE 12.1 Sources of Folate or Folic Acid

Your target intake is 400 micrograms (µg) per day. You can get that by choosing fruits, green vegetables, beans, legumes, and enriched grains and cereals. Note that unenriched ("all natural") cereals lack folate.

Food	Amount	Folate or folic acid (µg)
NATURAL FOODS		
Spinach	1 cup cooked	230
Lentils	1/2 cup cooked	180
Asparagus	6 spears	135
Broccoli	1 cup cooked	100
Romaine lettuce	1 cup shredded	65
Avocado	1/2 medium	60
Chickpeas	1/2 cup canned	60
Kidney beans	1/2 cup canned	50
Orange	1 medium	50
Peas, green	2 tbsp	30
Peanut butter	2 tbsp	25
Egg	1 large	25
FORTIFIED AND ENRICHED FOODS		
Cheerios	1 cup	335
PowerBar	1	240
Flour, enriched	1/2 cup	180
Oatmeal, instant	1 packet	150
Bread, whole wheat	2 slices	30
UNFORTIFIED CEREALS		
Puffins original	3/4 cup	0
Trader Joe's low-fat granola	3/4 cup	0

National Institutes of Health Office of Dietary Supplements, http://ods.od.nih.gov; USDA National Nutrient Database for Standard Reference, www.ars.usda.gov.

brain damage in the fetus at the time of conception and can reduce the risk of some types of birth defects. Folate is the natural form of this B vitamin found in food. Folic acid is the synthetic form found in supplements and enriched or fortified foods. The recommended intake is 400 micrograms of folate (or more precisely, dietary folate equivalents) per day.

Nutrition During Pregnancy

Each athletic woman experiences a pregnancy unique to her. Some feel fine, eat well, exercise regularly, and breeze through the nine months of pregnancy. Others experience fatigue, nausea, low-back pain, and other discomforts. Some gain more weight than anticipated. Others gain according to the standard guidelines. Eat according to your appetite, and trust that regularly scheduled meals and snacks will contribute to the weight gain appropriate for your body, the development of a healthy baby, and the enjoyment of a comfortable exercise program. You will become fitter and may reduce the risk of giving birth by cesarean section if you exercise, but your weight changes will likely be similar with or without purposeful exercise (Brik, Fernandez-Buhigas, and Martin-Arias 2018).

Your best bet for nutrition during pregnancy is to follow the nutrition guidelines in the first two chapters of this book as well as to read some of the pregnancy books suggested in appendix A. Your diet should focus on folic acid (see table 12.1 for sources), calcium-rich foods, dark green or colorful vegetables, fresh fruits such as oranges and other citrus fruits, whole grains, and foods rich in iron and protein. Athletes who enter pregnancy with low iron stores are at high risk for anemia. Pregnancy is already tiring enough!

For about two-thirds of women, tastes change during pregnancy. You may develop a strong aversion to meat, vegetables, or coffee. If you can hold down nothing but a few crackers, rest assured that your baby will still manage to grow on the nutrients you've stored up from your prepregnancy diet. If your intake is very limited because of nausea that lasts for more than three months, you might want to consult with a registered dietitian who can suggest ways to balance your diet.

If you experience unusual cravings, such as for salt, fat, or red meat, it's possible that nature is telling you that those foods have nutrients you need. Giving in to food cravings, in moderation, tends to be harmless, so listen to your body and respond appropriately. Try to resolve your cravings for sweets with the healthier choices, such as oatmeal raisin cookies, vanilla Greek yogurt, or dried pineapple and dates instead of candy. The reality may be that only one food will do the trick: the food you crave! Eating a healthy prepregnancy diet ensures that you start off well nourished so your body can survive the strange cravings and morning sickness.

Nutrition After Pregnancy

If you are a new mother who worries that you'll never lose the weight gained during pregnancy, be patient and remember that life has seasons. The first year after pregnancy may not be the season to be as lean or as athletic as desired. Pregnancy lasts for 9 months, and many women need an additional 9 to 12 months to return to their prepregnancy physiques (figure 12.1). Don't try to crash diet now.

Your better bet is to focus on eating well and trusting that healthy eating will contribute to the return of your appropriate weight. But this process is often confounded because motherhood brings its own set of nutrition challenges and frustrations. When your baby cries, your life stops, and so do many healthy eating habits. Fatigue, stressful life changes, family adjustments, and lack of energy to shop for and cook food can also take their toll on the quality of your diet. You may also lack the mental energy you need to maintain your exercise program.

The stresses and frustrations that accompany motherhood can interfere with your weight-loss plans and may even contribute to weight gain. If you are now home all day with readily available food, you may comfort yourself with candy, cookies, and other treats. Physical exhaustion, lack of time, and child-care responsibilities may thwart your intentions to exercise. If this is the case, you might want to pay a babysitter (or take childcare turns with another mom) so you can have time for self-care. This may help you feel better physically, improve your health status, and feel better about yourself.

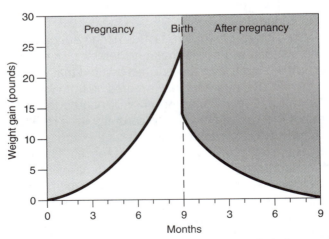

FIGURE 12.1 Pregnant women usually gain 25 to 35 pounds during pregnancy and may need nine or more months to return to their prepregnancy weight after delivery.

Do not expect postpregnancy weight to melt away with exercise—even if you do 45 minutes a day for five days a week (Lovelady 2011). Yes, regular exercise both during and after pregnancy can help curb undesired weight gain, but the factors mentioned earlier can affect your weight more than the lack of exercise (Haakstad and Bo 2011). If you fear that you'll end up at a higher weight for the rest of your life, take note of a survey of new moms. Most of these women, who were all runners, reported that they returned to running five weeks after delivery and were at their prepregnancy weights in five months (Lutter and Cushman 1982). Most athletes will return to their prepregnancy weight within six months (Bo et al. 2018). Yes, there can be a lean life after pregnancy, as verified by the many mothers you see around you who are lean. For now, love yourself from the inside out, enjoy your baby, be proud of your accomplishment, and be gentle on yourself.

WOMEN AS GATEKEEPERS FOR FAMILY NUTRITION

Many of my active clients are health- and weight-conscious parents who are frustrated by their children's eating practices. As Janine, a triathlete and parent of two girls (11 and 14 years old), vented, "I wish I could get my kids to eat better and exercise more. They love junk food, spend hours texting their friends, and weigh more than they should. Mealtimes are becoming World War III." Janine tried hard to teach her children about the importance of nutrition and health, but her messages fell on deaf ears.

I recommended that Janine not focus on "good" versus "bad" foods, but rather, teach her children to enjoy all kinds of food and appreciate how good nutrition helps a body do wonderful things. It is normal for children to want food with little nutritional value, but it is also pretty normal for them to want good-for-you foods, too. Balance—not restriction—should be the key message. Otherwise, kids sneak eat.

Despite popular belief, kids (and their parents) do not need to eat a perfect diet to have a good diet. Most children can meet their nutrient needs within 1,200 to 1,500 calories if they eat a variety of wholesome foods. Hence, there is space for "fun foods," in moderation. (Some active children can actually have trouble getting adequate calories if parents strictly limit treats.) One way to reduce your child's intake of not-so-good-for-you foods is to offer a healthy "second lunch" or "early dinner" after school and before sports. Enjoying peanut butter on crackers, an english muffin pizza, cereal with milk, a fruit smoothie, or a sandwich is preferable to the standard routine of munching on candy bars, cookies, and chips. A healthy second lunch is particularly important for kids who eat poorly at school.

To help put an end to food wars, I highly recommend Ellyn Satter's book, *Secrets of Feeding a Healthy Family.*

Children's Growing Bodies

Nina, a fitness runner and the mother of a 12-year-old swimmer, felt dismayed every time she saw her daughter in a bathing suit. "Sarah is pudgy, even though we try to keep her active." I reminded Nina that every child's body is unique; some are petite, some are larger, and some are in the middle. That is normal and OK. Although Nina was unhappy about her child's physique, I warned her to express her concern from the point of health, not beauty. Conveying the message "You're too fat" (which the child translates to mean "I'm unlovable") can be emotionally damaging. Sarah was undoubtedly more than aware of her excess body fat; helping her accept and appreciate her body would be an important step for her mom to take.

Although dieting is standard among swimmers and participants in other sports that emphasize leanness (figure skaters, dancers, gymnasts, runners), the pressure to acquire the "perfect" body can lead to trouble if the dieter has a poor self-image and low self-esteem. All too often, diets are about feelings of being imperfect or inadequate rather than weight alone. Dieting increases the risk of developing a full-blown eating disorder.

As a parent and role model, Nina needed to downplay body size as a way to evaluate self-worth and teach Sarah to love herself from the inside out. I advised Nina to never comment about the size of large children; Sarah could conclude that she must be thin to be valued and loved. This is particularly important for girls during puberty who are coping with body changes while struggling to be the best at their sports. Their efforts to control weight may lead to unhealthy dieting, frustration, guilt, despair, and failure.

Helping Your Overfat Child

Nina felt at a loss about how to help her daughter Sarah lose weight. I told her that childhood weight issues are complex and a topic of debate among parents and pediatricians alike. We know that restricting a child's food intake does not work. Rather, it tends to result in sneak eating, binge eating, guilt, and shame—the same stuff that adults encounter when they "blow their diets." But this time, the parents become the food police—an undesirable family dynamic.

Despite Nina's best intentions to prevent creeping obesity, I warned her against putting Sarah on a diet, depriving her of french fries, or banning candy. Dietary restrictions don't work—not for adults and not for kids. If diets did work, then the majority of people who have dieted would all be lean, and the obesity epidemic would not exist.

Diets for children cause more problems than they solve. They disrupt their natural tendency to eat when hungry and stop when content. Instead, they overcompensate and stuff themselves through "last-chance eating" (e.g., "It's my last chance to have birthday cake, so I'd better eat a lot now because when I get home, I'm restricted to celery sticks and rice cakes"). I suggested that Nina delicately ask Sarah whether she was comfortable with her body. If she admitted discontent and expressed a desire to learn how to eat better, Nina could then arrange for a consultation with a registered dietitian who specializes in pediatric weight management.

If you, like Nina, are the parent of a chubby child, you should know that children commonly grow "out" before they grow "up." That is, they often gain body fat before embarking on a growth spurt. Talk to your pediatrician to determine whether the problem is real. You can also assess your child's weight with growth charts available at www.cdc.gov/growthcharts.

You might be rightly concerned about your child's weight; we're seeing more and more medical problems linked to childhood diabetes, high cholesterol, and high blood pressure. But your concerns about your child's weight might reflect your own anxiety about having an "imperfect" kid. Yes, you say you want to spare your child the grief of being fat—but be sure to also examine your own issues. If you are very weight conscious and put a high value on how you look, you may be feeling blemished if your child is overfat. Often, a child's weight problem is really the parent's issue. You may want a "perfect child."

Be sure to love your overfat child from the inside out—and not judge her from the outside in. Little comments such as "That dress is pretty, honey, but it would look even better if you'd just lose a little weight" can be interpreted by your child as "I'm not good enough." As a result, self-esteem can take a nosedive and contribute to anorexic thinking (e.g., "thinner is better"), and dieting can go awry (see chapter 17 for information on eating disorders).

So, what can you do to help overfat kids slim down? Instead of maligning them and trying to get them thin by restricting food, get them healthier by helping them see the benefits of being more active. This could mean encouraging them to watch less TV, planning enjoyable family activities (unlike boot camp), and perhaps even creating a walking school bus with the neighborhood kids (a parent or high school student picks up the kids in the neighborhood as they walk together to school). As a family, you might want to sign up for a charitable walking or running event. As a contributing member of society, make your voice heard about the need for safe sidewalks, health clubs that welcome overfat kids, and swimming pools that allow children (and adults, for that matter) to wear T-shirts and shorts instead of embarrassing bathing suits.

Foodwise, provide your kids with wholesome, nourishing foods as well as semiregular "fun foods." (Otherwise, they will go out and get them.) Encourage your children to eat breakfast. Plan structured meals and snacks; take dinnertime seriously. Your job is to determine the *what*, *where*, and *when* of eating; the child's job is to determine *how much* and *whether* to eat. (Don't force your child to finish his peas or stop him from having second helpings.) If you interfere with a child's natural ability to regulate food, you can cause a lifetime of struggle. Trust your children to eat when hungry and stop when content—so they can have plenty of energy to enjoy an active lifestyle. For additional information, read *Your Child's Weight: Helping Without Harming* by Ellyn Satter.

WOMEN, WEIGHT, AND MENOPAUSE

Even elite athletes gain a little weight with age, and nonelite folks have been known to gain a lot. The trick to weight management is to stay active and eat quality calories that promote good health. Yet, many women fear midlife weight gain. As Mary, an avid tennis player, complained, "No matter what I do, I can't seem to stop gaining weight." She was frustrated about her expanding waist and frightened about runaway weight gain. She fearfully asked, "Are women doomed to gain weight in midlife?"

The answer is no. Women do not always gain weight during menopause. Yes, women ages 45 to 50 commonly get fatter and thicker around the middle as fat settles in and around the abdominal area. But the majority of these changes are caused by aging, a lack of exercise, and a surplus of calories—not simply a drop in estrogen (Kapoor, Collazo-Clavell, and Faubion 2017). In a three-year study of more than 3,000 women (initial age 42 to 52 years), the average weight gain was 4.6 pounds (2.1 kg). The weight gain occurred in all women, regardless of their menopause status (Sternfeld et al. 2004). Let's explore a few of the culprits that affect weight in middle-aged women.

Menopause occurs during a time when a woman's lifestyle becomes less active. If her children have grown up and left home, she may find herself sitting more in front of a TV or computer screen than running up and down stairs, carrying endless loads of laundry. A less-active lifestyle not only reduces calorie needs but also results in a decline in muscle mass; when women (and men) age, they tend to lose muscle mass unless they do regular strength training. Muscle influences the metabolic rate, so less muscle means a lower metabolic rate and fewer calories burned.

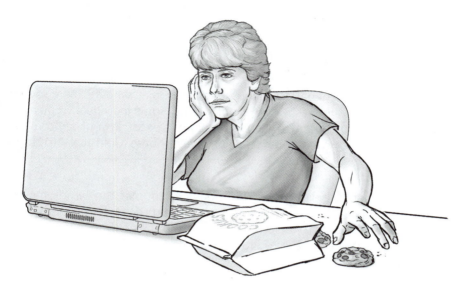

Another problem is that sleep patterns commonly change in midlife, often as a result of night sweats and partners who snore. Many women end up feeling exhausted most of the time. Exhaustion and sleep deprivation can easily drain motivation to routinely exercise, and this perpetuates more muscle loss and increases the drop in metabolism.

Sleep deprivation itself is also associated with weight gain. Adults who sleep less than seven hours per night tend to be heavier than their well-rested counterparts. When you are sleep deprived, your appetite grows. The hormone that curbs your appetite (leptin) is reduced, and the hormone that increases your appetite (ghrelin) becomes more active (Taheri et al. 2004). Hence, you can have a hard time differentiating between being hungry and being tired. In either case, cookies and chocolate can be very tempting.

Menopause may also coincide with career success, including business meals at nice restaurants, extra wine, plush vacations, and cruises. That can mean more calories and less exercise. By midlife, most women are tired of dieting and depriving themselves of tempting foods; they may have been dieting since puberty. The "No, thank you" that prevailed at previous birthday parties now becomes "Yes, please."

The best way to minimize, if not prevent, weight gain is to exercise regularly, eat wisely, limit calories from alcohol, get enough sleep, and maintain an active lifestyle. Research suggests that women who exercise do not gain the weight and waist of their nonexercising peers (Sternfeld et al. 2004). The optimal exercise program includes both aerobic exercise (to enhance cardiorespiratory fitness) and strengthening exercise (to preserve muscles and bone density).

FACT OR FICTION

Soy foods help prevent hot flashes.

The facts: A study of more than 3,300 pre- and perimenopausal women found no consistent patterns suggesting the women who ate more soy food had fewer hot flashes and night sweats. Some individual women did experience benefits, so there is no harm in boosting your soy consumption to see whether you have a positive response (Gold et al. 2012).

Despite popular belief, taking hormones to counter the symptoms of menopause does not contribute to weight gain. If anything, hormone replacement therapy may help curb midlife weight gain (Davis et al. 2012).

If you have gained undesired fat, do not diet. If you have been dieting for 35 to 40 years of your adult life, you should have learned by now that dieting does not work. Rather, you need to learn how to eat healthfully. This means fueling your body with enough breakfasts, lunches, and afternoon snacks to curb your appetite and energize your exercise program. Then, eat lighter dinners. Think *small calorie deficit.* Consuming 100 fewer calories after dinner (theoretically) translates into losing 10 pounds (4.5 kg) of fat per year.

To find peace with food and your body, read chapters 16 and 17, and consider meeting with a registered dietitian (RD) who specializes in sports nutrition. This professional can develop a personalized food plan that fits your needs. To find a local RD, go to www.scandpg.org. In addition, ask yourself, *Am I really overweight?* Maybe there is just more of you to love. Your body may not be quite as perfect as it once was at the height of your athletic career, but it can be good enough. I encourage you to focus on being fit and healthy rather than on being thin at any cost. No "perfect" weight will ever do the enormous job of creating midlife happiness.

CHAPTER 13

ATHLETE-SPECIFIC NUTRITION ADVICE

Throughout this *Sports Nutrition Guidebook*, I have offered general sports nutrition guidance for both casual exercisers and competitive athletes The following sport-specific or situation-specific information applies to niche athletes who are on teams, in power sports, in weight-class sports, or in ultradistance or extreme sports; who compete in winter sports; or who are injured, older, or getting back to exercise after gastric bypass surgery.

NUTRITION FOR TEAM SPORTS

Whether it's the soccer, hockey, lacrosse, tennis, or football team, when groups of athletes get together, they can easily end up at pregame tailgate parties and postgame celebrations that don't quite fit into an optimal sports diet. Add in travel, tournaments, and disrupted sleep, and nutrition can easily fall by the wayside. Yet, with strong leadership from their captains and coaches, teams can indeed win with good nutrition—especially if they are competing against teams with suboptimal fueling practices—when they make a commitment to each other to plan ahead and eat responsibly and, if the athletes are of drinking age, knock off the alcohol until the end of the season.

Here are a few factors to consider for teams that want to get to the winner's circle (Holway and Spriet 2011):

• Most team sports are stop-and-go sports; they involve bursts of high-intensity play followed by pauses with low activity. Athletes in these demanding sports can easily become glycogen depleted and dehydrated. Hence, all athletes need to be responsible and make the effort to fuel themselves optimally.

• Even with home games, someone needs to plan for food and fluids before, during, and after games or tournaments, as well as at half-time. Is this the job of the parents, athletes, team captain, team manager, or coach? Good communication can prevent problems.

- When traveling, a one-size-fits-all team menu is unlikely to work because each athlete has personal nutritional needs, goals, and food issues. Buffets with many options can meet the needs of most of the players most of time—including vegans and players with celiac disease or nut allergies.

- If the team is staying at a sport camp or a residence away from home, someone needs to review the menu and arrange for proper meals. If the menu is too "healthy" and too low in fat, the athletes resort to smuggling food into their living quarters. To reduce complaints, menus need to include enough "fun foods," special dinners, and ice cream socials, as well as a good supply of wholesome yet popular snacks (e.g., nut butter and honey sandwiches, baby carrots with hummus dip, corn chips with guacamole, yogurt, oatmeal raisin cookies, shelf-stable chocolate dairy or soy milk, dark chocolate–covered almonds) that are readily available, particularly on travel days.

- Teams that are lucky enough to have a sports dietitian will benefit from individual counseling, team talks, fact sheets (including information on popular sports supplements), supermarket tours, and cooking lessons. Ideally, this person will be available to chat with the players in informal settings, such as at meals. Having a skilled team sports nutritionist helps the coach and trainers stay within their scope of practice and focus on what they do best—coach!

- During preseason training with double workouts, athletes can easily become depleted and dehydrated, and lose weight. During the competitive season, athletes may have more time to eat but need fewer calories because of reduced training. This can lead to undesired weight gain. Nutrition education can help manage weight issues.

- When dehydration is a concern, the sports dietitian can set up weigh-ins before and after practices to identify players who lose more than 2 percent of their body weight (at which point performance can take a dive). When budget is a concern, the athletes can enjoy a homemade sports drink (see recipe in chapter 25) for a fraction of the cost of commercial sports drinks.

- The off-season is a good time for athletes to lose undesired body fat and build muscle. Some athletes get lazy; they gain fat and lose muscle. Making a plan for off-season weight management can prevent problems that affect the entire team at the start of preseason training.

The information in this book can help you establish nutrition policies and procedures for hydration, supplementation, and nutritional recovery after practices and games, and weight management (including body fat measurement and eating disorders). All athletes should know the policies and live by the same rules.

NUTRITION FOR POWER SPORTS

Power athletes include those who compete in middle-distance running, canoeing, kayaking, rowing, track cycling, and swimming. They train hard, exhaust themselves during workouts, and need to pay particular attention to their sports diets during training and while competing. Here are a few tips (Stellingwerff, Maughan, and Burke 2011):

• To train at high intensity, you need to start the workout well-fueled. If you start with low muscle glycogen, you will be unable to train at your best, and that means you'll be unable to compete at your best. A carbohydrate-based sports diet is particularly important the day before and after a high-intensity training workout or event. By staying well-fueled and adequately refueling afterward, you'll get the most out of your training program.

• To maximize muscle strength and mass, eat 20 to 30 grams (more precisely, 0.15 g/lb or 0.3 g/kg body weight) of protein at each meal and snack, spreading the protein evenly throughout the day so the muscles have a continual supply of amino acids for building and repairing tissue.

• Drink adequate fluids to reduce the risk of becoming dehydrated. If you are unable to swallow fluids during intense workouts and competitive events that last more than 45 minutes, at least try to swish and spit. Just rinsing your mouth with water or a sports drink can offer performance benefits (Rollo and Williams 2011).

• If you have more than one competitive event in a day, you will want to refuel as soon as tolerable after the first event to optimize recovery for the second event. The ideal target is about 0.5 gram of carbohydrate per pound per hour (1 g carbohydrate/kg/hour) for the first four to six hours (ACSM 2016). This means that you need to plan ahead so you'll have proper recovery foods ready and waiting. Sweet foods with a moderate to high glycemic effect may help maximize the restoration of depleted glycogen stores.

• Buffering agents, such as sodium bicarbonate and beta-alanine, may lead to performance benefits, but be sure to experiment with them during training.

NUTRITION FOR SPORTS THAT EMPHASIZE LOOKS AND WEIGHT

Gymnastics, figure skating, dancing, diving, rowing, and weight-class sports emphasize leanness and how your body looks. This can create a lot of pressure to attain the "perfect" body. You not only have to achieve a very low weight but also have to do so while trying to improve your performance. That's a tough order and can feel overwhelming (Sundgot-Borgen and Garthe 2011).

The pressure to be lean as well as fears about being judged by leanness can easily lead to extreme dieting, disordered eating behaviors, and dangerous weight-control methods (sweat suits, saunas, dehydration) that can not only hurt your performance but also hurt your health and, tragically, even lead to death. You might learn the hard way that weight loss will not improve your performance if it comes at too big a dietary deficit. Meeting with a sports dietitian can be a wise investment to help you accomplish your goals. Here is some food for thought.

- Enduring a very low-calorie diet is very difficult, mentally and physically. If you are starving, you'll undoubtedly be in a bad mood. With proper nutrition education, you can learn how to lose weight without starving yourself or using harmful dieting practices (see chapter 16). Ideally, you can lose weight in the off-season, at the rate of 0.5 to 1 pound (0.25 to 0.5 kg) per week. You should not lose more than 2 percent of your body weight through dehydration (3 pounds for a 150-pound athlete; 1.5 kg/68 kg athlete).

- Your nutrient targets include eating 0.7 to 1.0 gram of protein per pound of body weight (1.4 to 2.0 g/kg), 2 to 3 grams of carbohydrate per pound of body weight (4.0 to 6.0 g/kg), and 15 to 20 percent of calories from fat (Sundgot-Borgen and Garthe 2011). By backing your training into a meal, you can save "recovery snack" calories.

- Many female athletes in aesthetic sports restrict their food intake to the point that they stop having regular menstrual periods; their bodies lack the fuel needed to fully function. This can lead to poor bone health and stress fractures that sideline them (see chapter 12), and all that hard work goes unrewarded.

- Although the female athlete triad (amenorrhea, decreased bone mineral density that leads to stress fractures, eating disorders) has been studied in women, male athletes can also experience problems with inadequate energy intake that leads to reduced health and performance (Teneforde 2016). Hence, Relative Energy Deficiency in Sport (RED-S) has become the comprehensive term that addresses this concern in both males and females. In a group of male cyclists, 28 percent were diagnosed with low energy availability (inadequate calorie intake relative to their energy needs) that contributed to lower testosterone and reduced bone mineral density in the spine The researchers noted the cyclists who both restricted the most and trained the most commonly underperformed—despite their very low percent body fat and "optimal" power-to-weight ratio (Keay, Francis, and Hind 2018).

• Regardless of whether you are male or female, you should focus on gradual weight loss because that is least likely to hurt your athletic performance. Plus, by eating more than the bare minimum, you'll consume a little more protein, essential dietary fat, carbohydrate, calcium, iron, zinc, and all the other nutrients needed for good health and top performance. Chapters 14, 16, and 17 address weight-management issues in greater depth.

NUTRITION FOR ULTRADISTANCE AND EXTREME-SPORTS ATHLETES

With the growth of ultra-endurance events and extreme sports, many athletes are pushing their bodies to the limit. They train for three to five hours a day to compete for hours on end. Their goals might be to test their limits and try to finish an Ironman triathlon (2.4-mile [3.9 km] swim, 112-mile bike [180 km], and 26.2-mile [42 km] run), a double-century bike ride (200 miles [322 km]), a 100-mile (161 km) mountain run, an English Channel swim (28-plus hours), a trans-Atlantic row (50 to 60 days), an Appalachian Trail hike (2,160 miles [3,476 km]), or any number of other ultradistance events. Clearly, nutrition is a critical factor in being able to finish an event of this type. These athletes put sports nutrition principles to the test! Following these nutrition pointers will give you ultraenergy so you can complete your event successfully:

• Practice your event-day fueling during training sessions. Your training should include creating and practicing your fueling strategy so you can learn which foods and fluids settle best during extended exercise. Lemon or cherry sports drink? Gels or "real foods" such as bananas, dried figs, and baked sweet potatoes? Canned liquid meal replacements or peanut butter and jelly sandwiches? By having a list of several tried-and-true foods, you need not worry about making the wrong food choice on event day.

Also consider the "taste bud burnout" factor. That is, how many gels per hour can you endure in a triathlon? When hiking, how many days in a row will you enjoy powdered eggs for breakfast? Will you get "sugared-out" on sports drink during the century bike ride? Think about variety, and how you can enjoyably and easily consume enough carbohydrate to fuel your muscles and your brain, and enough protein to repair and protect your muscles. Use the strategies discussed in chapters 6 through 10.

• Optimize your daily training diet. All too often, in the midst of juggling work and school, family and friends, and sleep and training, endurance athletes have little time left to plan menus, shop for food, and prepare well-balanced sports meals, nor do they muster the energy to choose nutritious snacks. Hungry and tired athletes commonly grab cookies, nachos, and other high-fat comfort foods that fill the stomach but leave the muscles unfueled. You must remember this: You won't be able to compete at your best unless you can stay healthy and train at your best. That means eating a good sports diet every day.

Your goals are to constantly be fueling up before workouts and then refueling afterward by eating carbohydrate-based meals and snacks on a regular schedule. By feeding your body evenly throughout the day (as opposed to skimping on wholesome meals by day and then overindulging in treats at night), you'll have steady energy all day, without lags. You need to develop an eating strategy that fits your training schedule. One triathlete devised the following routine:

○ He drank 16 ounces (480 ml) of juice (i.e., carbohydrate) before his morning swim. He refueled afterward while commuting to work by eating a big bagel with peanut butter, a banana, and chocolate milk (in a travel mug).

○ At lunchtime, he ate a hot dinner-type meal from the cafeteria at work.

○ At lunchtime, he bought his afternoon snack, a bran muffin, yogurt, and orange juice.

○ At lunchtime, he also bought his evening meal (a turkey sub and a fruit salad), which he kept in the office refrigerator.

This food plan prevented him from haphazardly resorting to "junk eating" whenever he felt hungry.

• Plan rest days. Rest is an essential part of a training program. Because ultradistance athletes commonly feel overwhelmed by their impending tasks, they tend to fill every possible minute with exercise. Bad idea. Rest days are essential not only for reducing the risk of injury and giving muscles time to refuel but also for allowing time to shop for food (and even cook a big pot of chili for the week, if so inclined). Remember, the *bad* things happen when you train, and the *good* things happen when you rest.

Take heed: Performance improves more with quality exercise than with an excessive quantity of exercise (i.e., pushing yourself to train longer and longer). Knowing this, one triathlete completed the Hawaii Ironman by training only once a day, either hard or long. He took one day of complete rest per week. He finished midpack; his competitors were flabbergasted!

• Drink enough fluids. Monitor your urine daily. You should urinate frequently (every two to four hours); the urine should be clear and of adequate quantity. Morning urine that is dark and smelly is a bad sign— dehydration. Drink more!

During training, you can estimate your event-day fluid needs by weighing yourself naked before and after an hour of event-pace exercise. For each pound (0.5 kg) of sweat loss, you should plan to drink at least an additional 16 ounces (500 ml) of fluid while exercising to prevent that loss. See chapter 8 for more information on fluids and how to keep yourself from becoming dehydrated.

- Develop a defined feeding plan for the event. You should know not only your fluid targets but also your calorie targets. By working with a sports nutritionist or exercise physiologist, you can estimate your energy needs per hour. Try to replace at least a third or a half, if not more, of the calories burned during the ultraevent as tolerated. For example, a cyclist may need to consume 450 calories per hour during an extended ride. This is the equivalent of 1 quart (1 L) of sports drink and five fig bars, or 1 quart of water and a peanut butter and honey sandwich. Pack snack bags that meet your calorie targets for a half-hour or hour. Eat and drink on a schedule. The goal is to prevent dehydration and hypoglycemia (low blood sugar). See chapter 10 for more information about fueling during exercise.

- Be flexible and open minded. Although you should have a well-defined eating and drinking program that ensures adequate carbohydrate and fluid intake, you also need to be flexible. After all, your tastes may change during 18 hours of exercise! Your initial approach to consume wholesome fruits, juices, and energy bars may deteriorate into the ever-popular Coke, candy bars, and potato chips. Listen to your body's requests during the event; hopefully, you'll have the desired fuel available. Many ultradistance athletes crave sweets, and that's OK. Sugar during exercise does a fine job of delaying fatigue. Your job is to survive the event; your daily training diet will help you thrive healthfully.

Should You "Go Keto"?

The very low-carbohydrate, high-fat ketogenic diet is currently popular among some ultra-endurance athletes, particularly those with intestinal issues that worsen with extended exercise. By teaching their bodies to burn body fat, they report being able to maintain energy to perform well while consuming just water and electrolytes and avoiding the gels, sports drinks, and other snacks that can contribute to their intestinal distress. To date, the research is mixed on whether or not this fat-burning diet does indeed *enhance* performance (Burke et al. 2017; McSwiney et al. 2018). Until we have more research to determine whether competitive athletes will benefit from "going keto," you need to evaluate whether this extreme diet fits into your lifestyle and is worth the effort. For more information, see chapters 6 and 16.

NUTRITION FOR WINTER ATHLETES

If you are a skier or a winter runner, winter hiker, or other type of winter athlete, you must pay careful attention to your sports diet. A lack of food and fluids can take the fun out of your outdoor activities Adequate preexercise fuel is essential for generating body heat. Cold weather itself does not increase energy needs, but you will burn extra calories if your body temperature drops and you start to shiver. Shivering is involuntary muscle tensing that generates heat. Hence, you should fuel up before embarking on winter exercise, particularly before you ski, run outside, or participate in an outside activity in extreme cold. These tips can help you fuel wisely for cold-weather workouts.

Winter Hydration

• Drink enough fluids. Becoming dehydrated is a major mistake made by winter athletes. A study comparing the hydration status of athletes who skied with those who played football or soccer reported that the skiers had the highest rate of chronic dehydration. Before a competition, 11 of the 12 alpine skiers showed up dehydrated (Johnson et al. 2010). This might be because cold not only induces diuresis (the need to urinate) but also blunts the thirst mechanism. Winter athletes may feel less thirsty despite significant urine and sweat loss and may not think to drink. Some winter athletes purposefully skimp on fluids to minimize the need to urinate. There's no doubt that undoing layer after layer of clothing (e.g., ski suit, hockey gear) can be a hassle. Yet, dehydration hurts performance and is one cause of failed mountaineering adventures.

• Winter athletes (especially those skiing at high altitude) need to consciously consume fluids to replace the water vapor that is exhaled via breathing. When you breathe in cold, dry air, your body warms and humidifies that air. As you exhale, you lose significant amounts of water. You can see this vapor ("steam") when you breathe.

• Unless you are hot, do not drink icy water (i.e., from a water bottle kept on your bike or the outside pocket of your backpack). Cold water can cool you off and give you the chills. The better option is an insulated water bottle or a bottle filled with hot sports drink and then covered with a wool sock to retain the heat. If winter hiking, keep your water bottle in an inside pocket and in your sleeping bag at night to prevent it from freezing.

• Dress in layers so you sweat less. Sweaty clothing drains body heat. As the weather becomes "tropical" inside your exercise outfit, make the effort to strip down. You'll stay drier and warmer. Simply taking off a hat is cooling; exposing your head can dissipate 30 to 40 percent of your body heat.

Winter Fuel

- Food's overall warming effect is known as thermogenesis (i.e., "heat making"). Thirty to sixty minutes after you eat, your body generates about 10 percent more heat than when you have an empty stomach. Hence, eating not only provides fuel but also increases heat production (warmth). You want to eat at frequent intervals; no skipping meals or snacks!

- Aerobic workouts can increase your metabolism 7 to 10 times above your resting level. Exercise is an excellent way to warm up in the winter.

- If you become chilled during winter exercise (or even when swimming, for that matter), you'll likely find yourself searching for food. A drop in body temperature stimulates the appetite and you experience hunger. Your body wants fuel to "stoke the furnace" so it can generate heat.

- For safety, always carry a source of emergency food (such as a few energy bars) with you in case you slip on the ice or experience an incident that leaves you static in a frigid environment. Winter campers, for example, commonly keep a supply of dried fruit, chocolate, or cookies within reach in case they wake up cold at 3:00 a.m. And of course, carry your cell phone.

Energy Needs

- When you first become slightly chilled (such as when watching a football game outdoors), you'll find yourself doing an isometric type of muscle tensing that can increase your metabolic rate two to four times. As you get further chilled, you'll find yourself hopping from foot to foot and jumping around. This is nature's way to get you to generate heat and warm your body.

- If you become so cold that you start to shiver, these vigorous muscular contractions generate lots of heat—perhaps 400 calories per hour. Such intense shivering quickly depletes your muscle glycogen stores, however, and drains your energy. This is when you'll be glad you have emergency food with you!

- Your body uses a considerable amount of energy to warm and humidify the air you breathe when you exercise in the cold. For example, if you were to burn 600 calories while cross-country skiing for an hour at 0 degrees Fahrenheit (−18 degrees Celsius), you might use about 150 of those calories to warm the inspired air. In summer, you would have dissipated that heat via sweat.

- If you wear heavy clothes and carry heavy equipment such as skis, boots, parka, or snowshoes, you will burn a few more calories carrying the extra weight. The U.S. Army allows 10 percent more calories for heavily clad troops who exercise in the cold; cold-weather rations offer 4,000 to 5,000 calories a day. Yet energy requirements vary according to the intensity of the cold, the wind, and the type of physical activity (slow winter hiking vs. cross-country ski racing). See table 13.1.

- Weight management can be an issue for winter athletes. Some lose weight easily because of the demand for calories and limited access to food. (Just how many times are you willing to remove your gloves to unpack, unwrap, and eat snacks?) Yet, other winter athletes gain weight. Long nights of darkness offer plenty of time to eat excessively. To limit winter weight gain, stay active! Exercise helps manage health, weight, and the winter blues.

- The tricks to enjoying exercising in winter are to invest in proper clothing, fuel adequately, and prevent dehydration.

Winter Recovery Foods

- To chase away chills, replenish depleted glycogen stores, and rehydrate your body, enjoy warm carbohydrate-rich foods with a high fluid content and some protein, such as hot cocoa made with milk, oatmeal cooked in milk and topped with nuts and maple syrup, chili, lentil soup with a toasted

TABLE 13.1 Energy Requirements for Physical Activity in Temperate, Cold, and Hot Environments

Note that athletes need additional fuel not only in cold environments to stay warm but also in hot environments to stay cool.

	ENVIRONMENT		
	Temperate 32°-86° F (0°-30° C)	Cold <32° F (0° C)	Hot >86° F (30° C)
Daily exercise	**DAILY CALORIES/LB (KG) BODY WEIGHT**		
Light	15-20 (32-44)	16-21 (35-46)	18-25 (40-54)
Moderate	21-24 (45-52)	21-25 (47-55)	25-28 (55-61)
Heavy	24-29 (53-63)	26-31 (56-68)	28-34 (62-75)
Example of energy needs of a 150 lb (68 kg) person	2,200-4,400 cal/day	2,400-4,700 cal/day	2,700-5,100 cal/day

Adapted from E.W. Askew, Nutrition and Performance at Environmental Extremes, in *Nutrition in Exercise and Sports*, 2nd ed., edited by I. Wolinsky and J. Hickson, (Boca Raton, FL: CRC Press, 1994). https://archive.org/details/DTIC_ADA275621.

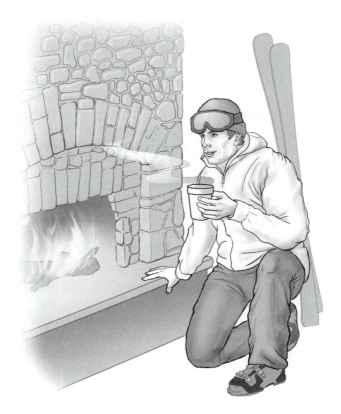

(low-fat) cheese sandwich, and pasta with meatballs. The warm food, added to the thermogenic effect of eating, contributes to rapid recovery.

• In comparison, eating cold foods and frozen fluids can chill your body. That is, save the slushy (ice slurry) for summer workouts; it will cool you off. In winter, you want warm foods to fuel your workouts. Bring out the mulled cider or thermos of soup!

NUTRITION FOR ATHLETES AT ALTITUDE

If you are a high-altitude skier, hiker, or mountaineer, you want to pay extra special attention to your diet. Lack of oxygen is exhausting enough without additional problems caused by inadequate food or fluids. Yet, altitude can dampen appetite so you may not feel hungry, even though your energy needs can be increased by lugging around heavy winter boots and clothing. If you start shivering, your energy needs will escalate.

You also may not realize how much water you are losing through your breath. Respiratory water losses are high because of the low humidity at altitude; cold air holds very little water. To maximize your enjoyment of your high-altitude adventure, pay attention to these tips:

- Make sure your iron stores are adequate by having your blood tested for serum ferritin at least a month before you go to altitude. Ferritin concentrations below 30 ng/ml suggest a suboptimal iron status that might hinder performance. If you do have low ferritin, talk with your doctor about iron supplementation before traveling to altitude so you'll have time to build up depleted iron stores. Iron is important for carrying oxygen from your lungs to your working muscles.

- Eat enough. Do not diet at altitude because your body needs energy to not only perform well but also to make red blood cells (to carry oxygen to your muscles). Although losing weight at altitude may be easier than at sea level (because of lack of appetite), the better time to diet is during the off-season or when you return home from your trip.

- Weigh yourself daily first thing in the morning so you can track weight loss. If the scale goes down, you may be underfed, underhydrated, or both. Adjust your diet accordingly.

- Plan to do just low-intensity exercise for the first few days; allow your body time to become familiar with altitude. Although you may be excited to start high-intensity skiing or hiking, overexercising at the start can lead to struggles by the middle of your trip. Total acclimatization can take four to six weeks. Be patient.

NUTRITION FOR INJURED ATHLETES

Being injured is one of the hardest parts of being an athlete. If you are unable to exercise because of a broken bone, knee surgery, or a stress fracture, you may wonder what you can eat to heal quickly. How can you avoid getting fat while you are unable to exercise? What supplements should you take? This section addresses these concerns and more.

To start, I offer this motherly reminder: Rather than shaping up your diet when you get injured, you should maintain a high-quality food intake every day. That way, you'll have a hefty bank account of vitamins and minerals stored in your liver, ready and waiting to be put into action. For example, a well-nourished athlete has enough vitamin C (important for healing) stored in the liver to last for about six weeks. The junk food junkie who sustains a serious sports injury through a bike crash, skiing tumble, or hockey blow and ends up in the hospital needing surgery or in a coma is at a big disadvantage.

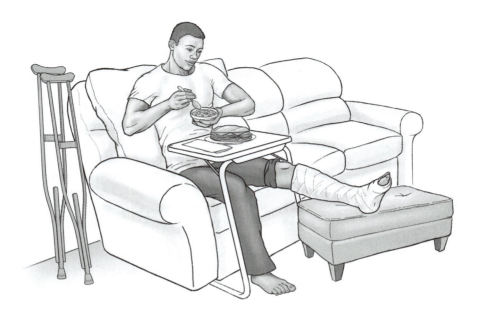

- A big barrier to optimal fueling for injured athletes is the fear of getting fat. Please remember that even injured athletes need to eat! A runner hobbled into my office on crutches saying, "I haven't eaten in three days because I can't run." He seemed to believe he only deserved to eat if he could burn calories through purposeful exercise. Wrong! Another athlete lost her appetite postsurgery. While part of her brain said, "What a great way to lose weight," her healthier side realized that good nutrition would enhance her recovery. The less you eat, the fewer healing nutrients you consume.

- Despite popular belief, the majority of the calories you eat are burned by your organs (e.g., brain, liver, lungs, kidneys, heart). Organs are metabolically active and require a lot of fuel. About two-thirds of the calories consumed by the average (lightly active) person support the resting metabolic rate (the energy needed to simply exist). On top of that, your body can require 10 to 20 percent more calories following trauma or minor surgery; major surgery requires much more; and walking with crutches increases energy needs. Yes, you may need fewer total calories because you are not training hard, but you definitely need more than your sedentary baseline.

- Your body is your best calorie counter, so respond appropriately to your hunger cues. Eat when hungry; stop when content.

FACT OR FICTION

Lack of exercise causes muscles to turn into fat.

The facts: If you are unable to train, your unexercised muscles will shrink, but not turn into fat. Wayne, a skier who broke his leg, was shocked to see how scrawny his leg muscles looked when the doctor removed the cast six weeks later. Once he started exercising, he rebuilt the muscles to their original size.

If you overeat while you are injured (as can easily happen if you are bored or depressed), you can indeed easily gain fat. Joseph, a frustrated football player with a bad concussion, quickly gained 15 pounds (6.8 kg) postinjury because he continued to eat lumberjack portions. But if you eat mindfully, your body can regulate a proper intake. Before diving into meals and snacks, ask yourself, Am I eating because I am hungry or bored? How much of this fuel does my body actually need?

When injured, some underweight athletes do gain weight. For example, Shana, a 13-year-old gymnast, perceived that her body was "getting fat" while she recuperated from a knee injury. She was simply catching up and attaining the physique appropriate for her age and genetics. She was not getting fat but maturing appropriately.

To enhance healing, choose a variety of quality foods that supply the plethora of nutrients your body needs to function and heal. Don't eliminate food groups; they all work together! Your body needs the following food groups.

• **Carbohydrate.** Consume from whole grains, fruits, and vegetables. These fiber-rich foods can be particularly helpful in managing constipation caused by postinjury pain medications and reduced exercise. By burning carbohydrate for fuel, the protein you eat can be used to heal and repair muscles. If you eat too few calories, your body will burn the protein for fuel, and that hinders healing.

• **Protein.** Consume from lean meats, dried beans, legumes, nuts, eggs, and low-fat dairy. Because you need extra protein postinjury or postsurgery, be sure to include 20 to 30 grams of protein at each meal and snack so your body has a steady stream of the tools that promote healing. A portion with 20 to 30 grams of protein equates to one of these: 3 eggs; 1 cup (230 g) of cottage cheese; 3 to 4 ounces (90 to 120 g, the size of a deck of cards) of meat, poultry, or fish; two-thirds of a 14-ounce (420 g) cake of firm tofu; or 1.25 cups of hummus. If you have a poor appetite (as commonly happens postsurgery), this amount of protein may seem overwhelming. Do your best, starting with 1 egg and then working up to 2 or 3; add a little chicken to the soup, then more. Greek yogurt can be an easy protein booster, as can commercial protein bars and powders, if needed.

Protein digests into the amino acids needed to repair damaged muscles. Although you might see ads for injury-healing amino acid supplements including arginine, ornithine, and glutamine, you can get the amino acids you need from food.

- **Plant and fish oils.** The fats in olive and canola oil, nuts, nut butters, ground flaxseed, flax oil, and avocado produce an anti-inflammatory effect. So do omega-3 fish oils. Eat at least two fish meals per week, preferably the oilier fish such as Pacific salmon, barramundi, and albacore tuna. Reduce your intake of highly processed and packaged foods with partially hydrogenated oils listed among the ingredients.

- **Vitamins.** By consuming a lot of colorful fruits and vegetables, you'll get more nutrition than in a vitamin pill. Fruits and veggies contain powerful antioxidants that knock down inflammation. Don't underestimate the healing powers of blueberries, strawberries, carrots, tomatoes, and pineapple. Make smoothies using tart cherry juice, pomegranate juice, and grape juice.

- **Minerals.** Many athletes, particularly those who eat little or no red meat, might need a boost of iron. Blood tests can indicate whether your iron stores are low. If they are, your doctor will prescribe an iron supplement. You might also want a little extra zinc (10 to 15 mg) to enhance healing.

- **Herbs, spices, and botanicals.** Anti-inflammatory compounds are found in curcumin (a component of the spice turmeric, used in curry), garlic, cocoa, green tea, and of course, fruits and vegetables. Some research suggests these foods can reduce inflammation, although more studies are needed to confirm their benefit for athletes. For therapeutic doses, you'd likely need to take high doses of these compounds in pill form. Yet, consuming these herbs and spices daily, in sickness and in health, would not be at all harmful and might lay a foundation for a quicker recovery.

NUTRITION FOR OLDER ATHLETES

As we age, changes at a cellular level contribute to the inevitable decline in performance that is seen even among elite athletes. If you are an older person who is "slowing down," fight back and stay active! Regular moderate to vigorous physical activity offers countless health benefits, including sleeping better, feeling better, and functioning better, to say nothing of preventing disease.

The 2018 Physical Activity Guidelines Advisory Committee Scientific Report (ODPHP, 2018) recommends 150 to 300 minutes a week, which translates into 30 to 60 minutes, five times a week. You don't have to train for a marathon, but keep that 5K on your radar screen. Staying in shape is easier than getting back in shape; just as not gaining weight (as can be done with the help of regular exercise) is easier than losing weight that creeps on year after year.

If you have arthritis, a healthy eating pattern rich in anti-inflammatory foods is a smart path. Anti-inflammatory foods consist of fruits and vegetables, tea, coffee, whole-grain bread and breakfast cereal, avocado, olive oil and canola oil, nuts, chocolate, and moderate amounts of red wine and beer. Include them in your overall healthy eating pattern. Claims that you should avoid tomatoes, eggplants, peppers, and other members of the nightshade family are not substantiated. And keep moving as best you can. The Osteoarthritis Action Alliance offers helpful information (https://oaaction.unc.edu).

As a masters athlete, you may wonder whether your nutritional needs differ from those of younger athletes. You may have slightly higher needs for protein, vitamin B_6, and vitamin D, so your best bet is to simply optimize your sports diet (and your exercise program) so you'll have every possible edge over the younger folks. Anti-inflammatory foods can help keep your immune system functioning well. Foods rich in nitrates (beets, spinach, arugula) might also give you a performance boost. Nitrates help lower blood pressure (which commonly increases with aging) and improve blood flow to muscles. See chapter 11.

Here are a few specific tips to help older athletes (and aging athletes—that is, all of us) create a winning food plan that's appropriate for every sport, including the sport of living life to its fullest:

• **Protein.** As you age, you want to optimize your protein intake—no skimping. Your muscles need a greater amount of amino acids to achieve the same muscle-building effect that occurs in younger athletes (Doering et al. 2016). You want to target 0.6 to 0.7 gram of protein per pound of body weight per day (1.4-1.6 g/kg/day). For a masters athlete who weighs 150 pounds (68 kg), this means 95 to 110 grams of protein per day. That's about 25 grams four times a day—more than you'd get from just oatmeal for breakfast and soup for lunch! Be sure to pace your protein intake and distribute it evenly throughout the day. For heart health, choose at least 7 ounces (200 g) of oily fish per week (one large serving or two smaller servings)—in particular, salmon, tuna, sardines, and barramundi.

Plan to refuel soon after you finish exercising; do not delay eating. If you are over 70 years of age, you may need 40 grams of protein postexercise to optimize muscle growth; this is much higher than the needs of younger men, who build muscle with just 20 grams of postexercise protein (Yang et al. 2012). A recovery smoothie with whey protein, which is high in the amino acid leucine and triggers muscle growth, might help you get the most from your workouts.

• **Fat.** Healthy plant and fish oils provide a health-protective anti-inflammatory effect. Given that diseases of aging such as heart disease, diabetes, and arthritis are triggered by inflammation, consuming canola, olive, avocado, walnut, and fish oils that reduce inflammation is a wise choice. See chapter 2 for information on healthy fat.

• **Calcium.** Even though your bones have stopped growing, they are constantly in flux, releasing and then redepositing calcium. In postmenopausal women, the balance between bone breakdown and bone formation shifts, resulting in bone loss and a higher risk of osteoporosis—particularly if the diet is calcium poor. By selecting a calcium-rich food at each meal (including soy or lactose-free milk products) as well sources of vitamin D (fortified milk, fortified cereal, sunlight, supplement) to enhance calcium absorption, you'll invest in bone health. Having strong muscles attached to your bones is also essential, so be sure to perform strengthening exercises such as lifting weights at least twice a week.

• **Fiber.** Eat enough fiber-rich foods to have regular bowel movements; this not only enhances comfort during exercise but also is an investment in good health. The fiber in oatmeal, for example, can reduce cholesterol and the risk of heart disease.

• **Vitamins.** The best all-natural sources of vitamins are colorful fruits and vegetables; eat a rainbow of produce. By keeping active and exercising, you can eat more calories—and more vitamin-rich fruits and veggies. These wholesome foods offer compounds that work synergistically and are more powerful than vitamin pills.

Supplementing with high doses of antioxidant vitamins such as C and E is popular among masters athletes, but research suggests that this can have a negative effect. The body responds to extra exercise by making extra antioxidants. See chapter 11 for more information on vitamin supplements.

• **Fluids.** The older you get, the less sensitive your thirst mechanism becomes. That is, you may need fluids but may not feel thirsty. To reduce the risk of chronic hypohydration, drink enough so that you void a significant volume of light-colored urine every three to four hours. During extended exercise, follow a hydration plan. See chapter 8 for more information on how to stay well hydrated.

The bottom line is to eat wisely by including protein-rich food in each meal, drink plenty of fluids, exercise regularly, lift weights, refuel rapidly, and enjoy feeling young. You may be getting older, but you don't have to act your age. Let wholesome food and enjoyable exercise be your winning edge!

NUTRITION FOR BARIATRIC ATHLETES

Without a doubt, exercise is an important part of a successful weight-maintenance program. Some people who have had bariatric surgery (e.g., gastric bypass or gastric sleeve operations) embrace exercise; an estimated 14 percent become "active" and another 6 percent, "highly active" (Wing et al. 2008). If you are among the highly active group, you may be spending several hours each day walking or working out in the gym. You might even be training for a marathon, Ironmen triathlon, or century bike ride. The following sports nutrition tips can help you reach your goals:

Note: Research on bariatric sports nutrition is very limited. I can only offer suggestions based on my experiences with bariatric athletes. You will need to learn by trial and error the best fueling practices for your unique and evolving body. As you become more and more active, you may need more than the standard prescription of 1,600 calories a day, particularly if you are exercising for more than an hour a day. These additional calories will not be "fattening," but rather, essential fuel that supports your exercise program, feeds your brain so you don't get light headed and dizzy, and staves off gnawing hunger.

Following are some of the beliefs and barriers that complicate a sports nutrition program for bariatric athletes, at least in the first year or two postsurgery. In time, you may be able to enjoy a more typical sports diet.

- **Fuel before you exercise.** "Why would I want to eat before I exercise?" asked one of my obese clients. "I'm trying to burn calories, not eat them!" Here's why: If you eat nothing before you exercise, you'll have less stamina and endurance. Your workouts will feel like drudgery. By consuming 100 to 300 calories, as tolerated, preexercise, you will be able to exercise harder and get better results from your workouts. You will also better enjoy your exercise program, and that's important. You need to sustain an active lifestyle for the rest of your life, so you'd better enjoy what you do.

- **Find carbohydrate sources you can tolerate.** If you are like most bariathletes, you live in fear of eating carbohydrate-containing foods or fluids that will cause you to "dump" (feel shaky or light headed or experience fecal urgency). You might also be afraid to reintroduce carbohydrate if you previously have struggled with a so-called carbohydrate addiction. Yet, as you build up your exercise program, you'll benefit from finding a fruit, energy bar, or sports drink that settles well in your intestinal tract. One long-distance runner described oatmeal as a "gentle carb" that he tolerated well before a workout, but he reported that refined sugar and white flour created intestinal problems within half an hour. He could enjoy dried fruits but not pasta. Clearly, each bariatric athlete (just like each non-bariatric athlete) needs to learn through trial and error which foods settle well and how much can be tolerated at one time.

• **Monitor your urine.** People who live in large bodies commonly sweat heavily during exercise and lose significant amounts of fluid. Monitoring urine is a good way to determine whether you have adequately rehydrated your body. Your goal is to void a significant volume of urine every two to four hours throughout the day. You may need to continually drink in sips throughout the day; carry a water bottle with you! See chapter 8 for more information about fluids.

• **Take your bariatric vitamin and mineral supplements.** Bariatric patients can easily develop nutritional deficiencies, particularly of iron, vitamin B_{12}, and vitamin D. An iron deficiency can significantly impair athletic performance. A bariatric walker complained about being tired all the time and not feeling good. He wondered whether he was training too hard or his body was missing important nutrients as a result of the bypass. I encouraged him to get a blood test to determine whether anemia contributed to his fatigue. Sure enough, that was the problem.

• **Set a reasonable weight goal that you can sustain**. A distorted body image and significant amounts of excess "flesh" can skew your weight goals. One cyclist who had weighed 350 pounds (159 kg) identified 170 pounds (77 kg) as his goal weight, despite having a body fat measurement of 8 percent fat at 220 pounds (100 kg). I helped him identify a healthy and sustainable weight that was in keeping with his genetics. He had failed to acknowledge that he had gained several pounds of muscle.

Although body fat measurements can help athletes assess whether they are losing fat and building muscle, little research exists on how to accurately measure the body fat of formerly obese athletes. Yet, a simple and relatively good tool is to routinely have skinfold measurements taken with calipers. The measurements need not be translated into percent body fat (the number would likely be inaccurate) but rather simply be compared from time to time. That is, if the thickness of the skinfolds remains the same, weight gain reflects an increase in muscle weight or water weight, not body fat. And excess skin can be mistaken for excess adipose (fat) tissue, creating confusion for the athlete.

- **Give yourself permission to take a rest day with no exercise.** Bariatric athletes commonly report exercising seven days a week; many are afraid to take a day off for fear of "getting fat." Some bariatric athletes are afraid that if they stop their exercise routine even for one day, they will not start again. They become rigid and compulsive exercisers, with no days allowed for rest. Unfortunately, this creates a high risk for becoming burned out, if not injured. For others, exercise becomes an excuse to eat more, to the point of becoming an exercise bulimic. One cyclist commented, "I've created a life where I have to bike so I can eat a pleasing amount of food . . . I've traded my food addiction into an exercise addiction." If that sounds familiar, seek help from a sports dietitian or therapist.

  Instead of allowing adequate rest, they become exhausted and experience overuse injuries. Plan at least one day off per week. You may feel hungrier on rest days. Bypass athletes need to learn that such hunger is a normal request for the carbohydrate needed to refuel depleted muscles. On rest days, you can appropriately eat about the same amount of food as on exercise days. If you weigh yourself after a rest day, be forewarned: The scale might go up, because for each gram of carbohydrate stored as muscle glycogen, the muscles also store about 3 grams of water. This rapid weight gain reflects water weight, not fat weight, and better fueled muscles.

- **Plan your time wisely.** Bariatric athletes commonly exercise at least an hour a day, if not more. One client reported waking between 4:00 and 5:00 a.m. to be sure to get exercise done before the start of a busy workday. You will need excellent time-management skills so you can have time to food shop, prepare food, and eat slowly—as well as exercise.

PART III

BALANCING WEIGHT AND ACTIVITY

CHAPTER 14

ASSESSING YOUR BODY: FAT, FIT, OR FINE?

By looking at portraits from past generations in art museums, you can see that nature has always wanted humans to have some body fat. In fact, the reference (as designed by nature) 24-year-old woman is about 27 percent fat, and the reference 24-year-old man is about 15 percent fat. Some of us have more fat than others—undesired bumps and bulges, muffin tops hanging over our pants, and flab on our thighs.

Our weight-obsessed society preaches that thinner is better, and consequently, many of my clients yearn to have low-fat bodies. Women strive to be slender yet strong. Men want to be muscular and trim. Although a certain amount of leanness is desirable for health and performance, obsessions about body fatness are unhealthy. One man did 1,000 sit-ups each day, hoping to get rid of the fat on his abdomen. A woman spent hours on the stair stepper, hoping to eliminate the fat on her thighs. Both came to me asking to have their body fat measured, and both were shocked to learn that they were leaner than they thought.

Scantily clad athletes commonly see themselves as too fat, but rarely too thin. Measuring body fat can thus offer a helpful perspective about where a person is in the scheme of fatness. Body-fat measurement allows you to quantify loss of body fat or gain of muscle as you embark on your diet and exercise program. This chapter addresses bodies, body fat, and body fatness; discusses methods of body-fat measurement; and offers perspectives on fatness in relation to fitness. Even overfat people can be fit, healthy, and at peace with their bodies.

BODY FAT: WHY DO WE HAVE IT?

Although excess body fat is excess baggage that can slow us down, we need a certain amount of fat for our bodies to function normally. Fat, or adipose tissue, is an essential part of the nerves, spinal cord, brain, and cell membranes. Internal fat pads the kidneys and other organs; external fat offers a layer of protection against cold weather. For the 150-pound (68 kg) reference man, essential fat makes up about 4 percent of body weight, or 6 fat pounds (2.7 fat kg). In comparison, the 125-pound (57 kg) reference woman has about 12 percent essential fat, or 15 fat pounds (6.8 fat kg). Essential fat is the minimum level of body fatness; we all should have more fat in addition to the essential fat. Table 14.1 further describes the various levels of body fatness. Keep in mind, no one best percentage of body fat exists for athletes. The best percentage is the one that allows you to feel good, perform well, eat appropriately, and enjoy quality of life. Even athletes gain fat as they age. Table 14.2 shows targets for athletic people as they age.

Women store essential fat in their hips, thighs, and breasts. This fat is readily available to nourish a healthy baby if a woman becomes pregnant. If you are a woman fighting the battle of the bulging thighs, you may be fighting a losing battle. The fat-storing enzymes are very active in women's thighs and hips compared with women's other fat storage areas—and compared with fat storage in men's hips and thighs. Moreover, the fat-releasing enzymatic activity is low in those areas, making fat loss difficult.

TABLE 14.1 Body Fat Percentages for Men and Women and Their Classifications

Description	Men % fat	Women % fat
Essential fat	3-5	11-13
Very low fat	5-10	12-15
Low fat	11-14	16-23
Average	15-20	24-30
Above average	>20	>30

Adapted by permission from A. Jeukendrup and M. Gleeson, *Sport Nutrition: An Introduction to Energy Production and Performance*, 2nd ed. (Champaign, IL: Human Kinetics, 2010), 316.

TABLE 14.2 Body Fat Percentages Change With Age for the Average Population

Age in years	Men	Women
Up to 30	9-15%	14-21%
30-50	11-17%	15-23%
50+	12-19%	16-25%

Adapted by permission from A. Jeukendrup and M. Gleeson, *Sport Nutrition: An Introduction to Energy Production and Performance*, 2nd ed. (Champaign, IL: Human Kinetics, 2010), 316.

The easiest time for women to lose hip and thigh fat is during the last trimester of pregnancy and while breastfeeding. At those times, the activity of the fat-storing enzymes drops, and the activity of the fat-releasing enzymes increases. In this way nature is protective of a woman's ability to care for her offspring.

BODY FAT AND EXERCISE

Myths and misconceptions surrounding the role of exercise in weight management are abundant. Here is information that might update your knowledge about body fat and exercise.

If I start an exercise program, will I automatically lose body fat?

To lose body fat, you need to create an energy deficit for the entire day. That is, by bedtime, you need to have burned off more calories than you consumed that day. Exercise can contribute to the calorie deficit, but exercise is often overrated as a way to reduce body fat (Aragon et al. 2017). Exercise is better used as a tool to prevent weight gain, maintain weight loss, and improve health (Schwartz et al. 2017). Exercise can relieve stress (which can reduce stress eating), boost your metabolism, and help you feel good about yourself, and it may increase your desire to feed yourself healthfully.

Many people do lose weight by adding exercise. That happens because they start a total health campaign that includes not only adding activity but also subtracting calories. After they work out, they tend to feel less stressed; they no longer unwind after a hectic day by mindlessly snacking as they did before starting the exercise program.

But some of my clients complain that they have lost no weight despite hours of working out. That often happens because they are rewarding themselves afterward with generous amounts of calories that replace all those they burned off. They may have exercised for 30 minutes and burned off 300 calories, but then in three minutes they consumed 300 calories of "recovery food." Despite popular belief, appetite tends to keep up with your exercise load (except in extreme conditions). The more you exercise, the hungrier you will become sooner or later, and the more likely you will be to eat enough to replace the calories you burned off (Schwartz et al. 2017). Nature does a wonderful job of protecting your body from wasting away, particularly if you are already lean with little excess fat to lose.

Another factor that influences the effectiveness of exercise as a means to lose weight relates to the toll of exercise on your total daily activity. Some avid exercisers are "sedentary athletes." They put all their effort into exercising hard for one or two hours per day but then do little spontaneous activity the rest of the day. For example, a group of moderately obese college-age students who participated in a 16-month aerobic exercise program had similar daily energy expenditures before starting the program as they did at the end of the program. This is because they had become more sedentary at other times of the day (Bailey, Jacobsen, and Donnelly 2002). This pattern is common among both casual and serious exercisers, many of whom claim to maintain weight despite their hard workouts.

If you do want to use exercise to promote weight loss, think about including exercise that builds muscle. Unlike aerobic exercise that burns calories primarily during the exercise session but very little thereafter, strength training builds muscles that boost your metabolism throughout the entire day and night. Muscle tissue actively burns calories. The more muscle mass you have, the more calories you burn just sitting around.

Will I lose more weight if I do low-intensity "fat burning" exercise instead of high-intensity exercise that burns carbohydrate?

Some people believe that the key to body-fat loss is doing fat-burning exercise, or low-intensity exercise that uses more fat than carbohydrate (muscle glycogen) for fuel. Wrong. The key to body-fat loss is to consume fewer calories by the end of the day than you burned. Studies have shown that burning fat during exercise does not affect loss of body fat (Zelasko 1995). But because you can sustain low-intensity exercise for longer than you can sustain high-intensity exercise, you can easily burn off more calories in, let's say, 60 minutes of jogging (600 calories) than in 10 minutes of fast running (150 calories).

High-intensity exercise may actually contribute to a lower percentage of body fat (Yoshioka et al. 2001). Research on 1,366 women and 1,257 men shows that those who performed high-intensity exercise tended to have less body fat than those who performed lower-intensity fat-burning exercise (Tremblay et al. 1990). Yet, a review of studies on CrossFit, Insanity, Gym Jones, and other extreme conditioning programs showed little or no effect on body fatness and indicates a need for more research (Tibana and Sousa 2018). If you choose to exercise harder, be sure to exercise wisely to reduce the risk of injury—warm up, stretch, and don't do too much too soon. Keep in mind that you may not enjoy high-intensity activity as much and end up exercising less as a result. But you might enjoy it even more than the less-challenging options. Just be sure the E in your exercise program stands for *enjoyment*, not *excruciating*.

Do men lose weight faster than women lose weight?

Nature seems to work hard to protect women's body-fat stores. In terms of evolution, nature wants women to have fat and be fertile; men are supposed to be lean hunters. In one study of previously sedentary normal-weight men and women who participated in an 18-month marathon training program, the men reported increasing their food intake by about 500 calories per day and the women reported increasing by only 60 calories, despite having added 50 miles per week of running. The men lost about 5 pounds (2.4 kg) of fat; the women lost less than 2 pounds (1 kg) of fat, despite reporting (with questionable accuracy) a larger calorie deficit (Janssen, Graef, and Saris 1989). Similarly, other studies suggest that normal-weight women fail to lose significant amounts of fat when they add exercise.

In a study of previously sedentary overweight males and females (average age 22 to 24) who did fitness exercise five times a week for 16 months with no dietary restrictions, the men lost 12 pounds (5.4 kg), and body fat dropped from 27 to 22 percent. They didn't eat extra to compensate for the additional calories they burned. The women, however, experienced no significant weight or body-fat changes; their appetites kept up with their calorie expenditures (Kirk, Donnelly, and Jacobsen 2002). As one of my female clients complained, "I've been running for 10 years, and I still haven't lost one pound." She's not the only one!

To reduce the fat around my abdomen and hips, should I do lots of sit-ups every day?

When you lose fat, you lose it everywhere, not just from the part of your body you are working most vigorously. Moreover, you need to create a calorie deficit for the entire day to reduce body fat. Muscle movement itself does not result in loss of body fat. For example, the man who did 1,000 sit-ups every day trying to burn off the fat in his abdomen certainly built strong abdominal muscles, but he failed to create a calorie deficit and lose abdominal fat.

Why do I get dimpled cellulite on my thighs—and how can I get rid of it?

Cellulite is fat that has a bumpy orange-peel appearance and often appears on the hips, thighs, and buttocks. The fat is deposited in pockets just below the surface of the skin. Although much is written about cellulite, little is understood about it. Some medical professionals believe that the dimpled appearance of cellulite may result from restrictions of the connective tissue that separates fat cells into compartments. If you overeat and fill the fat cells, the compartmental restrictions may cause the fat to bulge.

Cellulite is more of a problem for women than it is for men because women have thinner skin and their fat compartments are larger and more rounded. Also, women tend to deposit fat in their hips, thighs, and buttocks, areas in which cellulite appears easily. In contrast, men tend to deposit fat around their waists. A genetic predisposition toward cellulite may exist. If a mother has cellulite, the daughter is likely to acquire it as well. Cellulite affects 80 to 90 percent of postpubertal women (Friedmann, Vick, and Mishra 2017). Cellulite generally appears as a person ages because the skin loses its elasticity and becomes thinner. You get rid of it by eating fewer calories; when you lose fat, you lose it everywhere, including the cellulite.

If you are exercising primarily to lose weight, I encourage you to separate exercise and weight. You should exercise for health, fitness, stress relief, and, most important, enjoyment. I discourage you from exercising primarily to burn calories. Under those conditions, exercise feels like punishment for having excess body fat. You'll likely quit your exercise program sooner or later because you are not having fun.

Your job is to find an exercise program that has purpose and meaning so that you will enjoy incorporating some type of exercise into your daily schedule for the rest of your life. Consider these examples:

- Jim bought a dog and is now walking the dog 3 miles (about 5 km) per day.
- David enjoys gardening in the summer and walking in the woods in the winter.
- Gretchen, a busy executive, takes a 30-minute walk at lunch to relieve stress and process her feelings.
- Sherri commutes to work by bicycle.
- Kevin joined a marathon-training program.

Although exercise without a calorie deficit fails to result in weight loss, we do know that exercise is important for maintaining weight loss and improving health. People who burn off 1,000 to 2,000 calories per week with purposeful exercise tend to be leaner and healthier than sedentary people. Again, find an exercise program that has purpose and meaning.

BODY IMAGE

Monique, a competitive high school swimmer, was sensitive about her bulky body and described herself as "feeling fat." As I measured her body fat, she anxiously awaited the decisive moment. "You are actually very lean, Monique," I said. "You simply have a lot of muscle and a big bone structure. You have very little excess fat."

Visual appearance and body weight are deceptive for athletes who tend to compare themselves with their teammates. Humans, like animals, come in different sizes and shapes, most of which are genetically determined. Although you can change your body to a certain extent by losing fat or building muscle, you can't do a complete makeover. Even if you lose the excess baggage, sometimes you still won't end up with the body you want. A bulldog will never become a Chihuahua.

If you are a woman who has large thighs (like all the women in your family), or if you are a man who hates your "love handles" (which all the men in your family have), you need to be realistic in your expectations. You can trim the fat on your thighs or around your waist a bit by creating a calorie deficit, but you are unlikely to get it to vanish. Rather than obsess about your body fat, I recommend that you let go of your dissatisfaction with your physique, accept yourself for the sincere and caring person you are, appreciate your body for all the wonderful things it does for you, learn to tolerate your body for what it is not, and focus on the relationships in life that really matter. You can waste a lot of mental energy fretting about undesired body fat.

Genetics plays a large role in how we look. Just as some of us have thick hair, others have thin hair. Some of us have blue eyes, and others have brown. No one seems to care about hair thickness or eye color, but our weight-obsessed society has made us all care about body fatness. As a result, too many self-conscious people feel inadequate because of repeated failures at transforming themselves into a shape they aren't meant to be.

FACT OR FICTION

Most active people feel good about their bodies.

The facts: Few athletes naturally possess their desired physique. Most of us are ordinary mortals, complete with bumps, bulges, fat, and fleshiness. About one-third of all Americans are truly dissatisfied with their appearance, women more than men. A woman will most commonly complain about her thighs, abdomen, breasts, and buttocks. A man expresses dissatisfaction with his abdomen, upper body, and balding scalp. Sometimes the problem is imaginary (such as when the skater with anorexia complains about her fat thighs); sometimes it is real and ranges from a mild complaint about love handles that hang over the running shorts to a major preoccupation with flabby thighs that results in relentless dieting and exercise.

Remember that your value as a friend, colleague, or lover does not depend on your physical appearance. Your beauty comes from the inside. Your concern about how you look can be a mask for how you feel about yourself. People who obsess about their imperfect bodies commonly have low self-esteem. Somehow, they believe they are not good enough.

Body Dysmorphic Disorder

Body dysmorphic disorder (BDD)—a preoccupation with an imagined defect in appearance or an excessive concern for a slight physical defect such as crooked teeth, baldness, or a long nose—is on the rise. People with BDD feel socially anxious, believing that everyone around them is seeing their perceived flaws and judging their appearance. Even lean athletes, men and women alike, are not immune to the epidemic of body dissatisfaction, despite their fitness. Many perceive themselves as having unacceptable bodies, and this perception can lead to the development of eating disorders. The best predictor of an eating disorder is a struggle with body image.

What you look like on the outside should have little to do with how you feel on the inside.

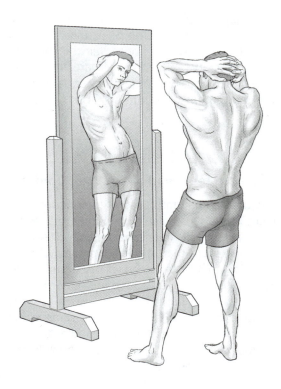

But in reality, many people think like this:

1. I have a defect (fat thighs) that makes me different from others.
2. Other people notice this difference.
3. My looks affect how these people see me—as repulsive and undesirable.
4. I'm bad, inadequate, and not good enough.

This type of thinking is common among young dancers who develop hips and thighs as they blossom from girls into women, runners who feel

Muscle Dysmorphia

Some men want to see how big they can get. They are obsessed with thoughts that they are too small and do not have enough muscle mass. This is called muscle dysmorphia, an obsessive–compulsive disorder that is a subtype of BDD. Muscle dysmorphia is sometimes called "bigorexia" because it is the opposite of anorexia (Leone, Sedory, and Gray 2005).

In most cases, these men are not small at all; they are "ripped" and may compete in bodybuilding competitions. Many lift weights for an extraordinary number of hours at the gym, stare at themselves in the mirror excessively, spend large amounts of money on supplements, and may take dangerous steroids and other drugs to bulk up. As one man commented, "Why should I be Clark Kent when I can be Superman?" (Olivardia 2002).

Not all athletes who want to build muscle have muscle dysmorphia. Just as lifting weights three times a week can be healthy, lifting weights for five hours every day means you likely have a problem. Here are some diagnostic questions you can ask yourself to determine whether this applies to you:

- Have your relationships with others been affected by your rigid exercise and diet regimens?
- Do you spend too much time exercising with the intent to bulk up rather than to improve your sports performance?
- Do you spend too much time thinking about your appearance?
- Do you devote too much money to enhancing your physical appearance?

pressure to be thinner, exercise leaders who believe that every student is scrutinizing their bulges, and numerous other people who believe they have imperfect bodies.

In traditional thinking, men are not supposed to be concerned about how they look because it could be seen as feminine or weak. Women, however, have grown up in a society with ads and social media messages that tell women they are not good enough as they are. (Color your hair. Wear make-up. Buy black clothing that makes you look thinner.) Although women historically have been the prime target for body makeovers, today's men are experiencing the same pressure. Both men and women struggle with body image issues.

If you believe your body image issues are taking control of your life, seek help from a therapist familiar with this disorder. Also refer to the resources in appendix A.

Learn to Love Your Body

Many people believe that the best solution to body dissatisfaction is to lose weight, pump iron, or do thousands of sit-ups. This "outside" approach to find happiness tends to be inadequate. Concern about what you look like is commonly a mask for how you feel about yourself, your self-esteem. Given that about 25 percent of your self-esteem is tied to how you look, you'll have a hard time feeling good about yourself unless you like your body and feel confident about your appearance. Weight issues are often self-esteem issues.

The best approach to resolving your body-shape issues is to learn to be grateful for, accept, and tolerate the body you have. You can slightly redesign the house that nature gave you, but you can't totally remodel it, at least not without paying a high price of restrictive dieting and compulsive exercising for the rest of your life.

If you are struggling with your body image, you need to think back to identify when you first got the message that something was wrong with your body. Perhaps it was a parent who lovingly remarked that you looked good in an outfit for a special occasion—but you'd look even better if only you'd lose some weight. Maybe it was the siblings who teased you about your flabby thighs. Then, you need to take the following steps to be at peace with your body and learn to like yourself and your body:

- Rename your disliked body part (e.g., rename "ugly jelly belly" a more loving "round tummy").
- Identify the parts of your body you do like.
- Give yourself credit for your attractive body parts with positive talk.

If you find yourself obsessing about the look of your body, give yourself permission to live your life in a healthier way. The Declaration of Independence From a Weight-Obsessed World section in this chapter provides a positive way to start accepting your body as it is. Dwelling on the negative will get you nowhere. Instead, be grateful for all the good things your body does for you. It rides bikes, lifts weights at the gym, goes canoeing, and lets you have fun. How could you enjoy sports without your body? Remember that healthy bodies come in many sizes and shapes, including fat but fit.

Declaration of Independence From a Weight-Obsessed World

I declare, from this day forward, I will choose to live my life by the following tenets. In doing so, I declare myself free and independent from the pressures and constraints of a weight-obsessed world.

- I will accept my body in its natural size and shape.
- I will celebrate all that my body can do for me each day.
- I will treat my body with respect, give it enough rest, fuel it with a variety of foods, exercise it moderately, and listen to what it needs.
- I will choose to resist our society's pressures to judge myself and other people on physical characteristics like body weight, shape, or size. I will respect people based on their depth of character and the impact of their accomplishments.
- I will refuse to deny my body valuable nutrients by dieting or using weight-loss products.
- I will avoid categorizing foods as either "good" or "bad." I will not associate guilt or shame with eating certain foods. Instead, I will nourish my body with a balance of foods, listening and responding to what it needs.
- I will not use food to mask my emotional needs.
- I will not avoid participating in activities that I enjoy (e.g., swimming, dancing, eating a meal) simply because I am self-conscious about the way my body looks. I will recognize that I have the right to enjoy any activity regardless of my body shape or size.
- I will believe that my self-esteem and identity come from within!

Courtesy of the National Eating Disorders Association, www.nationaleatingdisorders.org.

To start improving your relationship with your body, close your eyes and imagine that you have your desired body. Visualize the confident carriage, verbal expression, and body language you would use. Open your eyes and assume those characteristics. With practice, you'll come to learn that appearance is only skin deep and that your real worth is the meaningful relationships you have with your family and friends. You'll be able to muster the courage to face intimidating situations. You can even put on that bathing suit and feel at peace!

DON'T PLAY THE NUMBERS GAME

Some people give too much power to the number on the bathroom scale. Jean, a dedicated exerciser, resorted to keeping her scale in the trunk of her car because it too easily ruined her day. Ivan, a marathoner, said, "One morning I got so mad at the scale. It told me I'd gained 3 pounds, and I'd been starving myself for half a week. I angrily jumped up and down on it until it broke. That's the last time I've weighed myself!" Ivan can laugh now when he recalls that story, but he wasn't laughing at the time.

If you worry about your weight, I advise against weighing yourself daily. You'll likely refer to yourself as being *good* when your weight drops and *bad* when it goes up. Nonsense. You are the same lovable person, regardless of a pound (or kilo) or two either way.

A scale measures not only fat but also muscle gain, water, food, intestinal contents, the coffee you drank just before weighing yourself, and so on. The scale often gives irrelevant information. For example, if you increase your exercise program, decrease your food intake, build up muscle, and lose fat, the scale may indicate that your weight has remained the same. You will feel thinner, look thinner, and your clothes will be looser, but you will not gain psychological rewards if you depend on the scale.

Some athletes play games with the scales and fool only themselves. For example, runners, racquetball players, and other athletes who perspire heavily often prefer to weigh themselves after a hard workout. During exercise, they may have lost 5 pounds (2.3 kg) of sweat, not fat.

The only time to weigh yourself (if you insist) is first thing in the morning. Get up, empty your bladder and bowels, and then step on the scale before you eat or drink anything. You'll be weighing your body, pure and simple. If you weigh yourself at the end of the day, you'll also be weighing your dinner, beverages, and other foods in your intestines.

Also, remember that weight, like height, is more than a matter of willpower. When it comes to height, you have likely accepted the fact that you can't force yourself to grow 6 inches (15 cm). But when it comes to weight, you may demand that your body lose an inappropriate amount of weight.

Certainly, if you are overfat, you can reduce to an appropriate level of body fatness. Weighing yourself weekly can provide positive reinforcement. But if you are already a lean athlete who is struggling to drop those final 5 pounds (2.3 kg) below an appropriate weight, you may feel like a failure and question your self-worth: Why can't I do something as simple as lose 5 pounds? (Because it's not simple! Nature intervenes and hinders inappropriate fat loss.)

Some athletes are in a difficult situation when it comes to meeting the weight demands of their sports. Wrestlers, gymnasts, ballet dancers, and figure skaters participate in sports systems that do not accommodate athletes as designed by nature. This circumstance raises ethical concerns. Should genetically stocky people be discouraged from ballet, figure skating, gymnastics, and other sports that favor thinness? Should rowers be encouraged to drop 15 pounds (7 kg) to reach a lower weight class? How can the governing bodies of such sports accommodate the fact that health is more important than weight? These are tough questions.

HOW MUCH SHOULD I WEIGH?

Although only nature knows the best weight for your body, the following guidelines offer a method to estimate the midpoint of a healthy weight range (plus or minus 10 percent, depending on whether you have large or small bones). This rule-of-thumb guide does *not* apply to everybody—especially people with muscular bodies, including bodybuilders and football players.

- **Women:** 100 pounds for the first 5 feet of height, 5 pounds per inch thereafter (45 kg for the first 152 cm, 0.9 kg/cm thereafter)
- **Men:** 106 pounds for the first 5 feet of height, 6 pounds per inch thereafter (48 kg for the first 152 cm, 1 kg/cm thereafter)

For example, a woman who is 5 feet 6 inches (168 cm) could appropriately weigh 100 + 30 = 130 pounds (45 + 14 = 59 kg), with a range of 117 to 143 pounds (53 to 65 kg). A man who is 5 feet 10 inches (178 cm) could appropriately weigh 106 + 60 = 166 pounds (48 + 27 = 75 kg), with a range of 149 to 183 (68 to 83 kg).

Although athletes commonly want to be leaner than the average person, heed this message: If you are striving to weigh significantly (more than 10 percent) less than the weight estimated by this guideline, think again. Pay attention to the genetic design for your body, and don't struggle to get too light. The best weight goal is to be fit and healthy rather than starved and skinny.

If you are significantly overfat, your initial target should be to lose just 5 to 10 percent of your current weight. If you weigh 200 pounds (91 kg), losing just 10 to 20 pounds (5 to 10 kg) is enough to improve your health status and significantly reduce your risk of heart disease, diabetes, and high blood pressure. Although you may want to lose more fat for cosmetic reasons, you should know that losing the initial few pounds, or kilograms, is a meaningful accomplishment.

Body Mass Index

Although some people believe that determining body mass index (BMI) is a good way to screen for overfatness in athletes, it is actually a poor one because it is a ratio of body weight to height; it accounts for body mass, not body fat. Hulky football players, weightlifters, and other power athletes who have lots of muscle mass easily get ranked as obese (BMI greater than 30); this is generally far from the truth.

In the general population, people with a BMI greater than 25 are considered to have excess body fat and to be at risk of developing heart disease, diabetes, and other medical concerns. Yet, in a study of 28 collegiate hockey players, the average BMI was 26 (overweight), but the average body fat was a lean 13 percent (Ode et al. 2007). The definition of overweight does not begin or end with BMI.

In my counseling practice, I use BMI to determine who is too thin. If you have normal musculature, an appropriate BMI is 18.5 to 24.9. When an athlete's BMI is less than 18.5, I need to rule out the possibility of anorexia. To determine whether you fit this underweight category, search the Web for "body mass index calculator" and you'll find many websites where you can assess your BMI.

Body-Fat Measurements

When I counsel athletes who have a poor concept of an appropriate weight, I measure their body fat rather than rely on scales and height and weight charts. The fat measurement helps put in perspective the proportion of an athlete's body that is muscle, bone, essential fat, and excess flab. A scale provides a meaningless number because it doesn't indicate the composition of the weight. Obviously, the muscle weight contributes to top athletic performance in most sports. The fat weight is the bigger concern because excess fat can slow you down.

Believe me, judging from the tension that radiates from the body of a weight-conscious athlete, I believe that getting your body fat measured ranks high on the list of anxiety-provoking life experiences. This number unveils the truth. Hulky football players are often humbled to learn that 20 percent of their brawn is flab. Weight-conscious gymnasts are often thrilled to learn that they are leaner than they thought they were.

If you want to have your body fat measured, you'll certainly want to have it done correctly by a qualified health professional to eliminate any possibility of being told that you are fatter than you really are. Inaccurate readings can send people into a tizzy. If you later want to be remeasured, try to have it done by the same person using the same technique to ensure consistency.

Keep in mind that body-fat measurements should include a conversation about an appropriate weight for your body. They say nothing about genetics. If you are far leaner than other members of your genetic family but still have a higher percentage of fat than you desire, you may already be lean for your body. For example, a 5-foot 6-inch (168 cm) walker lost 50 pounds (23 kg), from 200 to 150 pounds (91 to 68 kg) and wanted to reach a seemingly appropriate weight goal of 130 pounds (59 kg). Because she couldn't seem to lose beyond 150 pounds (68 kg) without severely restricting her intake, I measured her body fat. She was 28 percent fat, at the higher end of average but far leaner than anyone else in her family. I

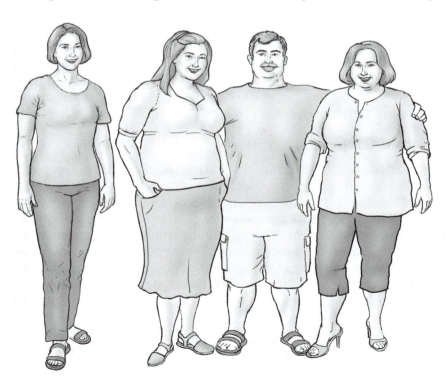

suggested that she be at peace with this healthier weight and remember that she was currently thin for her genetics. The best weight for her body was the weight she could achieve and maintain with a healthy lifestyle and healthy eating pattern.

When it comes to measuring body fat, no simple, inexpensive method is 100 percent accurate. Common methods such as air displacement (e.g., Bod Pod), skinfold calipers, and electrical impedance scales (e.g., Tanita and Seca brands) can all potentially produce inaccurate measurements. The following information evaluates these options to help you decide the best way to estimate your ideal weight should you want to quantify the fats of life.

Bod Pod

The Bod Pod is a podlike chamber that has a top that swings open and a seat inside. The person sits inside, scantily clad. (Standard clothing takes up space and alters the reading, so the person should wear spandex clothing and a bathing cap). The technician closes the top of the Bod Pod and then takes air-pressure measurements that determine body volume from air displacement. These measurements are then translated into percent body fat.

When using the Bod Pod, be sure to follow the instructions to refrain from eating, drinking, and exercising two hours before the measurement. A group of athletes were measured to be 21.3 percent body fat before running on a treadmill for 30 minutes. When they were tested after exercising they measured 19.6 percent body fat. That 2 percent drop was not caused by a loss of body fat, but rather to inaccuracy related to elevated body temperature (Otterstetter et al. 2012). In general, Bod Pod measurements may underestimate body fatness by 2 to 3 percent (Ackland et al. 2012).

Skinfold Calipers

Skinfold calipers are more convenient and less sensational than other methods of body-fat measurement. The calipers are large pinchers that measure the thickness of the fat layer at specific body sites. Skinfold calipers are the most accurate of affordable ways for consumers to measure body fat (Peterson et al. 2007). However, health professionals well trained in the technique are the most qualified to use this method. Active people often obtain their measurements from students or novice technicians who may be using imprecise or poorly calibrated calipers at crowded health fairs or fitness events. Little errors can translate inaccurately into high body-fat readings.

Even accurate measurements commonly translate into erroneous information because of inappropriate conversion equations. To be most accurate, the measurements from runners, wrestlers, bodybuilders, and gymnasts should be plugged into sport-specific conversion equations. Such equations are seldom used for the average athlete who gets tested at a fitness center or health fair.

Skinfold caliper measurements are an excellent way to measure changes in body composition (fat loss, muscle gain). I often record on a monthly basis the measurements of people losing a significant amount of weight through regular exercise. By comparing the numbers (measurements in millimeters, with or without converting into percent fat), the dieters can monitor changes. Athletes recovering from anorexia may appreciate periodic skinfold measurements to see that they are rebuilding muscle, not just gaining fat. As with other methods to assess body fat, this use of calipers may not give a 100 percent accurate picture, but it does a good job of showing trends, particularly when the same technician measures the person each time, using the same calipers and same conversion equations.

Bioelectrical Impedance Analysis

Measuring body composition by bioelectrical impedance is a simple procedure that takes just minutes to perform. You just step on a "scale" (such as Tanita or Seca) or hold a device (e.g., Omron) that sends an imperceptible electrical current through the body. The amount of water in the body affects the opposition to the flow of the current (impedance). Because water is found only in fat-free tissue, the current flow can be translated into percent body fat. As a result, it's relatively accurate if you are hydrated appropriately, but for sweaty athletes it is often less accurate than skinfold calipers. If you measure yourself after you exercise, you'll likely register a lower percentage of fat than you would preexercise because hydration affects the reading (Demura et al. 2002). As one of my clients reported, "I can be anywhere between 9 and 14 percent body fat, depending on when I use my Tanita scale."

Other factors that may affect the accuracy of the measurement include ethnic background, premenstrual bloat, food in the stomach, and carbohydrate-loaded muscles (water is stored along with the carbohydrate). The calculations are based on the assumption that the standard person is 73 percent water. Research has shown that young people tend to be 77 percent water, and older folks, 71 percent. If you are improperly positioned during the test (say, with part of your arms touching your body), you will also get an inaccurate reading. This error can easily happen in crowded exhibitions.

What's the Use?

Until researchers find the definitive, affordable, and easy method to measure body fat, here's my advice. Consider body-fat measurement as

TABLE 14.3 Body-Fat Measurements Across Devices

Device	Body-fat measurement*	Price (USD)
Omron HBF-510W: hand-to-foot BIA	26.1%	$90
Tanita BF-350: foot-to-foot scale	21.7%	$800
Tanita BF-522: foot-to-foot scale	21.7%	$365
DXA (researchers' gold standard)	21.06%	At least $25,000
Skinfold calipers: medical grade	19.5%	$250
Omron HBF-306C: hand-to-hand BIA	18.4%	$50

*This is the average measurement for a group of subjects across all devices.

Selected data from ACSM 59th Annual Meeting and 3rd World Congress abstract. J.T. Barnes, J.D. Wag-ganer, J.P. Loenneke, R.D. Williams, Y. Arja, G. Kirby, and T.J. Pujol, 2012, "Validity of bioelectrical impedance analysis instruments for the measurement of body composition in collegiate gymnasts," *Medicine & Science in Sports & Exercise* 44(5S).

a comparative tool to reflect changes in your body as you lose fat, gain muscle, shape up, and slim down. It is only one part of your health and performance profile and should not be a defining factor.

Don't expect more accuracy than is possible. The standard error is plus or minus 3 percent. Hence, if you are measured at 15 percent, you might be 12 percent or 18 percent. That doesn't take into account another 3 percent biological error because of individual variations in body fatness.

Just as weighing yourself on different scales results in different values, having your body fat measured by different people using different methods also results in different body-fat numbers. In a study done on collegiate gymnasts (Barnes et al. 2012), body fat ranged from 18.45 to 26.1 percent, with the least expensive method (Omron) being the least accurate compared to dual-energy X-ray absorptiometry (DXA), a gold standard method used primarily by researchers (table 14.3).

Your best bet is to see how the measurements change over time. Have the same person measure you at regular intervals to help you assess trends in your body-fat changes. But the measurements likely will tell you nothing you didn't already know from looking at yourself in the mirror or from the fit of your clothing.

LISTEN TO YOUR BODY

I strongly recommend that instead of entrusting your fate to an unreliable number, you listen to your body. Each person has a set-point weight at which the body tends to hover. You may slightly overeat one day and slightly undereat the next, but your weight will stay more or less the same. If you drop below this natural weight, your body will start to complain. You may fight a nagging hunger, become obsessed with food, and feel chronically fatigued. On the other hand, if you are above your set point, you will feel uncomfortable and flabby.

My experience in counseling athletes of all ages and weights indicates that you likely do know your comfortable weight zone. As Tricia, a 5-foot 2-inch masters swimmer, acknowledged, "I can diet down to 110 pounds (50 kg), an appropriate weight for the average person of my height. But I don't stay there. My body prefers to be between 117 and 120 (53 and 54 kg). That's heavier than most people my height, but that's what's normal for me and where I fit in with the rest of my family. Everyone is heavyset."

She had learned through years of unsuccessful dieting that she would never be able to fit her ideal image of perfectly thin. She has now accepted her build, learned to tolerate her body fat, and recognizes that she can healthfully participate in sports regardless of the few extra pounds. Weight, after all, is more than a matter of willpower, and happiness does not come from thinness. Your best weight is the weight that you can achieve and maintain with a healthy lifestyle.

CHAPTER 15

GAINING WEIGHT
THE HEALTHY WAY

To listen to all the ads for diets and diet foods, one might think that the only people who struggle with weight concerns are those who want to lose body fat. Yet a significant number of people, primarily teenage boys and young men, with a sprinkling of young women, struggle to gain weight. In a survey of 400 young men aged 13 to 18 (grades 7 to 12), 25 percent had deliberately tried to gain weight in the past 12 months (O'Dea and Rawstorne 2001). They wanted to bulk up by building bigger muscles so they could be stronger, have a better body image, improve their sports performance, and better protect themselves in sports that involved physical contact (football, soccer, rugby, hockey, boxing).

For those struggling to gain weight, eating can be a task, food a medicine, and the food bills an economic drain. Many skinny athletes devour doughnuts, ice cream, and french fries to help them pump in calories, less expensively but unhealthfully. They often wonder about weight-gain drinks and protein shakes, believing that ordinary food is not good enough. That is not the case.

FACT OR FICTION

A 13-year-old boy is too young to start lifting weights to bulk up for, say, football.

The facts: A well-supervised strength training program with a special emphasis on technique and safety (to prevent stress on immature bones and ligaments) can help boys in early adolescence grow stronger and prevent injuries. This differs from a powerlifting program, and it will not contribute to bulkier muscles until boys have enough male hormones to support muscular development. (This corresponds with the growth of adultlike pubic hair.) Boys generally bulk up after they have finished their growth spurts. Many need to be reminded that patience is a virtue!

If you are feeling self-consciously thin, dislike your skinny image, and seem to eat nonstop in the hope of putting a little meat on your bones, the information in this chapter, along with the protein information in chapter 7, can give you the knowledge you need to reach your goal healthfully. If your family and friends tell you that you "look great" but you don't believe them, you might want to read the body image information in chapter 14. Perhaps the problem is not your body but a distorted relationship with your body.

INCREASING YOUR WEIGHT

Theoretically, to gain 1 pound (0.5 kg) of body weight per week, you'd need to consume an additional 500 calories per day above your typical intake. Nature easily confounds this mathematical approach; some people are hard gainers and require more calories than other people do to add weight. In one landmark research study (Sims 1976), 200 prisoners with no family history of obesity volunteered to be gluttons. The goal was to gain 20 to 25 percent above their normal weights (30 to 40 lb [14 to 18 kg]) by deliberately overeating. For more than half a year, the prisoners ate extravagantly and exercised minimally. Yet only 20 of the 200 prisoners managed to gain the weight. Of those, only 2 (who had an undetected family history of obesity or diabetes) gained the weight easily. One prisoner tried for 30 weeks to add 12 pounds (5 kg) to his 132-pound (60 kg) frame, but he couldn't get any heavier.

A varied response was also seen in another study of identical twins who were overfed by 1,000 calories for 100 days. Some twin pairs gained only 9.5 pounds (4.3 kg) each, whereas others gained 29 pounds (13.2 kg). Twin pairs gained a similar amount of weight, suggesting strong genetic control (Bouchard 1990).

This discrepancy mystifies researchers. What happened to the excess calories that didn't turn into fat? Some say the body adjusts its metabolism to maintain a predetermined genetic weight (Leibel, Rosenbaum, and Hirsch 1995). Others look at increases in fidgeting and greater spontaneous movement in daily life (Levine, Eberhardt, and Jensen 1999).

If you are a hard gainer, take a good look at your genetic endowment. If other family members are thin, you probably have inherited a genetic predisposition to thinness. You can alter your physique to a certain extent with diet, weight training, and maturing, but you shouldn't expect miracles. A Kenyan marathoner will never look like a hulky Polish bodybuilder, no matter how much eating and weightlifting he does.

Among my clients, I've observed that hard gainers are fidgeters. They twiddle their fingers, swing their legs back and forth while sitting, and seem unable to sit still. All this involuntary movement burns calories. In comparison, the people who complain about their inability to lose weight generally sit calmly. I tell the fidgeters to mellow out. Chronic fidgeting might burn an extra 300 to 350 calories per day, if not more.

The technical term for this spontaneous movement is nonexercise activity thermogenesis, or NEAT. NEAT includes not only fidgeting but also pacing while you talk on the phone and standing (not sitting) while you talk with a teammate. If you overeat, activation of NEAT helps you dissipate excess energy by nudging you to putter around the house more, choose to shoot some hoops, or (yikes!) feel motivated to vacuum and clean the house. Your level of NEAT can predict how resistant you'll be to gaining weight (Levine, Eberhardt, and Jensen 1999).

Researchers don't understand the source of this increased activity, but they do know that people (such as athletes) with higher $\dot{V}O_2$max (a measure of athletic potential) are genetically predisposed to spend more time being active throughout the day. Hence, the natural ability to be active for long periods might be connected to both NEAT and leanness. In contrast, unfit people (with a lower $\dot{V}O_2$max) tend to perform less spontaneous movement, and that can lead to weight gain (Novak et al. 2010). Stay tuned for more information on the genetics of activity.

EXTRA PROTEIN TO BUILD MUSCLES?

Most people who want to bulk up believe that the best way to gain weight is to lift weights (true) and eat a very high-protein diet (false). Although you do want to eat an adequate amount of protein, your body doesn't store excess protein as bulging muscles. The pound of steak just doesn't convert into bigger biceps. You need extra calories, and those calories should come primarily from extra carbohydrate rather than extra protein. Carbohydrate fuels your muscles so they can perform intense muscle-building exercise. By

FACT OR FICTION

Eating extra protein will help a 12-year-old boy grow faster.

The facts: No amount of extra protein will speed the growth process. Boys generally grow fastest between the ages of 12 and 15. After this growth spurt, they have enough male hormones to add muscle mass and start to grow beards ("peach fuzz"). This growth spurt lasts longer in boys than it does in girls. After the growth spurt, boys continue to grow slowly until about age 20.

overloading the muscle not with protein but with weightlifting and other resistance exercise, the muscle fibers increase in size.

You are most likely to gain weight if you consistently eat larger-than-normal meals. I often counsel skinny athletes who swear they eat huge amounts of food. Aaron, a swimmer, swore that he ate at least twice what his friends did. But he ate only two meals per day. Because he swam both before and after school, he lacked time to enjoy a hearty breakfast and afternoon snack. He found time to eat only lunch and dinner. Granted, he did eat a lot at those meals, but that merely compensated for the lack of breakfast and snacks.

Aaron gained 3 pounds (1.4 kg) within three weeks of starting to eat three meals per day and an additional snack (actually, a second lunch) on a consistent basis. "I now look at food as my weight-gain medicine and have chosen to become more responsible and plan ahead so I have food with me at the right times. There are days when I'm rushed and almost forget about gathering my breakfast on the go—two energy bars and two juice boxes on my way to school. I've learned to put a big note on my swim bag, and that helps me remember to pack my sports breakfast. I'm enjoying the benefits—more energy, less morning hunger, plus a few more pounds of good weight."

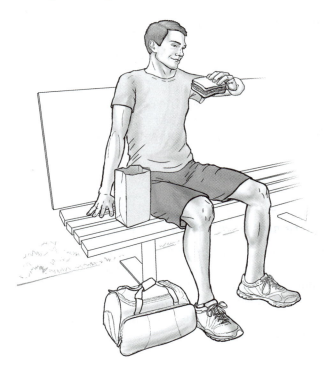

Keith, a 6-foot 4-inch high school basketball player, expressed a different complaint about his efforts to gain weight. He felt embarrassed whenever he ate with his friends because he'd eat twice what they did. A large pizza was no challenge. When I calculated his energy needs, he began to understand why he wasn't gaining weight. He needed about 5,000 calories per day to maintain his weight, plus more to gain weight. The pizza was 1,800 calories. Two pizzas would have been more appropriate.

I told Keith to feed his body what it needed and stop comparing his food intake with that of his shorter friends. I suggested that he explain to any teasers that his body was like a limousine that needed more gas to go the distance. I also suggested he snack on peanut butter and jelly sandwiches for between-meal snacks.

BOOSTING YOUR CALORIES

The trick to gaining weight is to eat larger-than-normal portions consistently for three or four meals per day and one or two snacks. If you have a busy schedule, finding the time to eat can be the biggest challenge to boosting your calories. You might need to pack a stash of portable snacks in your gym bag if you do most of your eating outside the home. To take in the extra calories needed to gain weight, you should eat frequently throughout the day, if that fits your lifestyle. Plan to have food on hand for every eating opportunity, or try these three tips: 1) Eat an extra snack such as a peanut butter sandwich with a glass of milk midmorning, 2) drink 100 percent fruit juice instead of water, and 3) choose calorie-dense foods.

If you eat foods that are compact and dense (e.g., granola instead of Cheerios), more calories can fit into your stomach with less volume. Keith became an avid food-label reader. He learned that 8 ounces (240 ml) of orange juice has 110 calories, whereas 8 ounces of cran-apple juice has 160 calories; a cup of green beans has 40 calories, a cup of corn, 140; a cup of Bran Flakes, 200 calories, a cup of granola, 780. He then chose more calorie-dense foods. That also saved him time needed for eating.

When you make your food selections, keep in mind that fat is the most concentrated form of calories. One teaspoon of fat (butter, oil, or mayonnaise) has 36 calories; the same amount of carbohydrate or protein has only 16 calories. Most protein-rich foods contain fat (such as the cream in cheese, the grease in hamburgers, and the oil in peanut butter), so these foods tend to be high in calories. Go easy on the bad-for-your-health saturated fat in meats, baked goods (butter cookies, pie crust, cakes), and ice cream.

Try to limit your intake of bad fat and focus on healthy fat, as found in peanut butter, walnuts, almonds, avocado, olive oil, and oily fish such as salmon and tuna. You should still eat a basic carbohydrate-rich sports diet; filling up on too much fatty food leaves your muscles underfueled.

The following foods and beverages can help you healthfully boost your calorie intake:

- **Cold cereal.** Choose dense cereals (as opposed to flaked and puffed types), such as granola, Grape-Nuts, and muesli. Top with nuts, sunflower seeds, ground flaxseed, chia seeds, raisins, bananas, or other fruits.

- **Hot cereal.** Cooking with milk instead of water adds calories and nutritional value. Add still more calories with mix-ins such as powdered milk, peanut butter, slivered almonds, sunflower seeds, wheat germ, ground flaxseed, walnut oil, and dried fruit.

- **Juices.** Apple, cranberry, cran-apple, grape, pineapple, and most of the juice blends (such as mango-orange-banana) have more calories than do grapefruit, orange, or tomato juice. To increase the calorie value of orange juice, use frozen concentrate and add less water than the directions indicate.

- **Fruits.** Bananas, pineapple, mangos, raisins, dates, dried apricots, and other dried fruits contain more calories than watery fruits such as grapefruit, plums, and peaches. Enjoy fruit smoothies.

- **Milk.** To boost the calorie value of milk, add 1/4 cup of powdered milk to 1 cup of 2 percent milk. (Powdered milk is an inexpensive protein powder.) Or try malt powder, Ovaltine, Carnation Breakfast Essentials, Nesquik, and other flavorings. Mix these up by the quart (or liter) so they are waiting for you in the refrigerator. You can also make blender drinks such as milk shakes and fruit smoothies. Fixing these kinds of drinks is far less expensive (and likely tastier) than buying canned liquid meal supplements. And they do the job!

- **Toast.** Spread with generous amounts of peanut butter (or any type of nut butter—almond, cashew), soft tub margarine (preferably made with canola oil), and jam or honey.

- **Sandwiches.** Select hearty, dense breads (as opposed to fluffy types) such as whole wheat (with added seeds), rye, and seven-grain. The bigger and more thickly sliced, the better. Stuff with lean meats and add hummus, low-fat cheese, or avocado for added calories. Sprinkle with olive oil. Peanut butter and jam remains the king of inexpensive, healthy, and calorie-dense sports sandwiches.

- **Soups.** Hearty lentil, split-pea, minestrone, and barley soups have more calories than brothy chicken and beef types, unless the broth is chock full of veggies and meat. To make canned soups (such as tomato and chowder) more substantial, add evaporated milk in place of water or regular milk, or add extra powdered milk. Garnish with Parmesan cheese and croutons. If you wish to reduce your sodium intake, be sure to choose the reduced-sodium soups or homemade varieties.

- **Meats.** Beef, pork, and lamb tend to have more calories than do chicken or fish, but they also tend to have more saturated fat. Eat them in moderation and choose lean cuts. To boost calories, saute chicken or fish in canola or olive oil, and add wine sauces and breadcrumb toppings.

- **Beans, legumes.** Lentils, split-pea soup, chili with beans, bean burritos, limas, and all forms of dried beans and legumes are not only calorie dense but also offer both protein and carbohydrate. Hummus (made with chickpeas) is an easy snack, dip, or sandwich filling.

- **Vegetables.** Peas, corn, carrots, winter squash, and beets have more calories than do green beans, broccoli, summer squash, and other watery veggies. Drizzle with olive oil and top with slivered almonds and grated low-fat cheese. Instead of steaming vegetables, add calories by stir-frying them in olive or canola oil.

- **Salads.** What may start out being low-calorie lettuce can quickly become a substantial meal by adding cottage cheese, garbanzo beans (chickpeas), sunflower seeds, avocado, assorted vegetables, chopped walnuts, raisins, dried cranberries, tuna fish, lean meat, croutons, and a liberal dousing of salad dressing made with heart-healthy oil, preferably extra-virgin olive.

- **Potatoes.** Add soft tub margarine and extra powdered milk to mashed potatoes. Although you might be tempted to add lots of butter and gravy for extra calories, think again. You'd also be adding saturated fat, which is unhealthy for your heart. Reduced-fat sour cream (or Greek yogurt) and low-fat gravies are better alternatives.

- **Desserts.** By selecting desserts with nutritional value, you can enjoy treats while nourishing your body. Try oatmeal raisin cookies, fig bars, chocolate pudding, strawberry shortcake, low-fat frozen yogurt, apple crisp, or other fruit desserts. Blueberry muffins, corn bread with honey, banana bread, and other sweet breads and muffins can double as dessert. See the recipes in part IV for ideas.

- **Snacks.** Instead of a small snack, think "second lunch" and "second dinner." A second lunch at 3:00 p.m. or second dinner at 10:00 p.m. is an excellent way to boost your calorie intake. Pack an extra sandwich. At dinner, cook enough for a second meal. If you don't feel hungry, just think of the food as the weight-gain medicine you need to take.

If you aren't interested in or able to eat a whole second meal, at least enjoy some snacks. Healthy snack choices include fruit yogurt, low-fat cheese and crackers, peanuts, sunflower seeds, almonds, granola, whole-wheat pretzels, english muffins, hummus with pita bread, whole-wheat bagels (with low-fat cream cheese and jelly), guacamole with (baked) corn chips, veggie pizza, baked sweet potato (with cottage cheese), peanut butter on crackers, milk shakes, instant breakfast drinks, hot cocoa, fruit smoothies, bananas, dried fruits, trail mix, and even sandwiches.

- **Alcohol.** For older athletes, moderate amounts of beer and wine can stimulate your appetite and add extra calories, particularly when consumed with snacks such as peanuts and popcorn. Because alcohol offers little nutritional value, do not substitute it for juices, milk, or other wholesome beverages. Do not drink if you are underage, and never drink alcohol shortly before an event. It has a dehydrating effect and can blunt your reflexes, create problems with hypoglycemia, and hurt performance. (See chapter 8.)

The sample menus in table 15.1 implement some of these suggestions. You can see how smart choices can accumulate into a hefty, carbohydrate-rich calorie intake that can help you meet your weight goals.

WEIGHT-GAIN DRINKS

Weight-gain drinks (with enticing names such as Muscle Milk, N-Large, Body Fortress, and Serious Mass) are high-calorie beverages that are more about convenience than necessity. A big jug of powder might cost $60 (if not more); the price for 1,000 calories ranges between $2.50 and $5.50, which is more than a few peanut butter and jelly sandwiches. The commercial weight-gain drinks do not offer an advantage over real food or your own homemade weight-gain drink. But if you lack the time or inclination to make extra sandwiches and smoothies, weight-gain drinks can be a convenient way to consume additional calories. The information in table 15.2 may inspire you to think twice before grabbing for commercial products.

The ingredients in weight-gain drinks vary from brand to brand, but all brands supply plenty of protein to help build muscle and most brands (check the Nutrition Facts label) contain plenty of carbohydrate to help fuel muscle-building exercise plus fuel the muscle-building process itself. The products are generally convenient, concentrated calories fortified with vitamins and minerals—and possibly other questionable ingredients as well.

TABLE 15.1   Sample 5,500-Calorie Weight-Gain Menu

Menu plan	Approximate calories
BREAKFAST	
16 oz (480 ml) orange juice	220
1 cup granola	450
1/4 cup raisins (40 g)	130
1 large banana	120
12-oz (360 ml) low-fat milk	180
Total	*1,100*
LUNCH	
4 slices hearty bread	520
One 5 oz (150 g) can tuna	120
4 tbsp light mayo	150
5 dates	100
2 oatmeal cookies	240
16 oz (480 ml) low-fat milk	250
Total	*1,380*
SECOND LUNCH	
1 average bagel	300
2 tbsp peanut butter	200
1 tbsp jam	50
16 oz (480 ml) chocolate milk	350
Total	*900*
DINNER	
One 12-inch (30 cm) cheese pizza	1,900
12 oz (360 ml) lemonade	200
Total	*2,100*
Total calories for day	**5,480**
60% carbohydrate (850 g)	
15% protein (230 g)	
25% fat (130 g)	

Note: For a 150-pound (68 kg) athlete, this provides 5 grams of carbohydrate and 1.5 grams of protein per pound of body weight (11 g carbohydrate and 3 g protein per kg), more than fulfilling the recommended targets.

TABLE 15.2 The Cost of Calories

Gaining weight can be expensive if you choose lots of commercial protein shakes or sports supplements. Believe it or not, you can get the same results with standard foods!

Food	Serving size	Calories	Price in USD[a]	Cost/100 cal
FOODS AT HOME				
Peanut butter and jelly sandwich	3 tbsp peanut butter, 2 tbsp jelly, 2 slices oatmeal bread	650	$0.95	$0.15
Granola and milk	1 cup granola, 1 cup 2% milk	500	$1.00	$0.20
Chocolate milk, 1% fat	Tall glass 16 oz (480 ml)	300	$0.60[b]	$0.20
Carnation Breakfast Essentials	1 packet mixed into 8 oz (240 ml) 2% milk	250	$0.80	$0.32
Welch's 100% grape juice	Tall glass 16 oz (480 ml)	280	$1.00[b]	$0.36
Muscle Milk, powder	2 scoops	310	$1.78/serving[c]	$0.57
DRINKS BOUGHT ON THE RUN				
Nesquik	16 oz (480 ml) bottle	300	$1.79 (at supermarket)	$0.60
Carnation Breakfast Essentials Ready to Drink	11 oz (330 ml) bottle	260	$1.75 (based on 4-pack)	$0.67
Ensure	8 oz (240 ml) bottle	250	$2.10 (based on 4-pack)	$0.84
Muscle Milk, ready to drink	14 oz (420 ml) bottle	230	$3.59 (at CVS)	$1.56

[a]Boston area prices from supermarket and convenience stores, December 2012.
[b]Based on half-gallon (2 L) price.
[c]Based on 5-pound (2.3 kg) tub of powder ($57).

(Remember, the sports supplement industry is poorly regulated.) Weight-gain drinks tend to be low in (saturated) fat, which offers an advantage over boosting your calories with french fries, cheeseburgers, and ice cream.

As for what to look for in a weight-gain drink, the most important factor is taste. If you enjoy your calories, you'll have an easier time sticking to your weight-gain program. Each brand touts the type(s) of protein it contains—whey, casein, egg, soy—and the type of carbohydrate—glucose, fructose, and glucose polymers (also called maltodextrins). Consuming a blend of protein and carbohydrate provides varying speeds of absorption, which creates a sustained-release effect—similar to what you get with standard foods. You have no need for more than 30 grams of protein per dose; your body can use only a limited amount of protein at one time (Phillips and van Loon 2011). (See chapter 7 for more information on meeting your personal protein needs.) Assuming that your meals include a balance of protein- and carbohydrate-rich foods, you are likely already meeting your goals for those nutrients: 0.7 to 0.9 gram of protein per pound of body weight (1.6 to 2.0 g/kg) and 3 to 5 grams of carbohydrate per pound of body weight (6 to 10 g/kg). For example, you'll get plenty of protein with the following choices:

- A cup of Greek yogurt with an energy bar and a latte for a breakfast on the run (30 g protein)
- A tuna sandwich (35 g protein) at lunch
- Peanut butter on graham crackers plus 16 ounces (480 ml) of chocolate milk for a "second lunch" (30 g protein)
- A 6-ounce (180 g) chicken breast at dinner (40 g protein)
- A bedtime bowl of cottage cheese (30 g protein)

The type of carbohydrate, protein, or weight-gain drink you consume as a supplement to your sports diet will likely have an insignificant long-term impact on your ability to reach your weight goals. The biggest impact comes from your genetics, training intensity, timing of fueling, and ability to consistently consume additional calories.

If you are a collegiate athlete, be sure to follow the National Collegiate Athletic Association (NCAA) guidelines regarding acceptable weight-gain supplements. Like the NCAA, I believe that proper nutrition based on scientific principles, not commercial supplements, lays the foundation for optimal performance. Generations of athletes have built muscles with hard work and real foods. You can, too.

If all efforts to boost your food intake fail to add weight, you could buy medical nutrition supplements such as Boost Very High Calorie (VHC) Complete Nutritional Drink, unflavored Benecalorie Calorie and Protein Food Enhancer, and Scandishake Weight Gain Shake Mix. These high-quality products would be free of questionable ingredients that could lead to a failed drug test. They are expensive but can be a helpful last resort.

EATING AT THE RIGHT TIMES

If you are serious about gaining muscle weight, you need to have the right foods available at the right times so you can eat strategically and optimize muscle growth. The following actions will help you reach your goals:

- Fuel up before you strength-train with a carbohydrate–protein snack, such as a yogurt or bowl of cereal with milk. The snack will digest into readily available glucose for fuel and amino acids to protect muscles.
- Refuel immediately afterward with protein to heal and rebuild muscles and more carbohydrate to refuel depleted glycogen stores. You want about three times more calories from carbohydrate than from protein.
- Eat frequently throughout the day. Eat at least every four hours: breakfast, lunch, a second lunch (if you train in the afternoon, split this meal into pre- and postexercise snacks), dinner, and an evening snack as desired. This even distribution of calories ensures that the muscles have a steady supply of glucose for fuel and amino acids for growth. When the amino acid levels in the blood are above normal, the muscles take up more of these building blocks; this enhances muscle growth. If you go for long periods without eating, your body will break down muscles for fuel; this happens to dieters and is counterproductive to reaching your goals.

You might be wondering how much of a difference meal timing really makes. The answer is quite a bit. A study of recreational male bodybuilders who consumed about 270 calories of carbohydrate–protein supplement immediately before and after midday exercise, as compared with a group taking the same supplement in the morning and evening (away from the workout), indicated significantly greater muscle growth at the end of the 10-week program—6 pounds versus 3.3 pounds (2.7 kg versus 1.5 kg) of muscle. That's almost twice as much gain. The bodybuilders who fueled before and after training were also able to bench press 27 more pounds (12 more kg) by the end of the study, as compared with 20 more pounds (9 more kg) for the group who fueled in the morning and evening (Cribb and Hayes 2006). Clearly, *when* you eat makes a difference.

Eating several protein-containing meals and snacks is preferable to gorging on one big dinner at the end of the day. As I mentioned earlier, your body can use only about 30 grams of protein at one time (see chapter 7). A simple way to ensure that a source of high-quality protein is readily available to be used by your muscles is to drink milk with meals and eat yogurt for snacks. Other examples of carbohydrate–protein combinations are chocolate milk, cereal with milk, a turkey sandwich, beans with rice, a fruit smoothie, an apple with cheese, soy nuts, baked chickpeas, a canned

FACT OR FICTION

Taking creatine supplements is a safe way to gain weight.

The facts: Creatine is a naturally occurring compound found in meat and fish. Creatine is also available in powder and pills. Research to date suggests that supplemental creatine causes no physical harm if it is taken in the recommended doses (and is from a reputable source that is not contaminated with unidentified substances). Yet, to date, no sports medicine organization has recommended the use of creatine in people under the age of 18. Teen athletes need to learn how to train hard and eat well.

Taking creatine does not result in muscle gain—but having a higher content of creatine in your muscles can help them perform better when you are lifting weights (or doing other brief, all-out exercise bouts) (Terjung et al. 2000). The muscles use creatine phosphate to generate energy for 1 to 10 seconds of intense work (such as occurs in weightlifting). This ability to do higher-intensity exercise can stimulate your muscles to grow bigger and stronger. But not everyone responds.

Teenagers are at an impressionable age. Taking a muscle-building, performance-enhancing substance establishes a risky attitude that could lead to the desire to take other dangerous substances down the road. Remember, the body you have at age 14 is not the body you will have when you are 15, 16, 17, or 18—or 28. Hence, I discourage the use of creatine in young bodies that are still growing and encourage teens to enhance their strength the all-natural way with a good sports diet and dedicated training. Take pride in your hard work. There are no shortcuts to excellent performance.

---

liquid meal (such as Boost or Carnation Essentials), or any number of commercial sports foods. The muscle-building supplement used in the previously noted study included about 32 grams of whey protein, 34 grams of sugar (glucose) for fuel, and 5.5 grams of creatine, known to enhance muscle mass and strength during resistance exercise (Cribb and Hayes 2006).

BALANCING YOUR WEIGHT-GAIN DIET

The best and simplest weight-gain diet follows a pumped-up version of the fundamental guidelines for healthy eating described in chapter 1. I suggest that you track your food for a few days to assess your typical intake; then figure out where you could plug in more calories (see Dietary Analysis and Nutrition Assessment in appendix A). Steve, a volleyball player, described to me what he typically ate, and together we listed ways he could consume more, without much effort, at certain times of the day. Table 15.3 shows what Steve typically ate as well as suggestions for how he could work more calories into his daily intake.

By adding more to his meals and snack, Steve could potentially pump his intake by 1,500 calories. Granted, that was a lot of additional food, and there was no guarantee that he would eat all of that every day, but at least he knew how to get more calories with little fuss or effort. He just needed to be responsible and set aside enough time to eat the extra calories.

If you are into the mathematical approach to weight gain, follow this more complex plan. Your muscles become saturated with glycogen when fed 3 to 5 grams of carbohydrate per pound (6 to 10 g/kg) of body weight, and your body uses less than 1 gram of protein per pound (2 g/kg) under growth conditions, so your primary dietary goal is to satisfy these requirements for carbohydrate and protein. Then you can choose the balance of the calories from a variety of (preferably healthy) sources of fat or carbohydrate. By tracking your calories with apps (such as MyFitnessPal), you can

TABLE 15.3 Working More Calories Into Your Diet

Typical intake	Calorie booster	Added calories
BREAKFAST		
1 bagel	Another bagel	+300
2 tbsp peanut butter	Another 2 tbsp peanut butter	+200
8 oz (240 ml) orange juice	Another 8 oz (240 ml) orange juice	+100
LUNCH		
1 sandwich	Another half sandwich	+200
8 oz (240 ml) milk	Another 8 oz (240 ml) milk	+100
1 cookie	Another cookie	+100
SNACK		
Nothing	Granola bar	+200
	Cran-apple juice, 12 oz (360 ml)	+200
DINNER		
Lasagna	Apple for dessert	+100
Salad		
Bread		
Milk		
		Total: 1,500 added calories

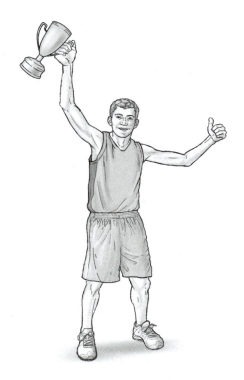

assess your intake. For example, if you are a 150-pound (68 kg) triathlete, you'd want the analysis to show that you consumed 450 to 750 grams of carbohydrate per day and, at most, 150 grams of protein per day.

PATIENCE IS A VIRTUE

By consuming the prescribed 500 to 1,000 additional calories per day, you should see weight gain. Be sure to include muscle-building resistance exercise (weight workouts, push-ups) to promote muscle growth rather than just fat deposits. Consult with the trainer at your school, health club, or gym for a specific exercise program that suits your needs. You may also want to have your body fat routinely measured to make sure your weight gain is indeed mostly muscle, not fat. Untrained men might gain about 3 pounds (1.5 kg) of muscle per month initially. The rate of gain in well-trained athletes is slower.

If you don't gain weight, look at your family members to see whether you inherited a naturally trim physique. If everyone is thin, accept your physique and concentrate on improving your athletic skills. Rather than drain your energy fretting about being too thin, capitalize on being light, swift, and agile. You will likely be able to surpass the heavier hulks that lack your speed.

Also keep in mind that most people gain weight with age. If you are still growing or are in your 20s, your turn to bulk up may still come. All too often, scrawny young athletes fatten up once they get out of school and start working. That's why I hesitate to encourage my clients to force-feed themselves. Doing so upsets the natural appetite-regulating mechanisms, and people lose the natural ability to stop eating when they are content.

Such was the case with Wes, a 30-year-old photographer and former football player. He reported with a sigh, "I was skinny all through high school. In college, my football coach insisted that I gain weight by eating extra buttered bread, piles of french fries, and mounds of ice cream. I developed quite a liking for these foods. I continued to eat them even after I'd reached my weight-gain goals. Voila—look at me now! I'm 60 pounds (27 kg) overweight and can barely walk, to say nothing of play football. I long for those days when I was lean and mean."

With a food plan that contained no fatty snacks or sugary soft drinks, Wes did lose weight over the course of a year. That fall, he coached an after-school football program. He advised the thin kids to be patient, eat healthfully, and develop smart lifelong eating habits.

I offer you the same advice. To gain weight, you need to choose larger portions of healthy foods at meals and snacks, eat on a regular schedule—no skipped or skimpy meals—and be responsible. You need to work hard to eat your fill consistently. You also have to work hard at weightlifting and other muscle-building exercise. And ultimately, your skills as an athlete will matter more than your weight.

CHAPTER 16

LOSING WEIGHT
WITHOUT STARVING

Weight loss is far more complex than the simple recommendation to "just eat less and exercise more." Both serious athletes and fitness exercisers struggle to either lose weight or keep off the weight they have lost. Why is weight loss so difficult? Are dieters just unable to comply with the demands of their diet, finding it difficult to limit their intake of the abundance of yummy food that pervades our environments? Do compounds in processed foods disrupt normal metabolic pathways? Does the body adapt to a reduced calorie intake? Does dieting ruin your metabolism? Does nature prefer women to have abundant body fat? What about obesogens in the environment (flame retardants in pajamas and furniture, BPA in canned goods, Teflon in cookware)—are they taking a toll on our weight? Does the balance of microbes in our guts impact weight? As you can see, we have to look at far more than just diet and exercise!

The purpose of this chapter is to address those questions and help you learn how to manage food to both lose body fat and maintain the weight loss. You'll learn how to listen to your body's hunger signals, eat wisely within your calorie budget, have the energy to enjoy exercise, and lose excess body fat without feeling denied or deprived. You might also decide that your larger, yet fit and healthy, body is fine at it's current size; not everyone is designed to live in a small body.

If you are a bodybuilder, wrestler, lightweight rower, or in another sport that requires that you make weight, the same rules that apply to fitness exercisers also apply to you. And remember: Not gaining weight in the first place in the off-season is often easier than losing weight preseason.

The best way to lose weight—and keep it off—is to seek professional advice that is tailored to your lifestyle and food preferences. This is far more effective than eliminating favorite foods or self-inflicting a miserable diet. I recommend that you meet with a registered dietitian (RD) or registered dietitian nutritionist (RDN), preferably one who is a board-certified specialist in sports dietetics (CSSD). This health professional has fulfilled specific educational requirements, has passed a registration exam, and is a recognized member of the largest organization of nutrition professionals in the United States: the Academy of Nutrition and Dietetics. Because some states lack specific standards defining who can rightfully call himself or herself a dietitian or nutritionist, you can protect yourself from self-taught nutrition gurus by seeking guidance from an RD or RDN. To find a local RD or RDN, use the referral networks at www.eatright.org and www.scandpg.org.

DIETS DON'T WORK

Because I'm a dietitian, most of my clients assume that I will put them on a diet. I don't. I teach them how to eat healthfully and appropriately. Athletes—and all people, for that matter—who go *on* a diet simply go *off* a diet. They have a high chance of not only regaining all the lost weight but also regaining proportionately more fat than muscle. That represents a lot of wasted (or is that waisted?) effort.

Dieting conjures up visions of rice cakes, salad with fat-free dressing, and yet another skinless chicken breast. Diets that are associated with extreme hunger can actually contribute to weight problems. The body rebels against hunger and the state of starvation by triggering binge eating, more commonly known as "blowing the diet," and dieters gain weight despite extreme efforts to lose it.

A study of 4,746 teens revealed that those who dieted in the fourth grade ended up heavier than their peers in high school. Dieting was associated with weight gain (to the classification of "overweight"), disordered eating, and eating disorders (Neumark-Sztainer et al. 2006). Another study of 370 male athletes (boxers, weightlifters, and wrestlers) who had to make weight for their sports suggested that they were at higher risk of becoming obese later in life, as compared with a group of nonathletes (Saarni et al. 2006). Dieting is simply the wrong way to try to lose weight.

To lose weight healthfully and to keep it off without dieting, you must pay attention to the following:

- **How much you eat.** There is an appropriate portion of any food.
- **When you eat.** Fuel during the active part of your day.
- **Why you eat.** Eat when your body requires fuel, not when you are simply bored, stressed, or lonely.
- **How much you sleep.** People who are tired often seek additional food for energy, when they actually just need sleep (Shlisky et al. 2012).

We can learn a lot about weight reduction from people who have lost weight and kept it off. According to the National Weight Control Registry

FACT OR FICTION

Being fat equates to being unhealthy.

The facts: Fitness is more important for health than is fatness. An estimated 30 to 40 percent of obese people have the same risk for heart disease and cancer as normal-weight people. They are free from metabolic complications and have normal blood pressure, cholesterol, and blood glucose levels. They have the same mortality risk as normal-weight people, and the fitter they are, the lower their health risks are (Ortega et al. 2012). Being fat but fit is far better than being fat and unfit, or being thin but unhealthy due to restrictive dieting. Don't let our weight-obsessed society ruin your health!

(a sample of more than 5,000 people who have lost more than 30 pounds [14 kg] and have kept it off for more than a year), there is not one weight-reduction food plan that is best for everyone. But the tricks to losing weight and keeping it off include eating breakfast, choosing fewer fried and greasy foods, eating consistently and maintaining the same eating patterns on weekends as on weekdays, exercising regularly, and weighing yourself regularly (once a week) (Wing and Phelan 2005).

Other studies find similar results and emphasize the need to change your daily lifestyle so that you get more sleep, watch less TV, eat more fruits and vegetables, cook meals at home (as opposed to frequently eating restaurant meals), and plan and track your food intake and exercise program (Fuglestad, Jeffery, and Sherwood 2012).

This chapter includes numerous food-management tips to help you achieve your weight-loss goals. But before attempting a weight-loss program, you might want to have your body fat measured (see chapter 14). All too often I counsel active people who weigh more than they desire, but their weight is primarily muscle with little excess fat. No wonder they struggle with trying to reduce! By knowing what percentage of your weight is excess body fat, you'll have a valid perspective from which to set an appropriate weight goal.

Avoiding Weight Gain

The best way to deal with weight loss is to not gain the weight in the first place. Three triggers that encourage excessive calorie intake are alcohol drinking, television watching, and sleep deprivation (Chapman et al. 2012). You can control these!

Exercise can protect against weight gain. A seven-year survey of about 6,100 male and 2,200 female runners who participated in the National Runners' Health Study indicated that those who ran more miles gained less weight (Williams 2007). While all the runners gained less weight than their sedentary peers, the men and women who ran more than 30 miles (48 km) per week gained half the weight of those who ran less than 15 miles (24 km) per week. Other benefits to running more miles each week included less weight gain around the waist in both men and women and less weight gain in the hips in women.

Another way to prevent weight gain is to not start dieting in the first place. Although this advice is likely too late for you now, if you are a parent, you can spare your kids the negative effects of dieting. Research consistently tells us that reducing diets are generally unsuccessful in the long run and contribute to weight gain, to say nothing of depression and disordered eating behaviors. A growing body of research suggests that intuitive eating is a healthier alternative to current strategies of dieting to lose weight (Denny et al. 2013). Eating intuitively means trusting that your body will tell you how much to eat so you will stop eating when you have satisfied your physiological need for fuel. This is how normal-weight people tend to eat—for physical, not emotional, reasons. Becoming trustful can be difficult for people who have been on the on-the-diet, off-the-diet roller coaster of starving followed by stuffing themselves. I hope the following information can help you arrive at a trusting relationship with food and your body.

Building Skills That Lead to Weight Loss

If diets worked, then everyone who has ever gone on a diet would be thin. That's not what happens; most dieters are heavy. The way to lose weight for the long haul is to learn how to eat—healthfully and appropriately. Chapters 1 and 2 offer guidelines for making healthy food choices. This chapter builds on that information to help you choose the right portions at the right times so you can lose weight without feeling denied or deprived. I'll teach you nutrition skill power, which is more sustainable than willpower. Such was the case with Roberta, a 42-year-old computer programmer, mother of two teenagers, and fitness runner.

"If only I had more willpower, I could lose weight," Roberta complained. "I've been trying to lose these same 8 to 10 pounds [4 to 5 kg] for 12—yes, 12—years. I'm the diet queen!" Feeling completely helpless, Roberta came to me as a last resort to help her achieve her weight goals.

When reviewing her dieting history, I noticed that Roberta needed a more realistic food plan. She would diet by trying to exist on coffee for breakfast, salad for lunch, yogurt for a snack, and fish with vegetables for dinner. Her intake was Spartan, to say the least, and it included a limited variety of food. I asked, "When you are not dieting, what do you eat?" She quickly listed her favorite foods (what she fed her children): cereal for breakfast, peanut butter and jelly sandwich for lunch, and pasta for dinner. Every time she went on her diet to lose weight, she denied herself these favorite family foods. She went to extremes to keep cereal and peanut butter out of her sight so that she wouldn't eat them. She deemed them too much temptation for her weak willpower, so she had her kids hide them from her.

I encouraged Roberta to stop looking at food as being fattening and instead start fueling her body appropriately with satisfying meals. Eating good food, after all, is one of life's pleasures. Given that she had liked cereal, breads, and pasta since childhood, she was naive to think she could stop liking them. Instead of trying to keep these foods out of her life, I encouraged her to eat them more often. I pointed out that her standard diet foods (salad, yogurt, and fish) had no power over her because she gave herself permission to eat them whenever she wanted. I encouraged her to include an adequate portion of cereal every day for breakfast (and even lunch, dinner, and snacks) to take the power away from that food.

If you, too, struggle with weight issues, you need to learn how to manage your favorite foods, not how to deny them. When you enjoy appropriate portions of whatever you like to eat, as often as you'd like, you no longer need willpower to avoid them. Nutrition skill power, not willpower, can result in permanent weight loss without feelings of denial and deprivation.

One skill that enhances your ability to eat appropriate food portions is to eat mindfully (not mindlessly). That is, chew your food s-l-o-w-l-y, taste it, and savor each mouthful. By doing so, you'll need far less to be satisfied, and you'll be content to eat smaller portions. By mindfully eating your favorite foods, you also defuse the urge to do last-chance eating. (You know, "Last chance to eat peanut butter before I go back on my diet. I'd better have another spoonful!") You can enjoy more peanut butter—even in a sandwich—when your body becomes hungry again. Nutrition skill power wins in the end.

A second skill that enhances weight loss is eating fewer processed and refined foods and more whole foods: fruits, vegetables, unrefined grains, and other fiber-rich foods. Fiber can assist with weight loss by promoting satiety and delaying the return of hunger, which contributes to eating less in subsequent meals. Calorie for calorie, fiber-rich fruits, veggies, and whole grains are more satiating than sugary sodas, lollipops, and Gummi Bears. You still need to limit calories, but you can feel fuller on calories from wholesome foods. Plus, processed foods can require less energy to digest, so your body assimilates more of their calories. These few extra calories add up over time.

A third weight-reduction skill is to include a protein-rich food in each meal. Like fiber, protein is satiating. As I mentioned in chapter 3, people who eat a high-protein breakfast tend to eat fewer calories at the end of the day.

By regularly choosing fruits, vegetables, beans, whole grains, fish, and low-fat dairy products, you'll not only lose weight but also reduce your risk of cancer, heart disease, and hypertension. The food plan that helps you manage your weight should be consistent with dietary guidelines for healthy eating. Don't go on a crazy diet only to regain the weight you lost because you failed to learn how to eat healthfully.

CALORIE AWARENESS

Most of my dieting clients are afraid to enjoy satisfying meals because they fear consuming too many calories. They believe that eating a real lunch, let's say, a tuna sandwich with a glass of milk, will make them fat, so they stick to cottage cheese and baby carrots. The problem is that self-created diets commonly are too limited and too low in calories. Dieters end up becoming bored with the limited food choices and too hungry with cravings for calorie-dense foods (Gilhooly et al. 2007). As a result, they blow the diet and splurge on the yummy meals they truly want to eat, and quickly regain any lost weight, plus more.

When working with dieters who have trouble regulating their food intake, I estimate an appropriate calorie budget so they become aware of how much is OK to eat to maintain or lose weight. Just as you know how much money you can spend when you shop, you might find it helpful to know how many calories you can spend when you eat. Ideally, you can intuitively choose the right number of calories by simply listening to your

What Exactly Is a Calorie?

A calorie, or more correctly, a kilocalorie, is a measure of energy. It is the amount of heat needed to raise 1 liter of water by 1 degree Celsius. (If you need to convert kilocalories to kilojoules, you can do so by multiplying the number of calories by 4.1868.) Exercise that raises your body temperature exemplifies how burning calories converts into heat.

body's hunger signals (see Hunger: A Simple Request for Fuel in chapter 17). But if you have been on and off many diets, you may have become disconnected from your body's request for fuel.

To best assess your body's energy (calorie) needs, you should meet with a registered dietitian or you can make a ballpark estimate of your calorie needs by using the following steps:

1. Estimate your resting metabolic rate—the number of calories you need simply to breathe, pump blood, and be alive (table 16.1)—by multiplying your healthy weight by 10 calories per pound (or 22 cal/kg). If you are significantly overweight, use an adjusted weight; a weight about halfway between your desired weight and your current weight. That is, if you weigh 160 pounds (73 kg) but at one time normally weighed 120 pounds (53 kg), use 140 (64 kg) as your adjusted weight.

For example, Roberta weighed about 130 pounds (59 kg) but could healthfully weigh about 120 pounds (53 kg). Hence, she needed approximately 1,200 calories (120 × 10) simply to do nothing all day except exist.

2. Add more calories for daily activity apart from your purposeful exercise. If you are moderately active throughout the day (excluding purposeful exercise), add about 50 percent of your resting metabolic rate (RMR). If you are sedentary, add 20 to 40 percent; if very active (in addition to your purposeful exercise), add 60 to 80 percent of your RMR. Roberta was moderately active throughout the day with her two kids and her job. She burned about 600 calories (50 percent × 1,200 cal) for activities of daily living. Her totals were as follows:

1,200 RMR + 600 cal daily activity
= 1,800 cal/day (without purposeful exercise)

TABLE 16.1 Resting Metabolic Rate: More Calories Than You Might Think to Be Alive

Organ	Calories per day*	Percentage of resting metabolic rate
Brain	365	21
Heart	180	10
Kidneys	120	7
Liver	560	32
Lungs	160	9
Other tissues	370	21

*Approximate number of calories burned by a 150-pound (68 kg) man while resting in bed all day.

3. Add more calories for purposeful exercise. For example, when Roberta went to the health club, she exercised aerobically for about 45 minutes and burned about 400 calories on the treadmill. Hence, this was her approximate total calorie need:

$$1,200 \text{ cal RMR} + 600 \text{ cal daily activity}$$
$$+ 400 \text{ cal purposeful exercise} = 2,200 \text{ total cal/day}$$

Note that the calories burned during exercise also include the RMR, so the estimate is actually higher than the calories burned only by exercise itself. While this does not significantly affect the fitness exerciser who works out for 45 minutes, the discrepancy adds up for a cyclist on an all-day bike ride.

Be honest and accurate in assessing your calorie needs. Athletes who exercise hard are often very sedentary the rest of the day as they rest and recover from their rigorous workouts. In a 13-week study with pudgy young men, those who did an hour of exercise a day did not lose more weight than those who exercised for only half an hour a day. The researchers noticed that the group that did twice the exercise ate more and moved less in the remaining 23 hours of the day (Rosenkilde et al. 2012). The more you exercise, the more sedentary you may become *unless you mindfully keep yourself moving.* I've counseled many marathoners and Ironman triathletes who were frustrated with lack of weight loss. They had fallen victim to the sedentary athlete syndrome.

To lose weight, subtract 10 to 20 percent (small deficits add up and can be easier to sustain) of your total calorie needs (Hills et al. 2013). Roberta deserved to eat about 2,200 calories per day to maintain her weight. Subtracting 10 to 20 percent of 2,200 calories (200 to 400 calories) left her with 1,800 to 2,000 calories for her reducing diet.

In the past, Roberta had tried to reduce on 1,000 to 1,200 calories per day. She was skeptical about my proposed reducing plan of 1,800 to 2,000 calories. "If I can't lose weight on 1,000 calories, why would I lose weight on 1,800?" she questioned. I reminded her that when she cut back too much, she'd get too hungry and blow her diet. She also lost muscle, slowed her metabolism, and consumed too few of the nutrients she needed to protect her health and invest in top performance. I reminded her that quick weight loss rapidly reappears. She could lose weight quickly, or she could lose weight for the long term. She had already failed many times at the "quick" diet. She agreed; it was time to try another approach.

A reasonable weight-loss target is 0.5 to 1 pound (0.25 to 0.5 kg) a week for a person who weighs less than 150 pounds (68 kg); 1 to 2 pounds (0.5 to 1 kg) a week is reasonable for heavier bodies.

Once you've established your total daily calories, divide them evenly throughout the day. Some people like having six small meals: breakfast,

FACT OR FICTION

Weight loss is mathematical. If you eat 500 fewer calories in a day, you will lose 1 pound (0.5 kg) of fat per week.

The facts: Weight loss is not as mathematical as we would like it to be. For example, obese people tend to lose fat relatively easily, but lean athletes can struggle to get below their set-point weight (Leibel, Rosenbaum, and Hirsch 1995). If you have no excess fat to lose, your body will conserve energy. I've had thin clients who claim they eat far less than they deserve yet maintain weight. They have cold hands and report that they are "always freezing"—just one way nature conserves calories.

snack, lunch, snack, dinner, snack. Others, like Roberta, find that eating four meals per day works well for them (see chapter 1).

Include at least three of the five food groups at each meal (see chapter 1) and two kinds of foods per snack. Too many dieters repetitively eat a single food, such as cottage cheese, for a meal. This practice limits their intake of the variety of vitamins, minerals, and other nutrients offered by a range of foods. They should instead strive for protein–carbohydrate combinations (e.g., cottage cheese plus banana plus crackers).

Roberta was initially skeptical when I suggested that she enjoy four meals each day; meals, after all, seemed "fattening." She complained, "I'm afraid I'll get fat from eating so much at breakfast plus *two* lunches." I reminded her that the purpose of the daytime meals is to ruin her appetite for dinner. By eating more during the day, she would be less hungry that evening, have more energy to exercise from 5:00 to 6:00 p.m., and be able to eat less (diet) at night. What seemed like more food was actually less. She'd simply trade her evening blown-diet calories of nutrient-poor food for wholesome foods earlier in the day.

If you hold the fear that meals are fattening, think again and remember these concepts:

- You won't gain weight from eating a substantial breakfast or lunch. You'll have more energy to exercise and burn calories.

- If you eat too much food at breakfast and lunch, you will be less hungry at night. You can then skimp at dinner and simply eat soup or salad. But don't have just soup or salad for lunch. It's not enough.

- If you skimp on daytime meals and develop a deep hunger, you'll be likely to overeat at night because of the strong physiological drive to eat.

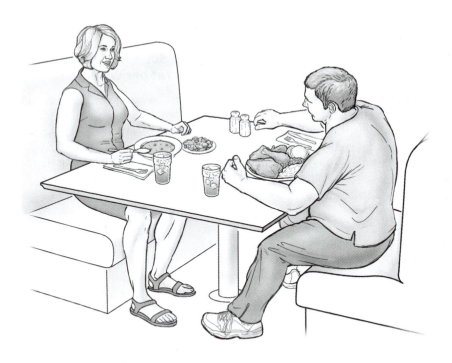

Become familiar with the calorie content of the foods you commonly eat, and then spend your calories wisely. Apps such as Lose It! and My Fitness Pal can be helpful, as can the other calorie-counting tools listed in appendix A. Be sure to count calories loosely (0, 50, or 100) and to consider them a general guideline and helpful tool for determining how much (rather than how little) food you can appropriately eat to satisfy your appetite without stuffing your stomach.

Calorie awareness can be a helpful bridge to put you in touch with your body's ability to tell you how much is OK to eat so that you feel satisfied. You can and should quickly replace calorie counting with listening to your body's signals for hunger and satiety. Calorie counting should not become an obsession. Your body can regulate food intake intuitively.

Roberta was an expert calorie counter. In fact, she expressed fear about becoming obsessed with counting calories. I encouraged her to start listening to her body and learn what, for example, 600 calories feels like. She could then use that feeling for future reference. For example, she could tell the right amount to eat at a restaurant by listening to her body's message of being pleasantly fed.

TEN STEPS FOR SENSIBLE FAT LOSS

Now that you know approximately how many calories you can target to lose body fat gradually, you need to learn how to eat those calories appropriately. Here are 10 steps for fat loss:

1. **Write it down.** Keep accurate food records of every morsel and drop for three days, if not more, to educate yourself about what and how much you actually eat. Research suggests that people who keep food records tend to lose weight. A handy place to keep food records is on your smartphone or on Internet food trackers. See the section Dietary Analysis and Nutrition Assessment in appendix A for apps and websites that can help you not only record your food but also calculate calories. Record why you eat. Are you hungry, stressed, or bored? Include the time and amount you exercise as well. Evaluate your patterns for potentially fattening habits such as skimping at breakfast, nibbling all day, overeating at night because you've become too hungry, entertaining yourself with food when you're bored, or rewarding yourself with chocolate when you're stressed.

Pay careful attention to your mood when eating. Roberta discovered that at times a hug and human comforting could have better nourished her than food did. She acknowledged that eating a tub of popcorn diverted her loneliness or anxiety and distracted her from her problems but did nothing to resolve the problem that triggered her eating.

If you eat for reasons other than to obtain fuel, you need to recognize that food should only be fuel. Food becomes dangerously fattening when it is eaten for entertainment, comfort, or stress reduction. And no amount of any food will solve your problems. Before you reach for extra food, ask yourself, Does my body need this fuel?

2. **Front-load your calories.** Roberta was surprised when I said that her diet breakfast of cereal with skim milk seemed too skimpy. She thought that diets were supposed to start at breakfast. I told her to start her diet at dinner. If you eat lightly during the day and excessively at night, experiment with having a bigger, higher-protein breakfast and lunch and a lighter dinner. You'll enjoy having less hunger—and more energy to get through your active day.

3. **Eat slowly.** Higher-weight people tend to eat faster than their normal-weight counterparts do. Because the brain needs about 20 minutes to receive the signal that you've eaten your fill, slow eating can save you many calories. For example, choose a broth-based soup for a first course before dinner at a restaurant. Hot soup takes time to eat and decreases your appetite for the entree. You'll be content to have a lighter meal.

Roberta had the bad habit of inhaling her meals in a matter of minutes. She'd eat nonstop, without enjoying the meal. I encouraged her to put her fork down frequently, taste the food, and eat it mindfully. After all, the best part of food is its taste. Don't miss out on one of life's pleasures!

Because Roberta had eaten quickly for most of her life, I suggested that she practice slowly eating at least one meal per day and then build up to two and then three meals. She discovered that lunchtime became more enjoyable once she gave herself permission to relax and enjoy both the meal and mealtime. She felt less tempted to eat dessert because the slowly savored lunch satisfied her appetite.

4. **Enjoy your favorite foods.** If you deny yourself permission to eat what you truly want to eat, you will be likely to binge. But if you give yourself permission to eat your desired foods in diet portions, you will be less likely to blow your reducing plan. If chocolate-glazed doughnuts are among your favorites, then have one or more every day until you get tired of them. Simply determine how many calories are in the doughnut (search online for "calories in doughnut"), and spend your calorie budget accordingly. When eating this treat, remember to chew it slowly, savor the taste, and fully enjoy it. You'll free yourself from the temptation to devour a dozen doughnuts in one sitting.

Roberta's downfall was chocolate-chip cookies. "I can go for four days without a cookie, but then I inevitably end up eating too many of them." I encouraged Roberta to budget a cookie (or two) into her lunch at least twice per week to prevent those unnecessary binges. When she did that, she discovered that she had fewer binges because she did not feel denied or deprived. Eating a bigger breakfast also helped abate the cookie cravings. By preventing herself from getting too hungry, she lost interest in sugary treats (see chapter 5).

5. **Avoid temptation.** Out of sight, out of mind, and out of mouth. If you spend a lot of free time in the kitchen, you might consider relocating to the den to relax, where food is less likely to be available. At parties, socialize in the living room, away from the buffet table and away from the snacks. At the market, skip the aisle with the cookies.

Roberta used to take walks that took her by a bakery. No wonder she'd succumb to temptation. I suggested that she walk down another street. This became the simple solution to what had been a major problem. She also learned to enter her house through the front door and go immediately upstairs to change her clothes and unwind from the day. Previously, she had entered the house through the kitchen door. She would then habitually open the refrigerator and graze for a few minutes while making the transition from working to being at home.

6. **Keep a list of nonfood activities you can do when you are bored, lonely, tired, or nervous.** Food is fuel, not entertainment, and not a reward for having survived another stressful day. Have strategies in mind that can save you calories: Call a friend, check your e-mail, take a bath, water the plants, listen to music by candlelight, surf the Web, work on a puzzle, go for a walk, take a nap, play with your kids, practice yoga, or meditate.

When Roberta felt tired and stressed, she would treat herself to food. I encouraged her to pause and ask herself before indulging: Is my body hungry—or am I just tired and stressed? Does my body need this fuel? If the answer was that she was tired, she talked herself into going to bed early. If the answer was that she was stressed, she learned to recognize that no amount of food would resolve the stress, so she shouldn't even start to eat. Making a phone call to her best friend or writing a page in her journal became her slimming alternatives.

When you overeat because you are stressed, you are only trying to be nice to yourself. Food alters your brain chemistry and may put you in a happier mood—for the moment, that is. Ultimately, this inappropriate coping skill will leave you even more stressed and depressed from the weight gain.

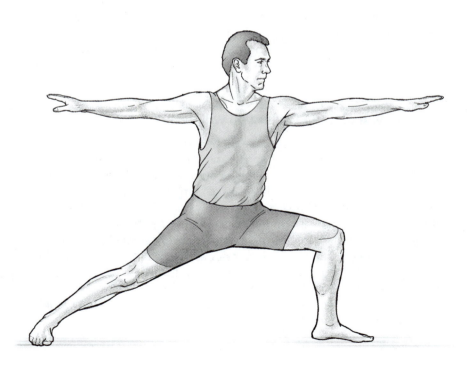

Learning how to manage stress without food is the obvious solution. Try dissipating stress by taking three deep, slow breaths—breathe in peace, breathe out stress. Yoga can be helpful, as can meditation. Calm your mind by sitting in a comfortable position and focusing on the word *ocean*. Slowly inhale on *O* and exhale on *cean*. Soon the calm vision of ocean waves will help soothe your nerves . . . and perhaps save you some calories.

7. **Make a realistic eating plan.** You don't have to lose weight every day. Rather, every day you can choose to lose, maintain, or even gain weight. For example, if you face a hectic schedule and wonder how you will survive the stresses of the day, give yourself permission to fuel yourself fully and have a maintain-weight day. You'll need the energy to cope. If you are going to an elegant wedding and want to enjoy the full dinner, go right ahead. A gain-weight day from time to time is part of normal eating. Your body will simply be less hungry the next day, and you'll naturally choose to eat a little less. (*Note:* Do not "save calories" for a big dinner by skimping on daytime food; doing so tends to backfire, and you'll inevitably end up seriously overeating in the evening.)

Roberta had always considered a diet to be a nonstop event that would last for weeks or months until she reached her target weight. I invited her to see weight reduction as a daily choice that depends on the energy level of the day. I also recommended that she plan in a treat once a week. Just as people need a day off from work, dieters need a day off from dieting. Roberta acknowledged, "Knowing that I can enjoy going out to eat for

FACT OR FICTION

The less you eat, the leaner you will be.

The facts: Generally, the less you eat, the more you will blow your diet, overeat because of extreme hunger, and gain weight. For example, if you knock off only 100 calories at the end of the day (the equivalent of two Oreo cookies or a spoonful of ice cream), you'll theoretically lose 10 pounds (5 kg) of fat a year, because 1 pound (0.5 kg) of fat equals 3,500 calories. If you eat 500 fewer calories per day than you normally do, you theoretically should lose 1 pound (0.5 kg) per week (but theory is often not reality and weight loss is not as mathematical as we would like it to be). Gretchen, a self-defined gym rat, tried to eat as little as possible. She'd knock off 1,000 calories and diet on 1,200 calories per day. She'd lose 2 pounds (1 kg) Monday through Thursday—but would inevitably regain it on the weekend.

Saturday breakfast helps me stay with my reducing program the rest of the week."

8. **Schedule appointments for exercise.** If you are a serious athlete and are trying to lose weight, you likely have a regular training program. But if you are a fitness exerciser and have trouble following a consistent exercise program, you might be helped by scheduling exercise time into your smartphone or appointment book. You want to exercise regularly to tone muscles, relieve stress, and improve your health, but you should not overexercise. If you exercise too much, you will likely end up injured, tired, and irritable. As I mentioned earlier, exercise should be for fun and fitness, not simply for burning calories. Be sure that you create enjoyable ways to live an active lifestyle.

Roberta would sometimes punish herself with extra-hard workouts on the stair stepper or longer walks to burn more calories. Although she did expend 500 to 600 calories per session, she'd end up so hungry that by the end of the day she would inevitably replace those calories, plus more. I encouraged her to stop using exercise as punishment for having extra body fat but to view it as something she does to improve her health and performance. Remember, exercise only contributes to weight loss if it culminates in a calorie deficit at the end of the day.

My clients commonly ask, "How much exercise is enough?" Enough for what? Enough to lose weight? You can lose weight without exercising; you just need to eat fewer calories. Enough for overall health and fitness? The 2018 U.S. Physical Activity Guidelines recommends accumulating at least 30 to 60 minutes of moderate to vigorous physical activity most days of the week (150 to 300 minutes per week). The classic Harvard Alumni Health Study found that the lowest death rates from cardiovascular disease occurred among those who burned more than 1,000 calories per week (Sesso, Pfaffenbarger, and Lee 2000).

9. **Make sleep a priority.** Getting too little sleep can make you feel hungrier. When you are tired, the signals to your brain to stop eating are very quiet, and the signals to eat more are very loud. Roberta often found herself tired and hungry at the end of her long day. She learned to go to bed earlier and reminded herself she needed to "snooze to lose." She knew that if she started eating, she would have great difficulty stopping.

10. **Think fit and healthy.** Every morning before you get out of bed, visualize yourself being fitter and leaner. This picture will help you start the day with a positive attitude. If you tell yourself that you are eating more healthfully and are losing weight, you will do so more easily. Positive self-talk is important for your well-being.

Roberta constantly reminded herself that she'd rather be healthier and leaner than allow herself to overeat. She took smaller portions. She made a daily eating plan and stuck to it. On her way home from work, she visualized herself eating a pleasant (but smaller) dinner, chewing the food slowly, savoring the taste, relaxing after dinner with a book rather than cookies, and following her food plan. By practicing this scene before she arrived home, she discovered that she was better able to carry through with her good intentions.

Roberta also reminded herself that when she ate well, she felt better, and exercised better. She also felt better about herself. After years of unsuccessful dieting, she liked feeling successful, perhaps even more than feeling thinner.

FAD DIETS

Every dieter wants to lose weight quickly, and a fad diet that promises instant success is appealing. Unfortunately, fad diets tend to work for only a short time because the dieter gets tired of being denied and deprived of favorite foods. Instead of hopping from one fad diet plan to another, you need to learn how to eat appropriate portions of the foods you like. You need to learn how to manage food—not how to eliminate foods by going on a diet.

I have clients who abandon my sensible weight-reduction advice, which is based on balance and moderation; they want to lose weight faster—and easier. A year or two later, they inevitably end up back in my office, heavier than when they first came. Here is a brief summary of some of the tempting fad diets that have failed to work for them, and likely for you, too:

• **Low-carbohydrate diet.** This food plan is inappropriate for athletes because it drastically cuts carbohydrate intake, an important source of fuel needed for intense exercise. While reducing your intake of sugars and refined grains (soda, snack foods) can be a step to reduce calorie intake, you want to retain (whole) grains, fruits, and vegetables as a part of your healthy eating pattern. As I have said before, carbohydrates are not fattening; excess calories (of any type) are the weight-gain culprit. In a 12-month study comparing a healthy low-carbohydrate (30 percent of calories) diet to a healthy higher-carbohydrate (50 percent of calories) diet, weight changes were similar (Gardner et al. 2018).

The seeming success of the Atkins and other low-carb diets demonstrates that a strong intake of protein and healthy fat can promote weight reduction because these types of foods are more satisfying than fat-free carbohydrate-based foods. When you feel less hungry, you can more easily eat fewer calories and thereby lose weight.

The bad news is that athletes generally need more carbohydrate to fuel their muscles for top performance. You cannot easily repeat days of hard exercise without carbohydrate serving as the foundation of each meal. If you are a casual exerciser, you may be able to exercise well enough with a reduced carbohydrate intake. But do you really want to live your life with limited pasta, bread, and cereal?

- **Paleo diet.** The paleo diet eliminates white sugar, white flour, and refined and highly processed foods that were not a part of the diets of cavemen. There's nothing wrong with that. My concern regards the questionable elimination of food groups, such as whole grains, legumes, and dairy.

If you are a recreational exerciser, you may be able to get enough carbohydrate from fruits and vegetables for your workouts. But if you are exercising hard and have a high demand for carbohydrate, you might want to try a modified paleo diet that limits processed foods but includes oatmeal, brown rice, low-fat yogurt, and other wholesome grains and calcium-rich dairy and soy foods. Again, the question arises: Do you really want to eat no pasta or birthday cake for the rest of your life?

- **Keto diet.** By minimizing intake of grains, fruits, vegetables, sugars, and starches to less than 50 grams (200 calories) of carbohydrate a day, the keto diet trains the body to burn fat as the primary fuel. This diet of 70 to 80 percent fat reduces hunger, which can help people lose weight, in the short term at least. But is this restrictive eating pattern sustainable? Is it giving your body all of the vitamins and minerals it needs for good health? What is happening to the gut microbes that thrive on fiber-rich fruits, vegetables, and grains? What happens when you leave Keto Jail: Do you binge on your favorite cookies and desserts and regain all of the lost weight? While some athletes might rave about it, I question whether this is a healthy eating pattern for the long term. We need more research.

- **Low glycemic–index diet.** The theory is that foods with a high glycemic index are fattening because they create a rapid rise in blood sugar, stimulate the body to secrete more insulin, trigger hunger and overeating, and promote fat storage. For most athletes and active people, this is not the case because fit people have a reduced insulin response (Archer 2018). Each person's response to a carbohydrate-containing food is unique, so just eat more foods closer to their natural state (apples instead of apple pie); they tend to have a lower glycemic index than highly processed foods (see chapter 6).

- **Intermittent fasting (also called alternate-day fasting or time-restricted eating).** Animal research suggests that alternating normal meals with extended amounts of time (such as 8 or 24 hours) without food might offer health benefits and contribute to weight loss, but long-term human research is limited. In a 10-week study on humans, 13 participants (ages 29 to 57 years) ate breakfast one and a half hours later than usual and dinner one and a half hours earlier than usual, increasing the overnight fast by three hours. They lived at home and were allowed to eat whatever they wanted. They lost a little body fat, but the majority complained that the time-restrictions interfered with social eating events and was incompatible with family life (Antoni et al. 2018).

These questions arise about time-restricted eating: Can you achieve the same health goals with standard healthy eating patterns? Yes. Are you learning how to eat in a way that you want to maintain for the rest of your life? Doubtful. Are you listening to your body's cues and learning how to eat intuitively? No. What happens once you have lost the weight? Do you go back to your former eating habits that contributed to the weight gain in the first place? Yes. Until more long-term research is conducted, here is my advice: Don't start a diet that you do not want to maintain for the rest of your life. The best diet is the one you don't know you are on.

• **Boot camps and exhausting exercise programs.** Doing exhausting workouts to burn more calories and melt away body fat may sound like a good idea. But what often happens is that the more you exercise, the more you want to eat. You may burn an extra 400 calories but then succumb to eating 500. Or, if you are able to restrict your caloric intake, your body will conserve energy in response to this perceived "famine" caused by the huge calorie deficit. Or, you are so tired that you veg out the rest of day, burning very few calories. Dieters who overexercise can easily end up injured, exhausted, and sick with a cold or the flu. Exercise should be for enjoyment, not punishment.

Yet, if you do want to do hard exercise as a part of your get-in-shape program, high-intensity intermittent exercise (HIIT) has been shown to help with fat loss. In a study of young men, those who sprinted on exercycles (8 seconds of hard exercise followed by 12 seconds of rest, for 20 minutes, three times a week for 12 weeks) lost belly fat, gained muscle, and even had fun (Heydari, Freund, and Boutcher 2012). Just make sure you honestly enjoy it.

The bottom line is that learning how to eat in moderation, without feeling denied or deprived, is the key to a successful diet. Your goal should be to learn how to lose weight by eating smaller portions of the foods that you always have and always will like. Diets that deny favorite foods have a very limited life. Plus, you end up feeling guilty if you "cheat" and have a bagel. Is living with guilt and self-anger for having eaten a bagel conducive to optimal health? Doubtful. In my value system, eating is not cheating.

WEIGHT-LOSS FACTS AND FALLACIES

Weight reduction is more complex than adding exercise and eliminating dietary fat (Academy of Nutrition and Dietetics 2016). Confusion abounds among athletes, exercisers, and obesity researchers themselves about the best way to lose body fat. The one-diet-fits-all approach to losing weight is not appropriate; different people have different histories. Some higher-weight people are genetically heavy; others are genetically lean. Some are men; others are women. Some are recently overfat; others have been fighting the battle of the bulge for years. Some have taken comfort in food since childhood; others have recently turned to food to smother tough emotions.

Despite these factors that contribute to the complexities of weight loss, people are forever searching for a simple method to shed excess body fat. This section addresses some of the weight-reduction misconceptions among athletes and fitness exercisers alike.

Is carbohydrate fattening?

No! As I explained in chapter 6, excess calories are fattening. Calories come from carbohydrate (4 cal/g), protein (4 cal/g), alcohol (7 cal/g), and fat (9 cal/g). Excess calories from fat are the main dietary demons. Your body can easily store excess dietary fat as body fat, whereas you are more likely to burn off excess calories of carbohydrate.

Excess calories from alcohol also quickly add up and can easily inflate your body-fat stores. So can the calories from the high-fat munchies that commonly accompany alcohol. But your body preferentially burns excess calories of carbohydrate for energy rather than stores them as fat.

Are high-protein, low-carbohydrate diets the best choice if you want to lose weight?

If you want to lose weight, your best bet is to eat smaller portions at dinner, so you create a calorie deficit by the end of the day. The fundamental type of food eaten, either protein or carbohydrate, seems to have less importance than total calorie intake. In a 12-month study comparing diets containing various amounts of carbohydrate, protein, and fat, the subjects lost similar amounts of weight (Gardner et al. 2018). The bottom line is that all calories count!

A high-protein, low-carbohydrate diet seemingly works because of several factors: Dieters lose water weight. Carbohydrate holds water in the muscles. When you deplete carbohydrate, you lose a significant amount of weight that's mostly water, not fat. People eliminate many calories when they eliminate carbohydrate. For example, you might eliminate not only the potato (200 calories) but also the butter (100 calories) on top of the potato, and this creates a calorie deficit. Protein tends to be more satiating than carbohydrate. High-protein eggs at breakfast stay with you longer than does a high-carbohydrate bagel with jam. By curbing hunger, you can more easily cut calories.

The overwhelming reason high-protein, low-carbohydrate diets do *not* work is that dieters fail to stay on them for a long time. (Do you really want to never eat warm rolls at a restaurant?) You should only start an eating plan you are willing to maintain for the rest of your life.

Do dieters lose only body fat when they lose weight?

About 25 to 30 percent of weight loss relates to loss of muscle, not just fat. To abate this loss of lean tissue, dieters can do the following: Create just a small calorie deficit (as opposed to starving themselves with a crash diet). Choose protein-rich meals and snacks. Include resistance exercise twice weekly in their training. Exercise helps maintain muscle mass and minimize muscle loss, but losing only body fat is unlikely.

Does eating fat make you fat?

If you eat excess calories, you will get fat. Weight control relies on a calorie budget, not only on a fat-gram budget. Fatty foods that fit into your calorie budget are not inherently fattening (McManus, Antinoro, and Sacks 2001). If you choose to spend 300 of your 2,000 calories on high-fat peanut butter instead of fat-free cottage cheese, you can still lose body fat.

Dieters who eat only fat-free foods fool only themselves. Sharon, a personal trainer, reported that she'd been known to eat a whole box of fat-free pretzels for a snack. Max, a bodybuilder, routinely polished off a half gallon (2 L) of fat-free frozen yogurt. And Nancy, a swimmer, used to eat at least six fat-free apples per day. No wonder they all complained that they hadn't lost weight even though they avoided foods containing fat. They were eating too many calories. Excess calories, regardless of the source, will ultimately be stored as fat (Hill et al. 1992).

Eating no fat to lose body fat can "work" if you eat fewer calories. For example, instead of having bacon, eggs, and buttered toast for breakfast (700 calories), Elliott switched to bran cereal, skim milk, and a banana (400 calories). He dropped weight because of the consistent calorie deficit.

Does food eaten after 8:00 p.m. readily turn into body fat while you sleep?

While overeating at night is a problem, the verdict is unclear as to whether night eating (within your calories budget) is inherently fattening. We do know that gymnasts and runners who undereat during the day and have their biggest meal at night tend to have more body fat than those who keep themselves better fueled (Deutz et al. 2000). The same holds true for more than 50,600 Seventh-day Adventists (Kahleova 2017).

If your body is truly hungry at night, you should honor hunger and eat. I recommend, however, that you fuel appropriately during the day, so that you are not hungry at 8:00 p.m. You'll not only have more energy for training but also reduce the risk of overeating at night. Remember that when you get too hungry, you can easily overeat. That urge to eat is physiological and has little to do with willpower.

Should you exercise on an empty stomach to burn more fat?

When you exercise on empty, you do burn more fat, but burning fat differs from losing body fat. You can hinder optimal training by exercising when hungry. See chapter 9 for information on the importance of preexercise food. I suggest that you fuel well for exercise, and focus on eating less at the end of the day, so that you lose weight while you are sleeping, not when you are exercising.

Will exercise kill your appetite?

Hard exercise may temporarily kill your appetite, but hunger will catch up with you within one or two hours. Temperature control regulates appetite to some extent. Therefore, if you feel hot after a hard workout, you may experience a temporary drop in appetite. But if you are chilled, such as after swimming, you may feel ravenous.

The effect of exercise on appetite varies according to gender. Regularly exercising male rats tend to lose their appetite and drop weight, whereas female rats increase their appetite, eat more, and maintain their weight (Staten 1991). Some human studies suggest that exercise makes food more attractive to women, but this might vary according to fitness and fatness (Howe, Hand, and Manore 2014). Studies of obese women who added moderate exercise to their sedentary lifestyles indicate that they did not eat more and hence lost weight. Diet and exercise studies of men suggest that the fatter they were, the more weight they lost (in comparison with their thinner peers) because their meals didn't compensate for the calories burned during exercise (Westerterp et al. 1992).

Is it true that the fatter a person is, the fewer calories he or she should eat?

This is plain wrong. Just as 18-wheel trucks need more fuel than do compact cars, large bodies need more calories than do smaller bodies. Contrary to popular belief, obese people rarely have slow metabolisms. Rather, they require significant amounts of food. A 250-pound (113 kg) person may need 3,000 to 4,000 calories per day to maintain weight. An appropriate reducing plan would be 2,400 to 3,200 calories. That's far more than the 800 to 1,000 calories offered by many quick weight-loss programs that fail in the long run.

My large-bodies clients repeatedly report that they don't have time for breakfast and commonly work through lunch. The fact is they choose to skip those meals. They may believe they don't deserve to eat, or they feel embarrassed to be seen eating. They eat meagerly during the day, and then succumb to excessive amounts of food at night. Of course, people who live in large bodies do deserve to eat. As one of my clients said, "Nancy, you are the only person who has ever told me it's OK to eat."

ATHLETES WITH WEIGHT LIMITS

If you are a jockey or lightweight wrestler, boxer, or rower, you are probably not fat. But you may have to lose a few pounds to achieve a lower weight standard for your sport or else be denied permission to compete. Use the information here and in chapter 13 to help you lose weight healthfully. You can reach your weight goals by following the sensible information in this book and abandoning tradition-bound dieting and dehydrating practices that are not backed by science (Morton et al. 2010).

The first step to attaining your weight class is to get a realistic picture of how much weight you need to lose by having your body fat measured (see chapter 14). If you don't have access to calipers or another means of measuring your percent body fat, give yourself the less professional pinch test. If you can pinch more than half an inch (1.5 cm) of thickness over your shoulder blade or hips, you can safely lose a little more weight.

The absolute minimum body fat percentage is 5 percent for men and 12 percent for women. The minimum recommended for wrestlers is about 7 percent body fat. If possible, do not try to achieve a weight that will result in your having to starve yourself to lose muscle or dehydrate yourself to lose water weight. Achieving an unrealistic weight is difficult and can hurt rather than enhance your health and performance.

Second, start to lose weight early in the season or, better yet, before the start of the season. That way you'll have the time to lose weight slowly

(0.5 to 1.0 lb [0.25 to 0.5 kg] per week) and more enjoyably. Your goal is to achieve and stay at your lowest healthy body-fat level.

To lose weight, follow the calorie guidelines outlined earlier in this chapter in Ten Steps for Sensible Fat Loss. No matter how much weight you have to lose, do not eat less than that required to sustain your resting metabolic rate. Most athletes need to eat at least 1,500 calories of a variety of wholesome foods every day to prevent vitamin, mineral, and protein deficiencies. Do not eliminate any food group. During the day or two before the event, choose low-fiber foods to reduce the weight of intestinal contents and restrict salty foods to reduce water weight.

If you are a numbers geek, here are more-specific guidelines:

- Meals plans should include 0.7 to 0.9 grams of protein per pound of body weight (1.5 to 2 g/kg) per day and 1.5 to 2.5 grams per pound of carbohydrate (3 to 5 g/kg)—or more, depending on the sport.
- Target 13.5 to 20 calories per pound per day (30 to 45 cal/kg/day). This is particularly important for women to prevent menstrual irregularities. Contrary to popular belief, you can eat carbohydrate.
- At least 15 to 25 percent of your daily calories should come from (healthy) fat.

Be sure to surround your workouts with food so that you fuel up and recover well to get the most out of your workouts. Your recovery meal should be one of your planned meals of the day (Sundgot-Borgen et al. 2013). Table 16.2 breaks down a reducing diet for athletes of a variety of weights and suggests appropriate meals and snacks.

Remember that water is not extra weight. Your body stores precious water in a delicate balance. If you disrupt this balance, you will decrease your ability to exercise at your best. Using diuretics, rubber suits, saunas, whirlpools, or steam rooms to dehydrate yourself is dangerous. And when replacing the fluid lost in sweat after training sessions, keep in mind that sports drinks, soft drinks, and juices all have calories. Ration these beverages wisely when refueling after exercise, and then drink water the rest of the day.

Losing weight rapidly before an event can be counterproductive because depleted muscle glycogen stores and dehydration can take their toll. The odds are against the starved wrestler who crash-diets to make weight and in favor of the well-fueled wrestler who routinely maintains or stays within a few pounds (or kilograms) of his competition weight during training.

In a study of wrestlers who quickly lost about 8 pounds (3.5 kg; 4.5 percent of their body weight), the wrestlers performed 3.5 percent worse on a six-minute arm-crank test designed to be similar to a wrestling competition.

TABLE 16.2 Reducing Diet for an Athlete in Training

Here's what a reducing diet (1 lb [0.5 kg] loss/week) for an athlete in training should offer in order to provide enough energy to train and minimize muscle loss.* No crash dieting, please!

Current Weight lbs (kg)	Calories /day to lose weight	Protein (g/day)	Carbohydrate (g/day)	Fat (g/day)
	13.5-20 cal/lb 30-45 cal/kg	0.7-0.9 g/lb 1.5-2.0 g/kg	1.5-2.5 g/lb 3-5 g/kg	15%-25% total calories
125 (57)	1,700-2,500	85-115	170-285	30-70
150 (68)	2,000-3,000	100-135	200-340	35-85
175 (80)	2,400-3,600	120-160	240-400	40-100

Note: When divided into a meal every four hours (e.g., breakfast, early lunch, late lunch, dinner), each meal contains approximately the following:

Current weight	Calories/meal	Protein/meal (g)	Carbohydrate/meal (g)	Fat/meal (g)
125 (57)	425-625	20-28	40-70	10-18
150 (68)	500-750	25-35	50-85	12-20
175 (80)	800-900	30-40	60-100	15-25

Note: For a 125-pound (57 kg) athlete, a day's intake might look like this:

Breakfast: 2 eggs, english muffin, Chiobani fruit yogurt, orange

Early lunch: 2 slices of bread, 2 ounces turkey, 1/4 cup hummus, lettuce and tomato, 1 slice cheese

Late lunch (divided into pre- and postworkout snacks): Clif bar, chocolate milk

Dinner: 3 ounces chicken, 1 cup rice, 2 stalks broccoli, 2 tbsp dark chocolate–covered raisins

*Based on Sundgot-Borgen (2013).

These results suggest that rapid weight loss before competition may be detrimental rather than result in a competitive advantage (Hickner et al. 1991). If you are a high school wrestler and worried that strict dieting will stunt your growth, note that you will catch up after the competitive season. Many wrestlers are short in stature not because of malnutrition but because of genetics. They tend to have short parents. Small people often select a low-weight sport because they are more suited to it than they are to football or basketball.

If you have resorted to dehydration to make your weight, you will need to follow an aggressive refueling program after the weigh-in. This can help minimize drops in performance (Slater et al. 2007). Choose high-carbohydrate, salty foods, and drink lots of fluids. For example, enjoy juice and pretzels. Be careful, though, to consume only the amount you can comfortably tolerate.

CHAPTER 17

DIETING GONE AWRY: EATING DISORDERS AND FOOD OBSESSIONS

For most active people, the *e* in *eating* stands for *enjoyment*. But for some, it stands for *evil*; for them, food is the enemy. These food- and weight-obsessed exercisers spend their days trying not to eat. They worry constantly about what they'll eat, when and where they'll eat, how much weight they'll gain if they eat a normal meal with their friends, how many hours they will need to exercise to burn off those calories, how many meals they should skip if they overeat by a few morsels, and so on. The endless fretting about food, weight, exercise, and dieting consumes them. But some of these people fail to understand that their anxiety is abnormal.

Here are five simple questions to help you determine whether your relationship with food is out of balance.* Give yourself 1 point for every "yes" answer. If you score 2 or higher, you would likely benefit from meeting with a sports dietitian for professional guidance.

1. Do you make yourself sick because you feel uncomfortably full?
2. Do you worry you have lost control over how much you eat?
3. Have you recently lost more than 14 pounds (6.5 kg) in a three-month period?
4. Do you believe yourself to be fat when others say you are too thin?
5. Would you say that food dominates your life?

*Source: J.F. Morgan, J.H. Reid, and J.H. Lacey, "The SCOFF questionnaire: Assessment of a new screening tool for eating disorders," *BMJ* 316, no 7223 (1999); 1467-1468.

WHY EATING DISORDERS HAPPEN

Eating disorders such as anorexia and bulimia commonly occur in people with low self-esteem; they believe they are not good enough. They believe that thinness will make them better and more loveable. The truth is that a thinner body does not make you better, just smaller. There is simply less of you to love. You are the same person, just anxious, obsessed, withdrawn, and exhausted. And when you severely restrict food, you lose muscle, strength, and stamina. This is not the way to become a star athlete.

The risk of developing an eating disorder seems to increase dramatically when an anxious athlete with low self-esteem is physically beautiful, has traits of perfectionism, and tends to be self-critical. Add to the scenario a mother who may have had (or still has) food and weight issues, and her daughter becomes a prime target for developing a full-blown eating disorder.

Athletes with eating disorders are less available to their friends. After all, when a person is constantly exercising and counting calories (calories eaten at meals, calories burned during exercise, calories saved by skipping lunch, calories about to be eaten at dinner) as well as counting fat grams and sit-ups, the brain has little energy left to manage bigger issues, such as life's problems and relationships. The anorexia or bulimia creates a smoke screen that masks the underlying issues.

One pathway to recovery is to see the eating disorder as being just one part of you. It is the part that tries to protect your other parts that don't like feeling lonely, rejected, or imperfect. For example, perhaps you had traumatic experiences in middle school. Your eating-disordered part can distract you from, and numb, feelings of pain, terror, and fear. It serves a purpose—it keeps you feeling more in control of your life. But it also keeps you miserable.

What Is Anorexia?

People with anorexia (more correctly, anorexia nervosa) tend to either consistently restrict food or restrict and then binge and purge. The American Psychiatric Association's definition of anorexia nervosa includes the following characteristics:*

- Intense fear of gaining weight or becoming fat, even though underweight
- Disturbance in the way a person experiences his or her body (i.e., claiming to feel fat even when emaciated), with an undue influence of body weight or shape on self-perception

- Weight loss to less than 85 percent of normal body weight or, if during a period of growth, failure to make expected weight gain leading to 85 percent of that expected
- Refusal to maintain body weight over a minimal normal weight for age and height
- Denial of the seriousness of the current weight loss

Historically, the absence of at least three consecutive menstrual cycles had been a part of the definition of anorexia, but this was removed in 2013. Some athletes with anorexia maintain normal menstrual cycles and fail to get the help they need, thinking they are not "sick enough."

*Adapted from American Psychiatric Association, *Diagnostic and Statistical Manual of Mental Disorders,* 5th ed. (Arlington, VA: American Psychiatric Association, 2013).

If you think that you or someone you know might have anorexia, look for these signs and symptoms:

- Significant weight loss
- Loss of menstrual periods
- Loss of hair
- Growth of fine body hair, noticeable on the face and arms
- Cold hands and feet and extreme sensitivity to cold temperature
- Wearing sweaters in summer heat because of feeling cold all the time
- Layers of baggy clothing to hide thinness (and keep warm)
- Light-headedness
- Inability to concentrate
- Low pulse rate
- Hyperactivity, compulsive exercise beyond normal training
- Recurrent overuse injuries and stress fractures
- Comments about being fat, distorted body image, expression of intense fear of becoming fat
- Food rituals such as cutting food into small pieces and playing with it
- Nervousness at mealtimes, avoiding eating with friends or in public
- Antisocial behavior, isolating from family and friends
- Excessive working or studying, compulsiveness, and rigidity
- Extreme emotions: tearful, uptight, oversensitive, and restless

What Is Bulimia?

The person with the purging type of bulimia nervosa may purge by self-induced vomiting and by misusing laxatives, diuretics, or enemas. With the nonpurging type of bulimia, the person uses other inappropriate compensatory mechanisms to prevent weight gain after a binge, such as fasting or exercising excessively. The definition used by the American Psychiatric Association includes these aspects:*

- Recurrent episodes of binge eating, characterized by one or both of the following:
    1. Eating, in a discrete period of time (e.g., within any two-hour period), an amount of food that is definitely larger than most people would eat during a similar time period and under similar circumstances
    2. Feeling out of control during the eating episode (unable to stop eating or control what and how much is eaten)
- Compensating for the food binge to prevent weight gain, such as inducing vomiting; misusing laxatives, diuretics, or other medications; or exercising excessively
- Evaluating self-worth according to body shape and weight
- Binge eating and purging, on average, at least once a week for three months

*Adapted from American Psychiatric Association, *Diagnostic and Statistical Manual of Mental Disorders,* 5th ed. (Arlington, VA: American Psychiatric Association, 2013).

If you think that you or someone you know might have bulimia, look for these signs and symptoms:

- Weakness, headaches, dizziness
- Frequent weight fluctuations because of alternating binges and fasts
- Swollen glands that give a chipmunklike appearance
- Difficulty swallowing and retaining food, damage to throat
- Frequent vomiting
- Damaged tooth enamel from exposure to gastric acid when vomiting
- Petty stealing of food or money to buy food for binges
- Strange behavior that surrounds secretive eating
- Disappearance after meals, often to the bathroom to "take a shower"
- Running water in the bathroom after meals to hide the sound of vomiting

- Extreme concern about body weight, shape, and physical appearance
- Ability to eat enormous meals without weight gain
- Compulsive exercise beyond normal training
- Depression
- Bloodshot eyes

What Is Binge Eating Disorder?

Binge eating disorder (BED) is a newly recognized eating disorder and is the most common eating disorder in the United States. In some aspects, it is similar to bulimia, but without unhealthy means to compensate for (i.e., purge) the influx of food. Among people with BED, up to two-thirds are higher than average weight.

Binge eating disorder is a serious condition characterized by repeated episodes of uncontrolled eating and weight gain. The eating can be a way to cope with depression, stress, or anxiety and can occur with people who have never learned how to deal effectively with their feelings. The definition used by the American Psychiatric Association includes these aspects:*

- Eating until uncomfortably full
- Eating large amounts of food when not feeling physically hungry
- Eating alone because of embarrassment about how much one is eating
- Feeling disgusted with oneself, depressed, or very guilty afterward

The binges occur, on average, at least once a week for three months.

*Adapted from American Psychiatric Association, *Diagnostic and Statistical Manual of Mental Disorders,* 5th ed. (Arlington, VA: American Psychiatric Association, 2013).

If you think that you or someone you know might have binge eating disorder, look for these signs and symptoms:

- Disappearance of large amounts of food or lots of empty wrappers and food containers
- Interest in new fad diets
- Stealing or hoarding food in strange places
- Grazing on food, but not through planned meals; skipping meals
- Noticeable weight fluctuations, both gain and loss
- Difficulty concentrating

EATING DISORDERS AND ACTIVE PEOPLE

Eating disorders among active people seem to be on the rise. Staff members at health clubs commonly express concerns about some of their clients, as do coaches about their athletes, especially athletes in sports that emphasize weight, such as running, gymnastics, and wrestling. Research indicates that eating disorders are widespread among athletes in all sports. An estimated 6 to 45 percent of female athletes and up to 19 percent of male athletes struggle with food, depending on their sport (Bratland-Sanda and Sundgot-Borgen 2013). Most people with eating disorders exercise compulsively, either to create a calorie deficit and be thinner or to burn off the calories consumed during a binge. Some report using exercise as a way to feel warmer; lack of fuel leaves them with chronically cold hands and feet (Carrera et al. 2012).

Many dieters abuse exercise to control their weight. On the outside, they appear to be healthy athletes, but in reality they could be better named compulsive exercisers. Many live in fear of becoming fat, and they constantly restrict their food intake in the hope of losing weight. They live with chaotic eating patterns and body hatred. Approximately half of all dieters report abnormal eating binges.

I estimate that at least 40 percent of my clients are obsessed with food, and they represent only a minority of people who seek professional nutrition guidance. Most food-obsessed people struggle on their own for years before asking for help because they are embarrassed that they can't seem to resolve their food imbalances. One 65-year-old woman, a regular at a health club, confided that I was the first person in 50 years to whom she had talked about her bulimia.

For these people, food is not fuel. It is the fattening enemy that thwarts their desire to be perfectly thin. Their goal is thinness at any price, and that price is often guilt, shame, mental anguish, physical fatigue, injuries that fail to heal, anemia, weakened bones, stress fractures, and impaired athletic performance. These athletes perform suboptimally because they eat poorly. One high school runner failed to connect her inability to finish track workouts with her one-banana-a-day diet. She thought she fell asleep in classes because she had stayed up too late studying, not because she was underfed.

If you struggle with anorexia, bulimia, or binge eating, I recommend that you seek help from a professional counselor experienced with eating disorders and obtain nutrition guidance from a registered dietitian. (See Eating Disorders in appendix A for websites that offer referral networks.) You (or your loved one) need not struggle alone. Be wise and make the

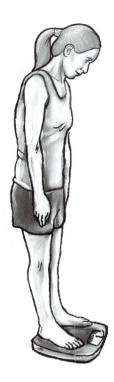

right decision to ask for help. Extreme eating disorders usually reflect an inability to cope with the day-to-day stresses of life.

For example, a woman in charge of fund-raising for a charitable organization smothered her stress with homemade chocolate-chip cookies warm from the oven. This treat certainly diverted her attention from her problems, but it didn't resolve any of them. Afraid of gaining weight, she'd burn off the calories with a long workout that was pure punishment. She became injured from the excessive exercise, panicked at her inability to exercise, tried to eat next to nothing, became ravenous, binged, and then resorted to self-induced vomiting to purge the calories because she could no longer exercise the way she desired. She came to me looking for help with food. I insisted that she also get psychological counseling to help her deal with stress and her feelings of being out of control.

Eating disorders affect all types of casual exercisers and competitive athletes, males and females alike, and perhaps even you or one of your friends. Some with a seemingly normal weight may not fit the weight criteria for anorexia, but they can have *atypical* anorexia. They have an abnormal relationship with food and spend way too much time thinking about food and weight. They fritter away each day, trying to get thinner.

In-depth interviews with women with subclinical or atypical eating disorders delineate these characteristic eating behaviors:

- They restrict their calorie intake to lose weight and eat a repetitive diet, with little or no variety in the types and amounts of foods they consume.
- They follow strict dietary rules and experience guilt and self-anger if they break one of their rules.
- They limit their intake of "bad foods" and usually choose low-fat or fat-free foods.

Almost all these women perceive themselves as slightly to very overfat and are preoccupied with weight (Beals and Manore 2000).

Active women seemingly adapt to the combination of intense calorie-burning exercise and restricted calorie intake. Nature perceives the big energy deficit as a "famine"; the body seems to shut down and conserve energy (similar to hibernation). Yet, research suggests that these women who maintain a stable weight may indeed get the calories they need, but through chaotic binge eating (Wilmore et al. 1992).

If you believe that your body is hibernating, and you believe you eat less than you "deserve" to eat given your exercise level, the solution is to increase your daytime calorie intake to an appropriate level, stop living in calorie deficit, and curb binge eating. You can do this gradually by adding about 100 calories (e.g., a yogurt) to your daily intake for four days; then adding another 100 calories (an orange) for the next four days, and so on until you approach your calorie requirements as outlined in chapter 16. A registered dietitian can be helpful in this process.

HUNGER: A SIMPLE REQUEST FOR FUEL

Being hungry all the time is not a personality quirk. Rather, hunger is the body's request for fuel. Hunger is a powerful physiological force that creates a strong desire to eat. Unfortunately, in our thin-is-in society, many active people fail to honor this simple request because they fear food as being fattening. The thought of eating elicits a sense of panic: "Oh, no, if I eat, I'll get fat. But if I stay hungry, I know I am not gaining weight." This is an unhealthy mind-set.

Athletes can eat without getting fat. Food, after all, is fuel. But problems arise when people deny themselves food (as happens with a strict reducing diet), when hunger becomes the norm. The result is an abnormal physiological state known as starvation.

Starvation has been inflicted on many people, including people in developing countries suffering through famines, poverty-stricken people at the end of the month when they have no money for food, and victims of World War II concentration camps. Starvation is also common among exercisers who are intent on losing weight.

What is the cost of starvation? What happens to the body and the mind when food is restricted and body weight is abnormally low? In 1950, Ancel Keys and his colleagues at the University of Minnesota studied the physiology of starvation (cited in Garner 1998). They carefully monitored 36 young, healthy, psychologically normal men who for six months were allowed to eat only half their normal intake (an amount similar to that consumed on a strict reducing diet or with anorectic eating). For three months before this semistarvation diet, the researchers carefully studied each man's behaviors, personality, and eating patterns. After the semistarvation diet, the men were then observed for three to nine months of refeeding.

As their body weight fell to 25 percent below baseline, the researchers learned that many of the symptoms that were thought to be specific to anorexia or bulimia were actually the result of starvation. The most striking change was a dramatically increased preoccupation with food. The subjects thought about food all the time, just as hungry dieters and people with anorexia do. They talked about it, read about it, dreamed about it. They even collected recipes. They dramatically increased their consumption of coffee and tea, and they chewed gum excessively. They became depressed; had severe mood swings; and experienced irritability, anger, and anxiety. They became withdrawn, had little interest in sex, and lost their sense of humor. They had cold hands and feet, they felt weak and dizzy, and their hair fell out. Their basal metabolic rates (the amount of food needed to exist) dropped by 40 percent as their bodies adapted to conserve energy. Perhaps these changes sound familiar.

During the study, some of the men were unable to maintain control over food; they would binge eat if the opportunity presented itself. During the refeeding period, many of the men ate continuously—large meals followed by snacking. Several ate until they were uncomfortably full, became nauseated, and then vomited. These abnormal eating behaviors lasted for about five months. By eight months, most of the men had regained their standard eating behaviors. On average, they initially regained 10 percent more than their original weights but then gradually lost that excess and returned close to their baseline weights.

So what can we learn from this starvation study?

- Preoccupation with food is a sign that your body is too hungry. Hunger creates a strong physiological drive to eat.
- Binge eating stems from starvation. If you worry about being unable to stop eating once you start, you have likely become too hungry. Eat a little more at breakfast and lunch to prevent extreme hunger.

- Weight is more than a matter of willpower. If you lose weight, your body will fight to return to a genetically normal level.
- Dieters who restrict to the point of semistarvation are likely to regain the weight they lost, plus more. If you have weight to lose, lose it slowly, not by starvation.

The Hunger Scale

If you have spent years dieting and not eating when you are hungry, then blowing your diet and stuffing yourself until you need to loosen your belt, you may feel troubled by the struggle to regulate your food intake. The hunger scale (table 17.1) can help you get back in touch with intuitive eating (i.e., eating like a child). Throughout the day, before, during, and after meals, pay attention to your levels of hunger, fatigue, contentedness, and fullness. Note that children eat when they are hungry and stop when they are content—and they rarely run out of energy.

TABLE 17.1 The Hunger Scale

1	3	5	7	10
Starved Light-headed Stomach growling	Thinking about food Moody, cold Bored	Content Pleasantly fed Satiated	Very full Uncomfortable "Ate too much"	Stuffed Painfully full Very uncomfortable

Stomach growling is a sign that you are *too* hungry. You should eat before you get to that stage. You might notice that you feel hunger in your head before you feel it in your stomach. Jessie, a computer programmer, complained that she snacked in the afternoon simply because she was bored. She didn't realize that feeling bored and unable to concentrate indicated needing fuel. I invited her to do this experiment: enjoy two graham crackers with peanut butter when she felt bored. She quickly discovered that this fuel boosted her blood sugar. She perked up, felt happier, and was able to work productively for the rest of the afternoon.

Your job is to listen to your body and eat until you are satisfied and feel pleasantly fed—not stuffed, not hankering for more because you are still hungry, and not stopping eating just because you think you should. The trick to feeding yourself appropriately is to eat slowly and mindfully, paying attention to the pleasant feeling of satiety that is midway between starved and stuffed.

To prevent hunger, you might find it helpful to know how many calories your body requires to maintain or to lose weight (see chapter 16). Then, the next time you get into a food tizzy, overeat, and wonder whether you are borderline bulimic, you can compare your intake to your requirements. You'll likely see a huge discrepancy between what you have eaten and what your body needs. Hunger is powerful. Avoid becoming too hungry!

THIN AT ANY COST

The restriction of food that accompanies the struggle to be perfectly thin creates health problems for casual exercisers and competitors alike. Eating too little food can greatly reduce the intake of vitamins, minerals, protein, and carbohydrate, placing athletes at risk of poor nutrition status. Food restrictions can also lead to health problems such as chronic fatigue, compromised immune function, poor or delayed healing, anemia, electrolyte imbalance, menstrual dysfunction, reduced bone density, and a much higher risk of stress fracture (Mountjoy et al. 2014).

I counsel many people with eating disorders and disordered eating who come to me believing that if only they were thinner, they'd be better athletes (and their overall lives would be better). I disagree. Their efforts to achieve their desired thinness reduce their energy and performance. They would be better athletes if they fed themselves better. Such was the case with Barbara, an avid cyclist. She came to me complaining about her inability to lose 5 pounds (2.3 kg): "If only I could shed this extra fat, I'd be so much faster climbing hills." She was severely restricting her food intake. I pointed out how few calories she was eating compared with what her body required. Once she started to eat adequately, she discovered that she could keep up with the other cyclists. Food works!

The following case studies are typical of the clients I treat. They may sound familiar and help those of you who constantly struggle with food and exercise.

The Stair-Stepper Mistress

Alicia, a 41-year-old teacher, had never been concerned about her weight and had never dieted until her 39th birthday. But in the previous two years, she had gained a few pounds because of the stress of a new job. Not liking the extra weight, she decided to join a health club. She forced herself through 60 minutes of stair stepping every morning before school, ate very little during the day, and would then devour any food in sight on arriving home from work. "I feel so guilty about the boxes of crackers, pretzels, and cookies I devour. After a binge, I won't eat dinner. Instead, I'll go back to the health club to burn off the excess calories. I'm exhausted all

Healing Mantras and Affirmations

If you are determined to start eating better, you might find the task easier said than done. Here are some mantras that have helped my clients as they strive to fuel their bodies appropriately:

- My body is hungry; that means it has burned off what I fed it, and it now needs more fuel. Hunger is simply a request for fuel.
- This food is fundamental, not "extra," not "fattening."
- One meal is not going to ruin my life forever.
- I need to be more flexible. I can always go back to my old ways, if I need to.
- My body is stronger when I fuel better, and I become a better athlete.
- I don't need to have a perfect diet to have an excellent diet.
- Starving my body will not solve any of my problems.
- Being happy and healthy is more important than any number on the scale.
- I have a choice: Do I want to be a person with anorexia or a well-fueled athlete?
- Everything will work out OK. I just need to keep focused on the big picture—I need to be healthy.

the time. I'm doing a poor job of teaching. I get easily irritated and feel like yelling at the students. I'm frustrated that I'm unable to do something as simple as lose a few pounds. I can't even eat normally now. I either starve or binge. I don't know if I should be seeing you or a therapist."

To help Alicia balance her food and exercise goals and to normalize her disordered eating patterns, I estimated how many calories her body required each day. She needed about 1,200 calories for her resting metabolic rate, 600 calories for moderate daily activity, and 500 calories for purposeful exercise, adding up to about 2,300 total calories per day. I also measured her body fat to determine whether she really had excess fat to lose. She was lean (18 percent fat); she agreed to take a vacation from dieting so she could better stabilize her eating.

Like many of my clients, she dieted too hard and unrealistically restricted her calories. She would burn off 500 calories at the health club but would not eat anything until lunch, when she limited herself to 250 calories of a frozen meal. No wonder she stuffed herself with food the minute she arrived home after school; she was starved! I advised her to stop dieting, start eating breakfast and lunch, and then enjoy a second lunch after school.

Alicia experimented with my recommendations to eat 2,300 calories, divided into four even-sized meals: breakfast, first lunch, second lunch (after school), and dinner. When she returned two weeks later, she reported with a big smile, "When I get home after school, I no longer act like a maniac in the kitchen, eating whatever I can get my hands on. I feel so much better because I'm not binge eating. Having a substantial high-protein breakfast and lunch gives me enough energy to have fun with my students. I'm less irritable—back to my old happy self. And, most important, I'm back in control of my food." Alicia had thought that dieting would help her lose weight, but instead she learned that normal, healthy eating is really the better path to weight management.

The Exercise Addict

Bill, a regional sales manager for a computer company, was addicted to exercise. He'd get up at 5:15 a.m. and arrive at the front door of the health club when it opened at 6:00. He'd do a stationary cycling class from 6:00 to 7:00 and then lift weights from 7:00 to 8:00. At lunchtime, he'd do a step-aerobics class at his company's fitness facility. After work he'd swim laps for an hour at his local YMCA. Because he exercised at three different locations, few people knew how much time he spent exercising, except his wife and family. They constantly complained that he was never home.

Holidays brought even more complaints. "Why do you have to exercise on Christmas morning?" his eight-year-old daughter complained when Bill announced that he was going for his two-hour Merry Christmas run, his present to himself. His family knew he would be incredibly irritable if he didn't run, so they waited patiently for his return before opening gifts.

Without question, Bill was addicted to exercise. He'd feel irritable, anxious, guilty, and depressed if he was unable to do at least four hours of exercise a day. He needed to do increasingly more exercise to achieve the same physical and emotional highs. Exercise was akin to his antianxiety medication. He'd exercise even when injured or sick. He had little energy for the rest of his life and was fearful that he would lose his job because of a steady decline in his work performance.

Bill's ability to exercise came to a halt when he experienced debilitating back pain. He could barely walk without severe anguish. While seeing the back doctor, he admitted that he needed help: "I can no longer exercise the way I'd like to, and I'm petrified of getting fat. I'm trying not to eat because I cannot exercise, but I end up sneaking food—and stealing my

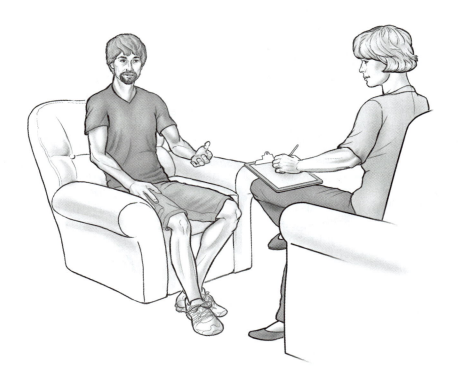

daughter's M&Ms." The doctor insisted that Bill make an appointment with me. To my eyes, Bill had a long way to go before anyone would consider him fat. He was 5 feet 10 inches (178 cm) tall and weighed 130 pounds (59 kg), but I listened to his fears. I reminded him that sick people in hospitals do little or no exercise, and they still eat and don't get fat; in fact, they commonly lose weight.

I worked with Bill on normalizing his eating and exercise practices, suggested reading material (such as *The Truth About Exercise Addiction: Understanding the Dark Side of Thinspiration* by Katherine Schreiber and Heather Hausenblas), and convinced him that meeting with a counselor would help keep his life from falling apart. With a doctor, therapist, and nutritionist on his treatment team, as well as a family therapist and the love of his wife and children, he evolved into a happier person. He learned to communicate his wants and needs so that he no longer felt the desire to run away from his problems. He came to understand that his underlying belief that he wasn't good enough was a misperception. He came to like and accept himself as the truly loving person he is.

How Much Exercise Is Enough?

Exercise should be a way to train and improve athletic performance, not a means of purging calories. If you are an exercise bulimic who spends too much time working out, note the following recommendations from the *2015-2022 Dietary Guidelines for Americans* as well as from the *Department of Health and Human Services' Physical Activity Guidelines for Americans*, 2nd edition (Piercy et al. 2018)

For health and fitness and to reduce the risk of disease, adults should participate in the following most days of the week:

- A minimum of 30 minutes a day of moderate activity to prevent chronic disease (or a total of 150 to 300 minutes per week) or 15 to 30 minutes a day (75 to 150 minutes a week) of moderate to vigorous aerobic activity
- At least twice a week, lifting weights or doing resistance training for muscle-strengthening
- At least 60 minutes a day of moderate to vigorous physical activity for youth ages 6 to 17

If you are an athlete training for a sport, you might spend more time than this. But consider getting help if you are a compulsive exerciser whose primary motivation is to burn calories. You are more likely to end up exhausted, injured, and unable to improve at your sport due to poorly fueled and rested muscles.

The Marathon Runner With Bulimia

Carol, a 29-year-old graduate student, had gained 12 pounds (5.4 kg) in the two years since she had started studying for her MBA. She tended to overeat when schoolwork became overwhelming and she felt as if she couldn't do all that was expected of her. "I binge at night and then vomit and go for a long run. I'm exhausted all the time and think of little else than what, when, and how I'll binge. I've stopped socializing with my friends at mealtimes because I'm afraid I'll overeat and be unable to purge. Instead, I spend my time studying and training for a marathon. I'm hoping the added exercise will contribute to weight loss. But I'm a foodaholic. When I finish my run, I inevitably end up at the corner store, where I buy at least two big muffins and heaven only knows what else. I just can't seem to control my food intake."

After listening to Carol's story, I recognized that she seemed addicted not only to food but also to schoolwork and exercise. She constantly pushed herself to meet self-imposed deadlines, weight goals, and exercise demands. She always felt stressed and overextended. She lacked a healthy balance in her life.

I asked if anyone in Carol's family had trouble with alcohol. She quietly admitted that her mother was an alcoholic. She seemed ashamed of this family secret. At least one-third of my clients with eating disorders grew up in families with some type of dysfunction, most commonly related to alcohol. The clients themselves may not be addicted to alcohol, but some are recovering alcoholics or drug abusers. Alternatively, they express other addictive behaviors such as overworking, overeating, overachieving, and overexercising. The traits and attitudes outlined in table 17.2 are characteristic of people who grew up in alcoholic or otherwise dysfunctional families.

Carol displayed all of the traits in table 17.2. She had a strong drive to be perfect and a desire for control. Since childhood she had tried to be perfect to compensate for her family's problems. Now, she was trying to eat the perfect diet, achieve the perfect weight, develop the perfect career, and maintain the perfect training schedule. She ran 10 miles (16 km) every day, despite blizzards, illness, or fatigue. She lived on calorie-free coffee, diet soda, and fat-free foods, until ravenous hunger overwhelmed her good intentions. After a binge, she'd vomit to bring a feeling of control back to her life and compensate for her imperfect eating.

I helped Carol get a better perspective on an appropriate weight by measuring her percent body fat (a lean 16 percent) and then asking how other people described her body. "They all think I'm crazy for wanting to

TABLE 17.2 Red-Flag Personality Traits

Personality trait	Common expression of trait
Drive for perfection	I've exercised for an hour every day for the past two years.
Desire for control	I never eat after 7:00 p.m.
Compulsive behavior	I work out for two hours every day, even if I have to get up at 4:00 a.m.
Feelings of inadequacy	I could have biked even faster if I'd lost more weight.
Difficulty having fun	Thanks for inviting me to the movie. I'll pass—I have to do my workout at the gym.
Trouble with relationships	My spouse complains that I spend too much time exercising and not enough time with my family.

lose weight," she said. We talked more about ways to resolve her distorted body image (see chapter 14). The problem wasn't her body, but her relationship with her body.

Carol agreed to start working with a coach who could help her create an appropriate training schedule that included rest days. She also expressed an interest in reading books about adult children of alcoholics (see Alcohol in appendix A), seeking guidance from a suitable counselor, and perhaps joining a support group such as Al-Anon or ACA (Adult Children of Alcoholics).

"For the past two years, I have tried to avoid food, thinking it was fattening," Carol wrote in a follow-up email several months later. "I've come to learn that food wasn't the problem. My inability to handle stress

What Is Normal Eating?

Normal eating is going to the table hungry and eating until you are satisfied. It is being able to choose food you like and eat it and truly get enough of it—not stopping eating just because you think you should. Normal eating is being able to give some thought to your food selection so you get nutritious food, but not being so wary and restrictive that you miss out on enjoyable food. Normal eating is giving yourself permission to eat sometimes because you are happy, sad, or bored, or just because it feels good. Normal eating is mostly three meals a day, or four or five, or it can be choosing to munch along the way. It is leaving cookies on the plate because you know you can have some again tomorrow, or it is eating more now because they taste so wonderful. Normal eating is overeating at times, feeling stuffed and uncomfortable. And it can be undereating at times and wishing you had more. Normal eating is trusting your body to make up for your mistakes in eating. Normal eating takes up some of your time and attention, but keeps its place as only one important area of your life.

In short, normal eating is flexible. It varies in response to your hunger, your schedule, your proximity to food, and your feelings.

For more about eating competence (and for research backing up this advice), see Ellyn Satter's *Secrets of Feeding a Healthy Family: How to Eat, How to Raise Good Eaters, How to Cook*. Also see www.EllynSatterInstitute.org/shop to purchase books and to review other resources.

was the problem. I'm now gentler on myself. I no longer strive to be the perfect student. For example, I took three days off from both school and running when I went on a ski weekend with my friends! I'm eating well and exercising healthfully rather than punishing myself with mega-miles to burn off calories. I feel better, enjoy better quality of life, and am at peace with myself and my body."

The Figure Skater With Amenorrhea

Emily, a 16-year-old student in a highly competitive figure skating program, was sent to me by her coach. Emily's mother made the appointment for her. Because she was chronically tired, Emily's ability to jump high and skate hard was compromised. Emily's first words to me were, "My coach and mother made me come here. They think I don't eat enough."

Emily weighed 92 pounds (42 kg). A year ago, she had weighed 110 pounds (50 kg), and at 5 feet 3 inches (160 cm), she could have appropriately weighed 115 pounds (52 kg). She was limiting herself to 1,000 calories per day but required about 1,800 calories, if not more. Because she was eating so little food, she had stopped menstruating (one sign of poor health), and her complexion was splotchy and grayish (a second sign).

With time and encouragement from her support team (a pediatrician, a therapist, and me), Emily gradually increased her energy intake. She made hard food choices and practiced eating healthfully so she could skate energetically. A key factor in her recovery was counseling to help her deal with her anxiety about food and weight. She routinely met with a psychologist skilled in handling eating disorders. She learned how to manage stress and

Athletes and Amenorrhea

If you believe you miss periods because you are too thin and are exercising too much, you may be wrong. Studies have shown no body-fat differences between athletic women who menstruate regularly and those who don't. But the question remains: Why are you amenorrheic when your peers, who have similar exercise programs and the same low percentage of body fat, are not?

You are likely eating inadequate calories to support your training program and are experiencing nutritional amenorrhea. Do not ignore this serious problem. Please read the information about how to overcome the energy imbalance that leads to amenorrhea (RED-S; see chapter 12.

also how to express her needs. Rather than withhold words and starve her feelings, she was able to end her silent cry for help.

Within three months of eating 1,800 calories per day, Emily started to menstruate, a good sign that she was adequately nourishing her body. She let go of her fantasy that a perfectly thin body would bring a perfect life. "I thought I'd be happier once I was thinner, but I was wrong. I've learned that happiness comes from loving myself from the inside out, not from the outside in."

HOW TO HELP

Perhaps you have friends, family, or teammates who struggle with food, and you wonder what you can do to help resolve the problem. Seeing a loved one seemingly waste away can be sad and scary. Often it's hard to tell whether the person is really struggling or just being a dedicated athlete. Even health professionals can have trouble distinguishing between the person who is lean and mean and the one who is experiencing anorexia.

An athlete with anorexia is generally a compulsive exerciser who trains frantically—out of fear of gaining weight—and never takes rest days. In comparison, a dedicated athlete trains hard with the hope of improving performance but also enjoys days with no exercise. Both push themselves to perfection—to be perfectly thin or to be the perfect athlete. Sometimes the two intertwine. Unfortunately, too many coaches, parents, friends, and teammates fail to confront the person who is devastatingly stressed by this struggle to achieve ultimate thinness. After all, how can anyone who is training hard and seems happy be sick?

If you suspect that your friend, training partner, child, or teammate has a problem with food, don't wait until medical problems prove you right. Speak up in an appropriate manner. Anorexia and bulimia are life-threatening conditions that shouldn't be overlooked. Here are 10 tips for approaching this delicate subject.

1. **Heed the signs.** You may notice that the person wears bulky clothes to hide her abnormal thinness or that her food consumption is abnormally restrictive and sparse in comparison to the energy she expends. Runners with anorexia, for example, may eat only a yogurt for dinner after having completed a strenuous 10-mile (16 km) workout. Perhaps you've never seen her eating in public, at home, or with friends. She finds some excuse for not joining others at meals. Or if she does, she may push the food around on the plate to fool you into thinking she's eating. You may also notice other compulsive behaviors, such as excessive studying or working.

Bulimic behavior can be subtler. The athlete may eat a great deal of food and then rush to the bathroom. You may hear water running to cover up the sound of vomiting. The person may hide laxatives or even speak about a magic method of eating without gaining weight. She may have bloodshot eyes, swollen glands, and bruised fingers (from inducing vomiting).

2. **Express your concern carefully.** Approach the person gently but persistently, telling him that you are worried about his health: "I'm concerned that your injuries are taking so long to heal." Talk about what you see: "I've noticed that you seem tired, and your race times are getting slower and slower." Give evidence for why you believe he is struggling to balance food and exercise, and ask if he wants to talk about it.

People who are truly anorexic or bulimic commonly deny the problem, insisting they're perfectly fine. Continue to share your concerns about the person's lack of concentration, light-headedness, or chronic fatigue. These health issues are more likely to be stepping-stones for the athlete to accept help, given that he undoubtedly clings to food and exercise as attempts to gain control and stability.

3. **Do not discuss weight or eating habits.** The athlete takes great pride in being perfectly thin and may dismiss your concern as jealousy. Avoid any mention of starving and bingeing as the issue. Focus on life issues, not food issues.

4. **Suggest unhappiness as the reason for seeking help.** Point out how anxious, tired, or irritable the athlete has been lately. Emphasize that she doesn't have to be that way.

5. **Be supportive, and listen sympathetically.** Don't expect someone to admit right away that there's a problem. Give it time, and constantly remind the person that you believe in him. Your support will make a difference in recovery. Offer a list of professional resources, including the books and websites listed in appendix A.

6. **Take care of yourself.** Seek advice from health care professionals about your concerns. You may need to discuss your feelings with someone. Remember that you are not responsible for the other person's health. You can only try to help. Your power comes from using guidance counselors, registered dietitians, medical professionals, or eating disorders clinics.

To help you understand more about these underlying issues, you might want to read the books for parents and loved ones listed at www.edcatalogue.com. These helpful resources can teach you what to say to your friend or loved one. Your job is to help the person by taking her to get professional guidance. This might mean finding a registered dietitian in your area who specializes in sports nutrition and eating disorders.

7. **Be open to hear a cry for help.** Although the athlete may deny the problem to your face, he may admit despair at another moment. If you don't know of a mental health counselor skilled in the treatment of eating

disorders, the resources and national organizations listed in appendix A can help you find an expert where you live. You can also call your local sports medicine clinic and ask to speak to a physician or nutritionist, your university health center or eating disorders program, or your local medical center and ask about setting up an appointment for the athlete, so he can be evaluated to determine the depth of the eating issues.

8. **Limit your expectations.** You alone can't solve the problem. It's more complex than food and exercise; an eating disorder is a psychological (not nutritional) diagnosis. You may feel frustrated about your unsuccessful efforts to resolve the problem. You may think, "If only my friend would eat normally, everything would be OK." Likely not. Food is just the symptom. The problem is that this person is unhappy. Remind your friend that no weight will ever be good enough to create happiness. Happiness comes from within, not from a number on the scale.

Share your concerns with others. Seek help from a trusted family member, medical professional, or health service. Don't try to deal with the problem alone, especially if you are making no headway and the athlete is becoming more self-destructive.

9. **Recognize that you may be overreacting.** Maybe there is no eating disorder. Maybe the athlete is appropriately thin for enhanced sports performance. But how can you know? To clarify the situation, insist that the person have an evaluation. If necessary, make the appointment, and take the athlete to the eating disorders clinic yourself. Only then will the athlete get an unbiased opinion of the degree of danger, if any.

10. **Be patient.** Recognize that the healing process can be long and arduous, with many relapses and setbacks, but your reward will be that you can make a critical difference in that person's life. People die from anorexia and bulimia.

PREVENTING EATING DISORDERS

Many people think, or feel pressured to believe, that by restricting their food intake to lose weight they will exercise better, look better, and enhance their overall performances. As I mentioned in chapter 16, dieting commonly precedes the onset of obesity, disordered eating, and eating disorders. Dieting is a risky behavior; it is not a solution to weight issues.

As a society, we must dispel the myths that diets work and that thinness equates to happiness and success, discourage the notion that the thinnest athlete is the best athlete, and love our bodies for what they are rather than hate them for what they are not. We must emphasize being fit and healthy as more appropriate goals than being skinny and be careful about how we acknowledge weight loss.

When Your Friends Lose Weight, What Should You Say?

When someone has lost weight, the knee-jerk response is to exclaim, "Wow! You look great!" This praise is intended to be positive, but it implies the following:

- The dieter looked horrible before.
- Physical size is more important than health.
- The person is somehow better or more valuable because of the weight loss.

Be it 2 pounds or 20 (1 kg or 10), the better way to acknowledge weight loss is to shift the focus away from physical weight change and focus instead on the praiseworthy aspect: the person's hard work and improved health status. Here are recommended phrases to share with people who are losing or have lost weight:

- "It looks like you've been working hard to lose weight." The dieter will be ever ready to talk about how proud she is of the hard work it took to lose weight. Listen to the story and be sure that the person is healthy.
- "You look smaller. Is there less of you to love?" The message is that your friend is not better for having lost weight, just smaller.
- "You look pleased with your weight loss. How do you feel about it?" The person may feel healthier and more energetic, but you may also hear him express frustration in not being quite thin enough yet.
- "You are looking fit. How are your workouts going? How is your energy level? How do you feel?" If your friend is losing weight appropriately, she will feel great.
- "You appear to be trading some of your excess fat for muscle." Acknowledge what you see, but don't suggest that dieting has made him a better person.

Regardless of the response, the goal is to help the dieter hold a solid appreciation of her value as a person. Beauty is in the sincere smile, the friendship offered, the positive qualities exhibited—not in being a size 2 instead of a size 12. People need to know they are loved from the inside out, not judged from the outside in. When dieters lose weight, they need to realize that there is simply less of them to love. They are not better or more likable. They are just smaller.

PART IV

WINNING RECIPES FOR PEAK PERFORMANCE

CHAPTER 18

BREADS AND BREAKFASTS

Agood sports diet starts at breakfast and can include yummy breads. May the recipes in this chapter give an energetic start to your day. *Note*: Recipes that you might expect to contain gluten but are actually gluten-free have "GF" after the recipe name.

Bread

Fresh from the oven, breads are one of the favorite forms of carbohydrate for active people. Here are baking tips to help you prepare the yummiest of breads:

- The secret for light and fluffy quick breads, muffins, and scones is to stir the flour lightly and for only 20 seconds. Ignore the lumps! If you beat the batter too much, the gluten (protein) in the flour will toughen the dough.

- Breads made entirely with whole-wheat flour tend to be heavy. In general, half white and half whole-wheat flour is an appropriate combination. Many of these recipes have been developed using this ratio. You can alter the ratio as you like. When substituting whole-wheat flour for white flour in other recipes, use 3/4 cup (105 g) whole-wheat flour for 1 cup (140 g) white flour.

- Most of these recipes have reduced sugar content. To reduce the sugar content of your own recipes, use one-third to one-half less sugar than indicated; the finished product will be just fine. If you want to exchange white sugar with honey, brown sugar, or molasses, use only 1/2 a teaspoon baking powder per 2 cups (280 g) of flour, and add 1/2 a teaspoon of baking soda. This prevents an "off" taste.

- Most quick-bread recipes instruct you to sift together the baking powder and flour. This method produces the lightest breads and best results. In some recipes, I direct you to mix the baking powder with the wet ingredients and add the flour last. My method is easier, produces an acceptable product, and saves time. Just be sure to sprinkle it on so it doesn't clump.

- To prevent quick breads from sticking, use cooking spray, or place a piece of waxed or parchment paper in the baking pan before pouring the batter. I've found that using paper is foolproof. After the quick bread has baked, let it cool for five minutes, tip it out of the pan, and then peel off the paper.
- To hasten cooking time, bake quick breads in an 8- × 8-inch (20 × 20 cm) square pan instead of a loaf pan. They bake in half the time. You can also bake muffins in a loaf or square pan, eliminating the hard-to-wash muffin tins.

RECIPE FINDER

Oatmeal suggestions — 361

Banana bread — 362

Date nut bread — 363

Peanut butter and dark chocolate chip muffins GF — 364

Carrot raisin muffins — 366

Molasses muffins with flax and dates — 367

Athlete's omelet — 368

Breakfast fruit salad with marmalade yogurt — 369

Honey nut granola — 370

Protein-packed scrambled eggs — 371

Fluffy oatmeal pancakes — 372

High-protein oatmeal pancakes GF — 373

See also: Extra-creamy potatoes and cheese (chapter 19); smoothie and milk shake recipes (chapter 25); and super-seedy granola bars, sweet and crispy almond bars, chia pudding, and banana ice cream (chapter 26).

OATMEAL SUGGESTIONS

Fresh from the stove top, oatmeal (or quinoa) is not only a healthy addition to your sports diet but also an easy-to-digest preexercise breakfast. If cooking first thing in the morning is not your cup of tea, prepare cook-free overnight oats the night before. Simply toss 1/2 cup (40 g) uncooked oats, 1 cup (240 ml) milk (or 2/3 cup [160 ml] milk and 1/3 cup [75 g] Greek yogurt) into an empty peanut butter jar, add extras as desired (such as chia, flax, maple syrup, salt), shake well, and let it sit in the refrigerator for at least four hours or overnight. In the morning, you'll have a pudding-like porridge you can grab for breakfast on the go.

The following oatmeal (or quinoa) suggestions will add variety to your breakfasts.

- Dried apricot pieces, honey, and a dash of nutmeg
- Raisins, cinnamon, and slivered almonds
- Sliced banana (cooked with the oatmeal), brown sugar, and peanut butter
- Dried cranberries, honey, and chopped pecans
- Diced apple (cooked with the oatmeal) or applesauce, walnut pieces, and maple syrup
- Pumpkin seeds, chia, or hemp hearts (sprinkled on top or cooked in)

Instead of adding sweetener, some people choose to add a little salt and eat the oatmeal (or quinoa) as a savory grain instead of a sweetened cereal. Because the diets of active people can accommodate some salt to replace what is lost in sweat, eating salted oatmeal is an acceptable practice—plus most athletes find that oatmeal tastes a lot better with salt.

BANANA BREAD

The key to success for this all-time favorite is using well-ripened bananas that are covered with brown speckles. Banana bread is a favorite for pre-marathon carbohydrate loading and for snacking during long-distance bike rides and hikes. Add peanut butter and you'll have a delicious sandwich that'll keep you energized for a long time.

3 large well-ripened bananas

1 egg

2 tablespoons oil, preferably canola

1/3 cup (80 ml) milk

1/3 to 1/2 cup (65 to 100 g) sugar

1 teaspoon salt

1 teaspoon baking soda

1/2 teaspoon baking powder

1 1/2 cups (210 g) flour, preferably half whole wheat and half white

Optional: 1/2 cup chopped nuts

1. Preheat the oven to 350 °F (180 °C).
2. Mash bananas with a fork.
3. Add egg, oil, milk, sugar, salt, baking soda, and baking powder. Beat well.
4. Gently blend the flour (and nuts) into the banana mixture. Stir for 20 seconds or until moistened.
5. Pour into a 4- × 8-inch (10 × 20 cm) loaf pan that has been lightly oiled, treated with cooking spray, or lined with waxed or parchment paper.
6. Bake for 45 minutes or until a toothpick inserted near the middle comes out clean.
7. Let cool for 5 minutes before removing from pan.

Yield: 12 slices

NUTRITION INFORMATION: 1,600 total calories; 135 calories per slice; 24 g carbohydrate; 3 g protein; 3 g fat

DATE NUT BREAD

Dates are an underappreciated fruit. These bite-sized nuggets of sweetness are nutrient dense and rich in phytochemicals (bioactive compounds that help fight inflammation). They are a positive addition to a sports diet!

Every year at Christmas, my mother made loaves and loaves of date nut bread. Perhaps you too want to share this treat with your friends and family.

8 ounces (175 g) dates, chopped
1 1/2 (360 ml) cups boiling water
2 tablespoons oil
1 egg
1/2 cup (100 g) sugar
1/2 cup (60 g) walnuts, chopped
1 teaspoon salt
2 teaspoons baking soda
2 1/2 cups (350 g) flour, preferably half whole wheat

1. Put the dates in a bowl and pour boiling water over them. Let stand until cool.
2. Preheat the oven to 350° F (180° C).
3. Add oil, egg, sugar, salt, and walnuts to the dates. Beat well.
4. Combine the baking soda and flour. Gently stir into the date mixture.
5. Pour into a greased or waxed-papered loaf pan. Bake for 45 to 50 minutes, or until a toothpick inserted near the center comes out clean.

Yield: 1 large loaf of 16 slices

NUTRITION INFORMATION: 2,800 total calories; 175 calories per slice (1/16 loaf); 32 g carbohydrate; 3 g protein; 4 g fat

PEANUT BUTTER AND DARK CHOCOLATE CHIP MUFFINS GF

Made with rolled oats that you make into flour in your blender or food processor (or oat flour that you purchase), this gluten-free recipe is also low in FODMAPs (see chapter 9). That means, if you have trouble with gas, bloating, and other digestive issues, this might be a good choice for you.

Even if you eat wheat and have no digestive issues, you'll enjoy this yummy recipe from the blog *For a Digestive Peace of Mind* by Kate Scarlata, RD, gut-health expert and author of *The Low-FODMAP Diet Step By Step*. As Kate says, it is healthy-ish and can pass as either a muffin or a cupcake.

Kate makes this recipe in a blender and pours the batter into the muffin tin. I prefer mixing the ingredients in a bowl. Take your choice!

2 eggs

3/4 cup (180 ml) milk, lactose free (low FODMAP) or regular

2 tablespoons oil, preferably canola

1/2 cup (100 g) brown sugar

1/2 cup (130 g) peanut butter, preferably all natural

1 teaspoon vanilla extract

1 1/2 cup (210 g) oat flour (pulverize oats in a blender until they look like flour)

1 tablespoon baking powder

3/4 cup (180 g) chocolate chips

Optional: 1/2 teaspoon salt

1. Preheat oven to 350 °F (180 °C).
2. Prepare 12-muffin tin with a light coating of oil or use paper baking cups.
3. Add the following ingredients in this order into a blender (or bowl): eggs, (lactose free) milk, vegetable oil, brown sugar, peanut butter, vanilla extract, oat flour, and baking powder.
4. Pulse blender (or mix well) until batter is creamy.
5. Fold in 1/2 cup (120) of the chocolate chips into batter.
6. Add batter evenly into the 12-muffin tin.
7. Distribute the extra 1/4 cup (60 g) chocolate chips evenly to the top of each muffin.
8. Bake for 12 to 15 minutes or until a cake tester comes out clean.

Yield: 12 muffins

NUTRITION INFORMATION: 3,000 total calories; 250 calories per muffin; 27 g carbohydrate; 7 g protein; 13 g fat

Courtesy of Kate Scarlata, RD. *For a Digestive Peace of Mind.*

CARROT RAISIN MUFFINS

These muffins are a favorite of Evelyn Tribole, RD, sports nutritionist and co-author of *Intuitive Eating: A Revolutionary Program that Works*. They're tasty from the oven and even tastier on the second day when the flavors have blended.

1 cup (140 g) whole-wheat flour

1 cup (140 g) white flour

3/4 cup (150 g) sugar

2 teaspoons baking powder

1 teaspoon salt

2 teaspoons cinnamon

1/2 teaspoon baking soda

3 eggs

1/2 cup (120 ml) buttermilk (or 1/2 cup milk mixed with 1/2 teaspoon vinegar and left to stand for 5 minutes)

1/3 cup (80 ml) oil, preferably canola

2 teaspoons vanilla extract

2 cups (220 g) finely shredded carrot

1 medium apple, peeled and shredded

1/2 cup (80 g) raisins

1/2 cup (60 g) chopped nuts

1. Preheat the oven to 350 °F (180 °C). Prepare 12-muffin tins with papers or cooking spray.
2. In a large bowl, stir together the flours, sugar, baking powder, salt, cinnamon, and baking soda.
3. In a separate bowl, stir together the eggs, buttermilk, oil, and vanilla; then add the carrots, apple, raisins, and nuts. Add to the flour mixture, and stir just until blended.
4. Spoon the batter into the muffin cups. Bake about 30 minutes or until a toothpick inserted near the center comes out clean.

Yield: 12 muffins

NUTRITION INFORMATION: 2,750 total calories; 230 calories per muffin; 37 g carbohydrate; 5 g protein; 7 g fat

Adapted with permission, www.EvelynTribole.com

MOLASSES MUFFINS WITH FLAX AND DATES

Flax is rich in substances that have been shown to protect against heart disease and cancer. It has a very mild taste and is good mixed into muffins and breads as well as sprinkled on cereal. This flax muffin recipe is one way to add a daily tablespoon of flaxseed to your breakfast and snacks. These muffins are remarkably sweet and moist, despite having no added fat. (The 3 grams of fat per muffin are from the health-protective fats in the ground flaxseed meal.)

1 egg

1/3 cup (115 g) molasses

1 cup (240 ml) buttermilk (or 1 cup milk mixed with 1 teaspoon vinegar)

3/4 cup (120 g) ground flaxseed meal

1/2 teaspoon salt

1 cup (175 g) chopped dates

1 1/2 cups (210 g) flour, preferably half whole wheat and half white

1 teaspoon baking soda

Optional: 1/2 teaspoon cinnamon, 1 teaspoon grated orange rind, 1 teaspoon vanilla extract

1. Preheat the oven to 350 °F (180 °C), and prepare 12 muffin cups with papers or cooking spray.
2. In a large bowl, mix together the egg, molasses, buttermilk, flax, and salt (and orange rind and vanilla extract), and add the dates to the batter.
3. In a separate bowl, mix together the flour and baking soda (and cinnamon).
4. Gently stir the flour mixture into the egg mixture.
5. Fill the muffin cups 2/3 full. Bake for 18 to 20 minutes or until a toothpick inserted near the center comes out clean.

Yield: 12 muffins

NUTRITION INFORMATION: 2,000 total calories; 165 calories per muffin; 30 g carbohydrate; 4 g protein; 3 g fat

ATHLETE'S OMELET

This recipe is a favorite from Gale Bernhardt, cycling and triathlon coach. What makes this an "athlete's" omelet is the added carbohydrate (rice)—and the compilation of nutrient-dense foods from a variety of food groups: veggies (spinach, pepper), fruit (tomato), protein (egg), dairy (cheese), and grain (rice). You can easily modify the omelet to suit your needs by adding diced, cooked (sweet) potato instead of rice; adding any and all vegetables that happen to be handy (e.g., onion, broccoli, mushrooms); and boosting the protein by adding cottage cheese, diced ham, or tofu into the scramble.

Before you dive into this omelet recipe, you'll need to have cooked some brown rice ahead of time so that it is chilled. (Alternatively, Gale suggests that you buy frozen brown rice.) Because the rice is chilled, the grains are firm and chewy in the omelet, creating a special texture. It's tasty for breakfast, lunch, dinner, and recovery meals.

> 1 teaspoon olive oil
> 2 whole eggs
> 1/2 cup (120 g) brown rice (precooked and chilled)
> 1/2 tomato, diced
> Handful of fresh spinach
> 1/4 sweet yellow bell pepper, diced
> salt and pepper, as desired
> *Optional:* 1/4 cup (60 g) shredded low-fat cheese

1. Lightly coat the bottom of a small skillet with the olive oil.
2. Stir the eggs together and set them aside.
3. On medium heat, lightly cook the vegetables until tender-crisp.
4. Add the eggs, rice (and cheese) at the same time. Cook the mixture until the eggs are firm and moist, but not hard. You can cook the egg mixture into a "pancake" (that you flip) or a folded omelet.

Yield: 1 serving

NUTRITION INFORMATION: 250 total calories (without cheese); 28 g carbohydrate; 15 g protein; 9 g fat

Courtesy of Gale Bernhardt.

BREAKFAST FRUIT SALAD WITH MARMALADE YOGURT

This fruit salad can be made with a mixture of fresh, canned, and dried fruits of your choice. Be creative, and buy fruits that may not be a part of your standard fare—mango, papaya, kiwi.

For the dressing, Greek-style yogurt works well because it is thicker and sweeter than regular yogurt and tastes rich and creamy. Vanilla-flavored yogurt also works well.

> 3 cups (480 g) cut-up fruit of your choice:
> Apple
> Banana
> Mango
> Pineapple (fresh or canned)
> Berries
> Dried apricots
> 1/2 cup (115 g) plain low-fat yogurt, preferably Greek style
> 1 tablespoon orange marmalade
> *Optional:* dash nutmeg or cinnamon, slivered almonds or chopped walnuts

1. In a small bowl, combine cut-up fruit.
2. Blend together the yogurt and marmalade.
3. Mix together the yogurt and the fruit (add seasoning and nuts), and serve.

Yield: 2 servings

NUTRITION INFORMATION: Dressing: 120 total calories; 60 calories per serving; 8 g carbohydrate; 5 g protein; 1 g fat

With fruit: 320 to 440 total calories; 160-220 calories per serving; 33 to 48 g carbohydrate; 5 g protein; 1 g fat

HONEY NUT GRANOLA

The nice thing about making your own granola is that you can avoid the unhealthy saturated fat found in commercially made granolas. Instead, this recipe offers healthy fat from nuts and canola oil, with a nice blend of carbohydrate-rich whole oats, dried fruits, and other add-ins of your choice to provide crunch and goodness.

Mixed with fresh fruit and yogurt, this recipe offers a delicious and healthy way to start the morning or to recover after a tiring workout. The milk powder and nuts add a protein boost.

> 3 cups (240 g) rolled oats (not instant oatmeal)
>
> 1 cup (120 g) chopped almonds
>
> 2 teaspoons cinnamon
>
> 1 cup (120 g) powdered milk
>
> 1/3 cup (115 g) honey
>
> 1/3 cup (80 ml) canola oil
>
> 1 cup (160 g) dried fruit bits (e.g., raisins, dried cranberries, chopped dates)
>
> *Optional:* 1 teaspoon salt, 1/2 cup (60 g) sesame seeds (untoasted), 1/2 cup (60 g) sunflower seeds (unsalted, untoasted), 1/2 cup (60 g) wheat germ, 1/2 cup (80 g) ground flaxseed meal

1. In a large bowl, combine the oats, almonds, cinnamon, and pow-dered milk (and salt, sesame seeds, and sunflower seeds, as desired).
2. In a saucepan or microwavable bowl, combine the honey and oil. Heat until almost boiling. Pour the honey mixture over the oat mix-ture and stir well.
3. Spread the mixture onto two large baking sheets.
4. Bake at 300 °F (150 °C) for 20 to 25 minutes, stirring every 5 minutes.
5. After the granola has cooled, add the dried fruit (and wheat germ and flaxseed meal, as desired). Store in an airtight container.

Yield: 10 1/2-cup servings

NUTRITION INFORMATION: 3,300 total calories; 330 calories per 1/2 cup; 40 g carbohydrate; 10 g protein; 14 g fat

PROTEIN-PACKED SCRAMBLED EGGS

Adding cottage cheese to eggs is a simple way to boost your morning protein. Plus, it makes the eggs creamy and yummier. You can use a blender to mix the ingredients, but honestly, no one will care if there's a curd of cottage cheese in the eggs; it just looks like egg white! Of course, you can be creative and add sauteed veggies and shredded low-fat cheddar cheese. Serve with whole-grain toast, oatmeal, (microwaved) sweet potato, or another source of carbohydrate to fill up your muscle glycogen stores.

Recipe courtesy of Judith Scharman Draughon, MSN, RDN, LD, author of *Lean Body Smart Life*.

> 2 eggs
> 1/4 cup (spoonful) cottage cheese
> *Optional:* 1/4 cup (30 g) grated (reduced-fat cheddar) cheese, sauteed onion, peppers, spinach

Yield: 1 serving

NUTRITION INFORMATION: 175 total calories; 3 g carbohydrate; 19 g protein; 10 g fat

Courtesy of Judith Scharman Draughon, *Lean Body, Smart Life.* www.foodswithjudes.com

FLUFFY OATMEAL PANCAKES

These pancakes are light and fluffy prizewinners, perfect for carbohydrate loading or recovering from a hard workout. For best results, let the batter stand for 5 minutes before cooking.

> 1/2 cup (40 g) uncooked oats, quick or old fashioned
>
> 1/2 cup (115 g) plain yogurt, buttermilk, or milk mixed with 1/2 teaspoon vinegar
>
> 1/2 to 3/4 cup (120 to 180 ml) milk
>
> 1 egg
>
> 1 tablespoon oil, preferably canola
>
> 2 tablespoons packed brown sugar
>
> 1/2 teaspoon salt, as desired
>
> 1 teaspoon baking powder
>
> 1 cup (140 g) flour, preferably half whole wheat and half white
>
> *Optional:* dash cinnamon

1. In a medium bowl, combine the oats, yogurt, and milk. Set aside for 15 to 20 minutes to let the oats soften.
2. When the oats are finished soaking, beat in the egg and oil, and mix well. Add the sugar and salt (and cinnamon); then add the baking powder and flour. Stir until just moistened.
3. Heat a lightly oiled griddle over medium-high heat (375 °F [190 °C] for electric griddle).
4. For each pancake, pour about 1/4 cup batter onto the griddle.
5. Turn when the tops are covered with bubbles and the edges look cooked. Turn only once.
6. Serve with syrup, honey, applesauce, yogurt, or other topping of your choice.

Yield: 6 6-inch (15 cm) pancakes

NUTRITION INFORMATION: 1,000 total calories; 330 calories per serving (2 pancakes); 57 g carbohydrate; 10 g protein; 7 g fat

HIGH-PROTEIN OATMEAL PANCAKES GF

These pancakes are not light-and-fluffy featherweights, but rather hearty, and packed with protein. As blogger, author of *Lean Body Smart Life* and recipe contributor Judith "Judes" Scharman Draughon, MS, RDN, LD (www.foodswithjudes.com) reports, they are quick and easy to prepare, a tried-and-true breakfast staple.

If you have celiac disease and are on a strict gluten-free diet, be sure you choose a gluten-free brand of cottage cheese (such as Daisy) and gluten-free rolled oats (such as Bob's Red Mill).

1/2 cup (115 g) cottage cheese

1 tablespoon raw honey or pure maple syrup

2 eggs

1/2 cup (40 g) rolled oats

1/4 teaspoon cinnamon

1/4 teaspoon baking powder

1/4 teaspoon salt

Optional: 1/2 teaspoon vanilla or almond extract

Optional toppings and mix-ins:

- Top with warm fruit, such as sliced peaches (fresh, frozen or canned) heated in the microwave oven (with a little bit of orange juice) or warm applesauce.
- Mix sliced banana, blueberries, diced peaches, or any fruit of your choice into the batter.
- Spread with nut butter, sliced banana, Greek yogurt, maple syrup, or a dash of cinnamon.

1. Blend the cottage cheese, honey, egg, oats, cinnamon, (salt and vanilla extract) in a blender or food processor on high for about 1 minute.
2. Stir in baking powder (and diced fruit).
3. Heat a lightly oiled griddle to medium low.
4. Pour batter onto the heated surface, making small 3-inch (7.5 cm) pancakes (to make them easier to flip). When the pancakes are golden on the bottom, flip them over and cook on the other side.
5. *Optional:* Top with the cooked peaches and enjoy!

Yield: 1 hearty breakfast of 6 3-inch (7.5 cm) pancakes

NUTRITION INFORMATION: 450 total calories (without fruit topping); 50 g carbohydrate; 32 g protein; 14 g fat

Courtesy of Judith Scharman Draughon. www.foodswithjudes.com.

CHAPTER 19

PASTA, RICE, AND POTATOES

Although some weight-conscious people mistakenly try to stay away from dinner starches such as pasta, rice, and potatoes, these carbohydrate-rich foods are important for a high-energy sports diet. The following cooking tips and recipes can help you add the right balance to your sports dinners.

Pasta

When trying to decide which shape of pasta to use for a meal, the rule of thumb is to use twisted and curved shapes (such as twists and shells) with meaty, beany, and chunky sauces. The shape will trap more sauce than straight strands of spaghetti or linguini will.

When trying to decide between white or whole-grain pasta, pay attention to the total fiber content of the meal. If you have whole-wheat pasta plus beans and lots of vegetables, your digestive tract might talk back to you during your next workout. Evaluate the fiber content of your overall healthy eating pattern, taking note that the *Dietary Guidelines for Americans* allow half of grains to be from enriched white flour. Choose the pasta that best suits your dietary needs.

Perfectly cooked pasta is tender yet firm when bitten into—*al dente*, as the Italians say. The quickest-cooking pastas are angel hair, alphabets, and little stars (stelline). Here are tips for cooking pasta perfectly:

- Allow 4 quarts (4 L) of water per pound (480 g) of dry pasta. Allow 10 minutes for the water to reach a rolling boil before adding pasta. (If you are rushed for time, you can cook the pasta in half the amount of water, and it will cook OK—in less time.) Plan to cook no more than 2 pounds (1 kg) of pasta at a time; otherwise, you may end up with a gummy mess.

- To keep the water from boiling over, add 1 tablespoon of oil to the cooking water.

- Add the pasta in small amounts to avoid cooling the water too much or causing the pieces to clump. When cooking spaghetti or lasagna, push down the stiff strands as they soften, using a long-handled spoon.
- If the water stops boiling, cover the pan, turn up the heat, and bring the water to a boil again as soon as possible.
- Cooking time will depend on the shape of the pasta. Pasta is done when it starts to look opaque. To tell whether it is done, lift a piece of pasta with a fork from the boiling water, let it cool briefly, and then carefully pinch or bite it, being sure not to burn yourself. The pasta should feel flexible but still firm inside.
- When the pasta is done, drain it into a colander set in the sink, using potholders to protect your hands from the steam. Shake the pasta briefly to remove excess water; then return it to the cooking pot or to a warmed serving bowl.
- To prevent the pasta from sticking together as it cools, toss it with a little oil or sauce.

Rice

Rice is the world's third-leading grain after wheat and corn. Brown rice is made into white rice when the fiber-rich bran is removed during the refining process. This also removes some of the nutrients, but you can compensate for this loss (if you prefer white to brown rice) by eating other whole grains such as oatmeal and whole-wheat breads at your other meals. Yet, learning to enjoy brown rice is an easy task.

Here are tips for cooking rice:

- For each cup (200 g) of rice, put 2 cups (480 ml) of water and 1 teaspoon of salt, as desired, into a saucepan. Bring to a boil, and then cover and turn the heat to low. Let the rice cook undisturbed until it is tender and all the water has been absorbed. Then, stir gently with a fork. (Stirring too much results in a sticky mess.) This method retains vitamins that otherwise could be lost in the cooking water.
- Because of its tough bran coat and germ, brown rice needs 45 to 50 minutes to cook; white rice needs only 20 to 30 minutes.
- Consider cooking rice in the morning while you are getting ready for work so you will only need to reheat it when you get home.
- When cooking rice, cook double amounts to have leftovers that you can freeze or refrigerate.

Use the following portion guides when cooking rice:

1 cup (200 g) uncooked white rice
= 3 cups cooked = 700 calories (3g fiber)

1 cup (200 g) uncooked brown rice
= 3 to 4 cups cooked = 700 calories (10g fiber)

Potatoes

Both white and sweet potatoes are carbohydrate-rich vegetables that offers more vitamins and minerals than plain rice or pasta. To help you include more potatoes in your sports diet, follow these tips:

- Potatoes come in different varieties. Some varieties are best suited for baking (russets), others for boiling (red or white rounds) and some do well any way (sweet). Ask the produce manager at your grocery store for guidance.
- Potatoes are best stored in a cool, humid (but not wet) place that is well ventilated, such as your cellar. Do not refrigerate potatoes because they will become sweet and off-colored.
- Rather than peel the skin (and remove some fiber), scrub the skin well and cook the potato, skin and all. Yes, even mashed potatoes can be made with unpeeled potatoes.
- One pound (480 g) of potatoes equals three medium or two large potatoes. A large "restaurant-size" potato has about 200 calories.
- To bake a potato in the oven, allow about 40 minutes at 400 °F (200 °C) for a medium potato, and closer to an hour for a large potato. Because potatoes can be baked at any temperature, you can adjust the cooking time to whatever else is in the oven.
- The potato is done when you can easily pierce it with a fork.
- To cook a potato in a microwave oven, prick its skin in several places with a fork, place it on a paper towel, and cook it for about 4 minutes if it is medium sized or 6 to 10 minutes if it's large. Cooking time will vary according to the size of the potato, the power of your oven, and the number of potatoes you are cooking. Turn the potato over halfway through cooking. Remove the potato from the oven, wrap it in a towel, and allow it to finish cooking outside the oven for 3 to 5 minutes.

RECIPE FINDER

Quick and easy pasta toppings	379
Angel hair Alfredo	380
Skillet lasagna	381
Gourmet vegetarian lasagna	382
Cauliflower macaroni and cheese	384
Pasta with mushrooms and asparagus	385
Quick and easy potato toppings	386
Oven french fries	387
Extra-creamy potatoes and cheese	388
Avocado potato salad	390
Quick and easy rice (or quinoa) ideas	391
Southwestern rice and bean salad	392

See also: athlete's omelet (chapter 18); honey-glazed sweet potatoes (chapter 20); chicken with pasta and spinach, savory African peanut stew, (chapter 21); shrimp and shells, tuna pasta salad (chapter 22); Boston baked beans and rice (chapter 23); Buddha bowl ideas, pasta and white bean soup with sun-dried tomatoes (chapter 24).

QUICK AND EASY PASTA TOPPINGS

The following pasta toppings are a change of pace from the standard tomato sauce straight from the jar.

- Steamed chopped broccoli
- Salsa, plain or heated, and then mixed with cottage cheese
- Red pepper flakes
- Low-fat salad dressings of your choice
- Low-fat Italian salad dressing with tamari, chopped garlic, and steamed vegetables
- Low-fat sour cream or Greek yogurt and Italian seasonings
- Italian seasonings and cottage cheese or Parmesan cheese
- Chicken breast sauteed with oil, garlic, onion, and basil
- Chili with kidney beans (and cheese)
- Lentil soup (thick)
- Spaghetti sauce with a spoonful of grape jelly
- Spaghetti sauce with added protein: canned chicken or tuna, tofu cubes, canned beans, cottage cheese, ground beef or turkey
- Spaghetti sauce with added fresh diced tomato and parsley

ANGEL HAIR ALFREDO

Who says Alfredo sauce goes only with fettuccini? You can make it with angel hair pasta—and shorten cooking time. Serve this with a salad or green vegetables and grilled chicken or fish.

1/4 box (4 oz, or 110 g, dry) angel hair pasta

1/3 cup (75 g) Greek yogurt

1/3 cup (35 g) Parmesan cheese

salt and pepper to taste

Optional: oregano, garlic, cooked vegetables such as broccoli
  or mushrooms

1. Bring a pot of water to boil. Add the angel hair pasta and cook until al dente, about 4 minutes. Drain the pasta, saving a little bit of the cooking water to thin the sauce, if needed.

2. Sprinkle the Parmesan on the pasta and then mix in the Greek yogurt. Add seasonings, as desired (salt, pepper, oregano, garlic salt, cooked vegetables).

Yield: 1 large serving, when served as an entree (or 2 smaller servings, as a side dish)

NUTRITION INFORMATION: 580 total calories; 86 g carbohydrate; 34 g protein; 11 g fat

SKILLET LASAGNA

This is a much quicker version of the classic Italian lasagnas, and it offers all the taste. Because it is so simple to make, you'll want to enjoy lasagna more often. For a vegetarian dish, replace the ground beef with crumbled tofu or textured vegetable protein. To fuel your muscles with more carbohydrate (only half the calories are from carbohydrate), serve this with crusty whole-grain rolls and fruit for dessert.

1/2 to 1 pound (240 to 480 g) extra-lean ground beef or ground turkey

One 26-ounce (780 ml) jar spaghetti sauce

3 cups (720 ml) water

8 ounces (240 g) egg noodles, uncooked

1 cup (230 g) cottage cheese, preferably low fat

1/4 cup (25 g) grated Parmesan cheese

1/2 to 1 cup (120 to 240 g) shredded part-skim mozzarella cheese

1. In a large skillet, brown the ground beef. Drain.
2. Add the jar of spaghetti sauce and the 3 cups of water. (Use some of the water to rinse out the jar.) Bring to a boil.
3. Stir in uncooked noodles. Bring to a boil, stirring occasionally. Reduce heat, cover, and simmer for about 10 minutes or until the noodles are done.
4. Add the cottage, Parmesan, and mozzarella cheeses; stir gently into the noodle mixture. Cover and cook for 5 minutes more.
5. *Optional:* Sprinkle with additional mozzarella before serving.

Yield: 4 hefty servings

NUTRITION INFORMATION: 2,100 total calories; 525 calories per serving; 60 g carbohydrate; 35 g protein; 16 g fat

Courtesy of Karin Daisy.

GOURMET VEGETARIAN LASAGNA

This "company is coming" lasagna has a wonderful flavor and is a nice variation from standard lasagnas. The sun-dried tomatoes and pine nuts make the difference—well worth the effort of buying them if you have none stocked.

15 lasagna noodles

1/2 cup (60 g) pine nuts (pignoli nuts)

8 to 9 sun-dried tomatoes

1 to 3 cloves garlic, peeled and finely chopped

1 teaspoon oil, preferably olive or canola

1 pound (480 g) ricotta cheese, part skim or nonfat

4 to 8 ounces (120 to 240 g) shredded low-fat mozzarella cheese

1 to 2 dashes nutmeg

1/4 teaspoon oregano

1 10-ounce (300 g) package frozen spinach, thawed and drained

1 28-ounce (840 ml) jar spaghetti sauce

Optional: 1/4 cup (25 g) grated Parmesan cheese

1. Cook the lasagna noodles in a large pot of boiling water according to the package directions. Drain and rinse with cold water and set aside.

2. Toast the pine nuts on the stove top in a nonstick skillet over medium-high heat for 2 to 3 minutes.

3. Place the sun-dried tomatoes in a small bowl and cover with boiling water. Soak oil-packed tomatoes for 5 minutes or dried tomatoes for 10 to 15 minutes. Drain, cool, and finely chop.

4. Saute the garlic in oil for 2 minutes. Do not brown.

5. In a large mixing bowl, combine the ricotta, mozzarella, nutmeg, oregano, spinach, sun-dried tomatoes, pine nuts, and garlic.

6. Pour enough tomato sauce into a 9- × 13-inch (23 × 33 cm) pan to coat the bottom. Layer on five lasagna noodles, cutting or folding to fit. Then add one-third of the ricotta mixture and then one-third of the remaining spaghetti sauce. Repeat twice, making three layers of ricotta. On the last layer, end with noodles and tomato sauce. Sprinkle with Parmesan, if desired.

7. Cover with foil. Bake for 30 to 40 minutes or until hot at 350 °F (180 °C).

Yield: 8 servings

NUTRITION INFORMATION: 3,600 total calories; 450 calories per serving; 53 g carbohydrate; 21 g protein; 17 g fat

Adapted from a recipe contributed by Linda Press Wolfe.

CAULIFLOWER MACARONI AND CHEESE

I've lightened up this family-favorite meal by adding diced cauliflower. Even kids are unlikely to notice the difference, especially if you use small shells for the pasta. The cauliflower hides inside the shell.

If you don't have time to bake the mac and cheese, skip those instructions. It tastes good even before it is baked.

Because this recipe includes chopping and grating, invite a friend or family member to help you cook. While you make the sauce, someone can grate the cheese, and another person can dice the cauliflower. The final result is a meal made with love.

> 2 cups (about half a box or 240 g) of uncooked small pasta, such as small elbow macaroni or small shells
>
> 2 cups (480 g) finely diced cauliflower
>
> 2 cups (480 ml) milk
>
> 3 tablespoons flour
>
> 1/4 teaspoon dry mustard
>
> 1/4 teaspoon garlic powder
>
> dash cayenne pepper
>
> salt and pepper to taste
>
> 5 ounces (150 g) shredded reduced-fat cheddar cheese
>
> *Optional:* 2 tablespoons low-fat cream cheese

1. Fill a pasta pot with water and bring it to a boil. While the water is heating, dice the cauliflower into small pieces.

2. Add the pasta to the boiling water, cook for about 5 minutes, and then add the diced cauliflower. Drain when the pasta and cauliflower are tender, 4 or 5 minutes.

3. In a large saucepan, whisk together the flour and milk, place over medium-high heat, and bring to a boil, stirring constantly.

4. Add the mustard, garlic powder, cayenne pepper, (low-fat cream cheese), salt, and pepper; mix well.

5. Add the grated cheddar cheese, stirring until melted, and then add the pasta and cauliflower.

6. Enjoy eating it as is, or pour the mixture into an oiled 8- × 8-inch (20 × 20 cm) baking pan and bake for 20 minutes or until bubbly at 350°F (180°C).

Yield: 5 servings (as a side dish)

NUTRITION INFORMATION: 1,250 total calories; 250 calories per serving (1/5 of the recipe); 43 g carbohydrate; 11 g protein; 4 g fat

PASTA WITH MUSHROOMS AND ASPARAGUS

Mushrooms add a meaty flavor to a meal and are a sneaky way to reduce meat intake without feeling deprived. Mushrooms left in the daylight can also produce vitamin D. How about leaving the mushrooms in the sun for a few hours and make this dish frequently in the winter?

2 cups uncooked pasta (about 1/2 lb, or 225 g) such as bow ties

1 pound (480 g) asparagus spears

1 tablespoon olive oil

1/2 pound (240 g) sliced mushrooms

1/4 cup (230 g) pesto

1/2 cup (120 ml) hot water (or cooking water)

Optional: grated Parmesan cheese

1. While bringing the pasta water to a boil, break off the tough lower ends of the asparagus, and then cut the spears into 1-inch (2.5 cm) pieces.
2. Start cooking the pasta, and in 5 minutes, add the asparagus pieces.
3. Meanwhile, in a small saute pan, add the olive oil and sliced mushrooms. Cook for about 7 minutes or until tender.
4. Drain the pasta when it is tender. Return the pasta and asparagus to the cooking pot along with the 1/2 (120 ml) cup of hot water.
5. Mix in the pesto and the mushrooms.
6. *Optional:* Top with grated Parmesan cheese.

Yield: 5 servings as a side dish

NUTRITION INFORMATION: 1,300 total calories; 260 calories per serving (1/5 of recipe); 38 g carbohydrate; 7 g protein; 9 g fat

QUICK AND EASY POTATO TOPPINGS

To spice up your potato, try the following toppings:

- Plain or Greek yogurt
- Low-fat sour cream, chopped onion, and grated low-fat cheddar cheese
- Low-fat cottage cheese and garlic powder or salsa
- Chili and grated low-fat cheddar cheese
- Cooked chopped spinach and crumbled feta cheese
- Soup broth or milk mashed into the potato
- Mustard (and Worcestershire sauce)
- White and flavored vinegars or low-fat salad dressing
- Soy sauce
- Pesto
- Herbs such as dill, parsley, and chives
- Steamed broccoli or other cooked vegetables
- Chopped jalapeno peppers
- Baked beans, refried beans, lentils, or lentil soup
- Applesauce

OVEN FRENCH FRIES

This healthy french fry recipe can be made with white or sweet potatoes and is a popular family favorite—and no one will realize it is low in fat. For added flavor, dip the fries in salsa, nonfat yogurt mixed with fresh herbs, or ketchup.

1 large baking potato (white or sweet), cleaned, unpeeled

1 teaspoon oil, preferably canola or olive

salt and pepper to taste

Optional: red pepper flakes, dried basil, oregano, minced garlic, Parmesan cheese; replace oil with prepared pesto

1. Cut the potato lengthwise into 10 or 12 pieces. Place in a large bowl, cover with cold water, and let stand for 15 to 20 minutes. (This soaking can be eliminated, but it shortens the cooking time and improves the final product.)
2. Drain the potato pieces, dry them on a towel, and then put them in a bowl or sealable bag. Drizzle them with the oil, and sprinkle with the salt and pepper, as desired. Toss to coat evenly.
3. Place the potatoes evenly on a shallow, oiled baking pan.
4. Bake at 425 °F (220 °C) for 15 minutes. Turn the potatoes over, sprinkle with the optional seasonings, as desired, and continue baking for another 10 to 15 minutes. Serve immediately. Be careful; the potatoes will be very hot.

Yield: 1 serving

NUTRITION INFORMATION: 260 calories per potato; 52 g carbohydrate; 4 g protein; 4 g fat

Courtesy of Ann LeBaron, RD.

EXTRA-CREAMY POTATOES AND CHEESE

Whether served with dinner (goes nicely with fish and a green vegetable), or enjoyed as leftovers for breakfast or lunch, cheesy potatoes are a welcomed sports food. They are easy to digest and offer a nice balance of protein and carbohydrate. If you want to get creative, add other vegetables (sliced carrots, spinach) for color and nutrients.

To accommodate vegan, gluten-free, and lactose-free diets, make these with lactose-free or soy milk and soy cheese, and thicken the sauce with 1/4 cup (35 g) (gluten-free) cornstarch. This recipe is one of several tasty high performance potato recipes highlighted on https://www.potatogoodness.com.

6 medium potatoes (about 2.5 lbs, or 1.2 kg), preferably russet or yellow, but whatever you have on hand

2 tablespoons butter or tub margarine

3 cups (720 ml) milk, 2 percent fat or as you choose

1/2 cup (70 g) all-purpose flour

1 teaspoon salt, as desired

1/4 teaspoon pepper, as desired

4 ounces (1 cup, or 120 g) shredded cheese, such as low-fat cheddar

Optional: 1/2 teaspoon nutmeg, 1/4 teaspoon garlic powder, dash of cayenne pepper, 2 tablespoons grated Parmesan cheese

1. Wash the potatoes, (peel them, if desired) and cut into thin (1/8 in., or 0.3 cm) slices.

2. In a medium-size saucepan, melt the butter with 1 1/2 cups (360 ml) of milk. To the remaining 1 1/2 cup (120) milk, stir in 1/2 cup (70 g) flour until all the lumps are gone.

3. Whisk the flour and milk mixture into the butter and milk mixture and cook until thickened. Season with salt, pepper, (and cayenne pepper, nutmeg, or garlic powder).

4. Prepare a 9- × 13-inch (23 × 33 cm) baking pan with cooking spay (or line with foil for easy cleanup). Preheat the oven to 400 °F (205 °C).

5. Spread a layer of potato slices on the bottom of the baking dish, top with 1/3 of the white sauce, and 1/3 of the shredded cheese. Make two more layers of potato and white sauce.

6. Cover with aluminum foil, and bake at 400 °F (205 °C) for 30 minutes covered.

7. Uncover and bake for an additional 20 to 30 minutes or until the potatoes are tender when poked with a fork.

8. If desired, broil on high for a minute or two until nicely browned.

9. Let stand 5 to 10 minutes before serving to let the sauce settle.

10. *Optional:* Sprinkle top with Parmesan cheese before baking.

Yield: 6 servings

NUTRITION INFORMATION: 1,900 total calories; 320 calories per serving; 44 g carbohydrate; 13 g protein; 10 g fat

This recipe is adapted from the contribution of food blogger Manuela Mazzocco of https://cookingwithmanuela.blogspot.com/.

AVOCADO POTATO SALAD

Here's a suggestion for a simple way to enjoy avocado so you get more heart-healthy monounsaturated fat, the "good fat" that helps protect against heart disease. This is just one of many ways to eat avocado beyond guacamole and sliced avocado on a sandwich. For other ideas, check out www.loveonetoday.com.

1 pound (480 g) potatoes, preferably red skinned

1/2 cup (115 g) mayonnaise, low fat or fat free

1 tablespoon cider vinegar

1 teaspoon Dijon mustard

salt and pepper to taste

1 large avocado

Optional: 1/4 cup (60 g) sliced scallion greens

1. Cut potatoes into 1-inch (2.5 cm) cubes and boil or steam for about 15 minutes or until tender when poked with a fork. Drain and let cool in a large mixing bowl.
2. In a small bowl, mix together the mayonnaise, vinegar, salt, and pepper (and sliced scallions).
3. Fold the mayonnaise mixture into the potatoes until well coated.
4. Peel and dice the avocado into 1/2-inch (1.3 cm) cubes. Gently fold in the diced avocado without mashing it.
5. Place the potato salad in the refrigerator to allow the flavors to blend, ideally for 2 hours or overnight. Serve cold.

Yield: 4 servings

NUTRITION INFORMATION: 900 total calories; 425 calories per serving (1/4 recipe); 27 g carbohydrate; 2 g protein; 12 g fat

Adapted from a recipe available at www.avocadocentral.com

QUICK AND EASY RICE (OR QUINOA) IDEAS

Here are a few rice suggestions for hungry athletes who need to refuel depleted muscle. For variety, try cooking rice (or quinoa) in these liquids:

- Chicken or beef broth
- Mixture of orange or apple juice and water
- Water with seasonings: cinnamon, soy sauce, oregano, curry, chili powder, or whatever might nicely blend with the menu

You can also combine rice (or quinoa) with these foods:

- Leftover chili
- Toasted sesame seeds and chopped nuts
- Steamed vegetables
- Chopped mushrooms and green peppers, either raw or sauteed
- Low-fat sour cream, raisins, tuna, and curry powder
- Raisins, cinnamon, and applesauce
- Soy sauce and diced scallions
- Honey, raisins, and toasted sliced almonds

SOUTHWESTERN RICE AND BEAN SALAD

This makes a nice side dish with barbequed chicken. If you do not have lime juice on hand, you can use lemon juice, rice vinegar, or white vinegar.

2 cups cooked rice, cooled (about 2/3 cup [130 g] when uncooked)

1 15-ounce (425 g) can black beans, drained and rinsed

1 large tomato, chopped

3 ounces (90 g) low-fat cheddar cheese, diced into small 1/4-inch (0.5 cm) cubes

Dressing:

1 tablespoon oil, preferably olive or canola

2 tablespoons lime juice, lemon juice, or vinegar

1 tablespoon taco seasoning mix (or 1 teaspoon cumin and 1/8 teaspoon cayenne pepper)

Optional: 2 tablespoons chopped cilantro; 1/4 cup diced onion, salt, and pepper

1. In a large bowl, combine the cooked rice, beans, tomato, and cheese (and cilantro and onion).
2. In a small bowl, whisk together the oil, lime juice, and taco seasonings. Pour over the rice mixture and mix well. Adjust the seasonings to the desired taste. Refrigerate until ready to serve.

Yield: 4 servings (as a side dish)

NUTRITION INFORMATION: 960 total calories; 240 calories per serving; 27 g carbohydrate; 15 g protein; 12 g fat

CHAPTER 20

VEGETABLES AND SALADS

Vegetables are perfectly delicious when served plain, without added flavorings. Or you can season them with herbs, spices, garlic, and onion. Whatever you do, carefully cook vegetables just until they are tender-crisp and still flavorful. Limp, overcooked veggies lose their appeal as well as some of their nutrients.

Most vegetables contain negligible amounts of protein and fat but offer carbohydrate, fiber, and abundant vitamins and minerals. Eating vegetables is an excellent way to boost your vitamin intake—and is preferable to taking vitamin pills. These "all-natural vitamins" work synergistically with other phytochemicals found in food to protect your health.

The first five recipes offer basic advice about cooking methods. Because you will choose your own vegetable combinations in the earlier recipes, nutrition information is provided only for the remaining recipes. Refer to tables 1.2 and table 4.1 for additional nutrition information.

RECIPE FINDER

Steamed vegetables	394
Stir-fried vegetables	395
Roasted vegetables	396
Microwaved vegetables	397
Grilled vegetables	398
Spinach salad with sweet and spicy dressing	399
Spinach salad with Asian dressing	400
Baked beets	401
Honey-glazed sweet potatoes	402

See also: carrot raisin muffins (chapter 18); southwestern rice and bean salad, skillet lasagna, gourmet vegetarian lasagna, cauliflower macaroni and cheese, extra-creamy potatoes and cheese, pasta with mushrooms and asparagus (chapter 19); sauteed chicken with mushrooms and onions, chicken with pasta and spinach, chicken, kale, and black bean quesadilla (chapter 21), fish and spinach bake (chapter 22); burger that's better for you (chapter 23); Buddha bowl ideas, kale and cannellini bean soup, pumpkin chili; chickpea, curry, and peanut butter soup (chapter 24); smoothie suggestions, beet-cherry smoothie (chapter 25); carrot cake (chapter 26).

STEAMED VEGETABLES

By steaming vegetables, you'll conserve the vitamins and minerals that otherwise would leech into the cooking water. The vegetables will not only have more taste but also more nutritional value. Following are examples of vegetables that lend themselves nicely to steaming:

- Broccoli
- Spinach
- Carrots
- Green beans
- Brussels sprouts

  Optional: Sprinkle vegetables with herbs before or after cooking. Add basil and oregano to zucchini and squash, ginger to carrots, and garlic powder to green beans. With carrots, add a teaspoon of honey afterward. Be creative!

1. Wash the vegetables thoroughly. Cut into the desired size.
2. Put 1/2 inch (just over 1 cm) of water in the bottom of a pan with a tight lid. Bring to a boil; then add the vegetables. Cover tightly. Or put the vegetables in a steamer basket and put the basket into a saucepan with 1 inch (2.5 cm) of water (or enough to prevent the water from boiling away). Cover tightly and bring to a boil.
3. Cook over medium heat until tender-crisp, 3 to 10 minutes, depending on the type and size of vegetables.
4. Drain the vegetables, reserving the cooking liquid for soup, sauces, or even for drinking as vegetable broth.

STIR-FRIED VEGETABLES

A large skillet is useful for stir-frying vegetables. The goal is to end up with vegetables that are cooked until tender-crisp and flavorful. By combining only two or three vegetables, you'll get more distinguished flavors. Plus, this makes it easier to time the cooking so they are all done at the same time.

Olive and canola oils are among the heart-healthiest choices for stir-frying. For a wonderful flavor, add a little sesame oil (available in the Asian food section of larger supermarkets or health food stores). If you are watching your weight, be sure to add only a little oil. The following are popular combinations:

- Carrots, broccoli, and mushrooms
- Onions, zucchini, and tomatoes
- Chinese cabbage and water chestnuts
- Sugar snap peas, Chinese pea pods, and green peas

  Optional: toasted sesame seeds, nuts, mandarin orange sections, pineapple chunks

1. Wash the vegetables and drain well (to prevent oil from spattering when the vegetables are added to the hot skillet, wok, or pan). Cut into bite-sized pieces or 1/8-inch (0.3 cm) slices. When possible, slice the vegetables diagonally to increase the surface area; this helps them cook faster. Try to make the pieces uniform so they cook evenly.

2. Heat a wok, or large frying pan over high heat until very hot, and then add 1 to 3 teaspoons of canola, olive, or sesame oil—just enough to coat the bottom of the pan. For an interesting flavor, try adding a slice of ginger root or minced garlic to the oil. Stir-fry for a minute to flavor the oil.

3. First add the vegetables that take the longest to cook (carrots, cauliflower, broccoli); a few minutes later, add the remaining veggies (mushrooms, bean sprouts, cabbage, spinach). Rather than stir constantly (as the name would imply), wait about 30 seconds between stirrings so the pan can regain its heat. Adjust the heat to prevent scorching.

4. Don't overcrowd the pan. Cook small batches at a time. The goal is to cook the vegetables until they are tender but still crunchy, 2 to 5 minutes.

5. *Optional:* Garnish the vegetables with toasted sesame seeds, toasted nuts (almonds, cashews, peanuts), mandarin orange sections, or pineapple chunks.

ROASTED VEGETABLES

If the oven is already hot because you are baking potatoes, chicken, or a casserole, you might as well make good use of the heat and bake the vegetables, too. Roasting vegetables evaporates much of their water, concentrates their natural sugars, and yields a rich, sweet taste and meaty texture. Here are popular combinations:

- Eggplant halves sprinkled with garlic powder
- Zucchini or summer squash halves covered with onion slices
- Carrot chunks
- Sweet potato slices and apples
- Winter squash, sliced into quarters and sprinkled with salt and pepper

1. Put the oven rack in the middle of the oven, and then heat the oven to 400 °F (200 °C).
2. While the oven is heating, cut vegetables into equal-sized chunks, rub with a little canola or olive oil, and spread them in a single layer on a rimmed baking sheet lined with foil and treated with cooking spray.
3. For best results, tightly cover the vegetables with foil (so they will first steam), bake for 15 minutes, uncover, and then finish baking for another 20 to 30 minutes or until tender.

Alternative way to bake vegetables:

1. Wrap the vegetables in foil, or put them in a covered baking dish with a small amount of water. (This actually steams them rather than roasts them.)
2. Bake at 350 °F (180 °C) for 20 to 30 minutes (depending on the size of the chunks) until tender-crisp.
3. When you open the foil or covered baking dish, be careful of escaping steam so that you don't get burned.

MICROWAVED VEGETABLES

Microwave cookery is ideal for vegetables because it cooks them quickly and without water, retaining a greater percentage of nutrients than with conventional methods. All vegetables cook fine in the microwave oven, but these are some nice options:

- Green beans
- Peas
- Broccoli
- Cauliflower
- Carrots

   Optional: Sprinkle vegetables with herbs (basil, parsley, oregano, garlic powder), soy sauce, or whatever suits your taste.

1. Wash the vegetables and cut them into bite-sized pieces.
2. Put them in a microwavable dish with a cover. If the vegetables vary in thickness (as stalks of broccoli do), arrange them in a ring with the thicker portions toward the outside of the dish.
3. Microwave until tender-crisp. The amount of time will vary according to your particular oven and the amount of vegetables you are cooking. You'll learn by trial and error. Start off with 3 minutes for a single serving; larger quantities take longer. The vegetables will continue cooking after they are removed from the microwave, so plan that into the time allotment.

GRILLED VEGETABLES

When grilling your entree (chicken, fish, meats), plan to save space for grilling vegetables as well. Grilled vegetables have a wonderful flavor; the heat evaporates their water content, and in the process, their flavor becomes more concentrated. Ideally, vegetables should be cooked over a medium-hot fire—you should be able to hold your hand 5 inches (13 cm) above the cooking surface for 4 seconds. Here are popular options:

- Asparagus
- Eggplant
- Mushrooms
- Onions
- Peppers

1. Slice vegetables such as summer squash, peppers, potato, and eggplant into "steaks." For smaller pieces of vegetables (cherry tomatoes, onion chunks, mushroom tops), use skewers or a grilling basket.

2. To prevent the outside of the vegetables from getting charred, first microwave the cut-up veggies for 1 to 2 minutes; then brush with olive oil. Put smaller pieces in a plastic bag, add a little oil, and shake to coat.

3. Arrange on the grill, skewer, or grilling basket. Cook until tender, turning with tongs or a metal spatula. Cook for 5 to 10 minutes.

SPINACH SALAD WITH SWEET AND SPICY DRESSING

Spinach is a powerhouse vegetable, rich in potassium, folate, beta-carotene, and many other nutrients. You can easily incorporate more spinach into your diet with tasty spinach salads. Here is one version.

1 10-ounce (300 g) package or large bunch fresh spinach, rinsed well and cut up

Optional: 1 cup (70 g) sliced mushrooms; 2 fresh tomatoes, cut into wedges; 2 hard-boiled eggs, sliced; 1/2 cup (60 g) broken walnuts

Sweet and Spicy Dressing

3 tablespoons olive oil

2 tablespoons red wine vinegar

1 tablespoon sugar

1 teaspoon salt, as desired

1 tablespoon ketchup

1. Place the spinach in a salad bowl (combine with the mushrooms and tomatoes, as desired).
2. In a jar, combine the olive oil, vinegar, sugar, salt, and ketchup. Cover and shake until well blended.
3. Pour the dressing over the salad, toss well, and then garnish with eggs and walnuts, as desired.

Yield: 4 large salads

NUTRITION INFORMATION: 480 total calories; 120 calories per serving; 7 g carbohydrate; 2 g protein; 9 g fat

SPINACH SALAD WITH ASIAN DRESSING

This recipe goes nicely with a simple baked fish or chicken meal and fresh whole-grain bread.

1 10-ounce (300 g) package or large bunch fresh spinach, rinsed well and cut up

Optional: 4 ounces (125 g) water chestnuts, sliced; 1/2 pound (240 g) mushrooms, sliced; 1/2 pound (240 g) bean sprouts; 1 can (11 oz, or 310 g) mandarin oranges; 1/2 teaspoon toasted sesame seeds

Asian Dressing

1 tablespoon soy sauce, light or regular

1/4 cup (60 ml) vinegar, preferably rice vinegar

2 teaspoons fresh lemon juice (or 2 teaspoons more vinegar)

1 teaspoon sugar

1/2 teaspoon grated ginger

1/4 teaspoon garlic powder

2 tablespoons sesame oil

1. Place the spinach in a salad bowl (combine with the water chestnuts, mushrooms, bean sprouts, and mandarin oranges, as desired).
2. In a jar, combine the soy sauce, vinegar, lemon juice, sugar, ginger, garlic powder, and sesame oil. Cover and shake until well blended.
3. Pour the dressing over the salad and toss well.
4. Garnish with sesame seeds, as desired.

Yield: 4 large salads

NUTRITION INFORMATION: 320 total calories; 80 calories per serving; 4 g carbohydrate; 2 g protein; 6 g fat

BAKED BEETS

Beets are rich in nitrates, a compound that might enhance performance when consumed about two and a half hours before hard exercise (see Endurance Enhancers in chapter 11). Although some athletes suffer through beetroot juice "shots," I suggest that you bake up a pound (480 g) of beets as a more enjoyable way to ingest their nitrates. Baked beets become sugary-sweet and yummy! Sort of like eating candy that's good for you.

1 pound (480 g) beets
2 to 3 teaspoons olive oil

1. Cut off the beet greens and tails; then scrub the beets and dry with a towel. (Cook the greens another time as you might cook spinach or collards.)
2. Peel the beets, as desired, and then cut them into quarters or eighths, depending on their size.
3. Line a rimmed baking sheet with foil. Put the beets in one layer on the foil. Drizzle with olive oil, and then mix them around to be sure they are evenly coated. Alternatively, put the beets in a large plastic bag, add the oil, and shake until the beets are evenly coated.
4. Place in a cold oven that you then heat to 400 °F (200 °C) and bake for about 30 minutes, or until easily pierced with a fork.
5. Let cool a bit, and then pop the beet chunks into your mouth (skin and all)!

Yield: 2 servings for dinner; 1 for ergogenic benefits, if tolerated pre-event

NUTRITION INFORMATION: 250 total calories; 125 calories per dinner serving; 23 g carbohydrate; 4 g protein; 4 g fat

HONEY-GLAZED SWEET POTATOES

Carbohydrate-rich and colorful, sweet potatoes offer lots of health-protective beta-carotene. Enjoy sweet potatoes with chicken, fish, and tofu meals, and plan to make extra so you'll have leftovers to enjoy cold as a preexercise snack. Sweet potatoes are healthier than a cookie—but just as sweet!

2 pounds (1 kg) sweet potatoes (about 4 medium)

1/4 cup (60 ml) water

2 tablespoons brown sugar

2 tablespoons honey

1 tablespoon olive oil

1. Preheat oven to 375 °F (190 °C).
2. Lightly coat the bottom and sides of a 9- × 13-inch (23 × 33 cm) baking pan with cooking spray; set aside.
3. Peel (if desired) and cut the sweet potatoes into 3/4-inch-thick (2 cm) chunks.
4. In a small bowl, stir together the water, brown sugar, honey, and olive oil.
5. Transfer the sweet potatoes to the baking pan and spread into a single layer. Pour the sauce over the potatoes and turn the potatoes to coat thoroughly.
6. Cover with foil and bake 30 to 45 minutes or until tender, stirring gently twice to ensure that they are coated.
7. When the sweet potatoes are tender, remove the foil and bake an additional 15 minutes or until the glaze is set.

Yield: 4 servings

NUTRITION INFORMATION: 1,050 total calories; 260 calories per serving; 55 g carbohydrate; 3 g protein; 3 g fat

Adapted from a recipe available at www.mayoclinic.com.

CHAPTER 21

CHICKEN AND TURKEY

The white and dark meat of chicken and turkey are excellent examples of muscle physiology. They represent two types of muscle fibers. The white breast meat is primarily composed of fast-twitch muscle fibers used for bursts of energy. Athletes such as elite gymnasts, basketball players, and others who do sprint types of exercise tend to have a high percentage of fast-twitch fibers.

The dark meat in the legs and wings is primarily composed of slow-twitch muscle fibers that function best for endurance exercise. Elite marathoners, long-distance cyclists, and other successful endurance athletes tend to have a high percentage of slow-twitch fibers. The dark meat of poultry contains more fat than the white meat because the fat provides energy for greater endurance; dark meat also has slightly more fat calories than light meat:

3 oz (90 g) chicken or turkey breast (white meat) = 120 calories

3 oz (90 g) chicken or turkey thigh (dark meat) = 150 calories

The dark meat also contains more iron, zinc, B vitamins, and other nutrients. I recommend that athletes who don't eat beef select skinless dark-meat poultry to boost their intake of these important nutrients. Because the highest source of fat in chicken is in the skin, be sure to remove the skin before cooking. This eliminates the temptation to eat it.

RECIPE FINDER

Quick and easy chicken ideas 405

Oven-fried chicken 406

Sauteed chicken with mushrooms and onions 407

Chicken with pasta and spinach 408

Green chili chicken enchilada casserole 409

Chicken salad with almonds and mandarin oranges 410

Chicken black bean soup 411

Chicken and white beans 412

Chicken, kale, and black bean quesadillas 413

Savory African peanut stew 414

Turkey cran-apple wrap 416

Turkey meatballs with tangy cranberry sauce 417

See also: skillet lasagna (chapter 19); stir-fried vegetables (chapter 20); fish in foil Mexican style, broiled salmon with mustard-maple glaze (chapter 22); burger that's better for you, meatballs by the gallon, enchilada casserole (chapter 23); pasta and white bean soup with sun-dried tomatoes, peanut butter soup with curry and chickpeas, kale and cannellini bean soup, pumpkin chili (chapter 24).

QUICK AND EASY CHICKEN IDEAS

For a basic chicken meal, put 1/2 inch (just over 1 cm) of water in a sauce-pan, add pieces of chicken (with or without bone, with or without skin), cover tightly, and bring just to a boil. Turn down heat; gently simmer over medium-low heat for 20 to 25 minutes or until the juices run clear when the chicken is poked with a fork. You may prefer to place the skinless chicken on a rack in a baking pan. Bake uncovered at 350 °F (180 °C) for 20 to 30 minutes or until the juices run clear when the meat is poked with a fork. For easy cleanup when baking chicken, use a baking pan treated with cooking spray, or line the pan with aluminum foil.

Here are ways to add variety to your chicken meals:

- Add seasonings to the cooking water: a low-sodium chicken bouil-lon cube, lite soy sauce, curry, basil, or thyme. Or replace cooking water with orange juice, white wine, or a can of stewed tomatoes.
- Cook rice along with the chicken (add extra water) and add veg-etables in the last 5 minutes.
- Make stuffing with the chicken broth and stuffing mix.
- Dice the cooked chicken and wrap it in a tortilla with salsa, shred-ded lettuce, and grated low-fat cheese.
- Spread a teaspoon of Dijon mustard on raw chicken, add a gener-ous sprinkling of Parmesan cheese, and bake.
- Spread a teaspoon of honey on raw chicken; then sprinkle on curry powder and bake.
- Wrap a raw chicken breast around a piece of string cheese sliced in half lengthwise, secure with toothpicks, and then bake.
- Marinate the chicken in a sealable bag with soy sauce, a shake of ground ginger, mustard, and garlic powder, and then bake or saute.
- Dip in olive or canola oil and then in sesame seeds, cracker crumbs, or cornflake crumbs, and bake or saute.
- Place a chicken breast on a piece of foil, cover with vegetables and seasonings of your choice. Wrap well by folding the edges of the foil together, and then bake at 375 °F (190 °C) for about 20 to 25 minutes. Be careful you are not burned by the steam that escapes when you open the foil packet.

OVEN-FRIED CHICKEN

Deep-fried chicken is popular with many athletes but is certainly not the healthiest of sports foods. This recipe offers a lower-fat alternative that will get a thumbs-up from even fussy eaters. The wire rack allows air to circulate on all sides; you'll get crisper chicken, and you won't have to turn it during cooking. Meanwhile, the pan lined with foil speeds your cleanup time.

1 box (5 oz, or 150 g) Melba toast

2 to 4 tablespoons olive or canola oil

1 egg

4 boneless, skinless chicken breasts

Optional: 1 tablespoon Dijon mustard, salt and pepper as desired

1. Heat oven to 400 °F (200 °C).
2. Place a wire rack in a shallow baking pan lined with foil.
3. Add the Melba toast to a heavy-duty plastic bag, seal, and crush with a rolling pin (or other hard object) into crumbs, leaving some crumbs as large as small corn kernels.
4. Pour the crumbs into a shallow dish and drizzle the oil over them. Toss well to distribute the oil evenly.
5. Beat the egg in a medium bowl. Add mustard, salt, and pepper if desired.
6. Dip each piece of chicken into the egg mixture, allow excess to drip off, and then place each coated breast in the crumbs. Sprinkle the crumbs over the chicken and press them in. Shake off excess crumbs and place the chicken on the rack.
7. Bake for 40 minutes. The coating should be deep brown, and the juices should run clear when the meat is cut.

Yield: 4 servings

NUTRITION INFORMATION: 1,200 total calories; 300 calories per serving; 12 g carbohydrate; 40 g protein; 10 g fat

Adapted from *Cook's Illustrated* magazine, May/June 1999.

SAUTEED CHICKEN WITH MUSHROOMS AND ONIONS

This simple recipe is tasty enough for an impromptu gourmet dinner. It includes common ingredients that are easy to keep stocked: (frozen) chicken breasts, (canned) mushrooms, onions, low-fat cheese, and wine. Enjoy it with (brown) rice, crusty whole-grain rolls, and a green vegetable.

1 to 2 tablespoons oil, preferably olive or canola

4 boneless, skinless chicken breasts

1 medium onion, diced

1 pint sliced fresh mushrooms or 2 6-ounce (180 g) cans sliced mushrooms, drained

1 cup (240 ml) dry white wine

2 ounces (60 g) Swiss cheese, preferably low-fat

Optional: 1 to 2 cloves garlic, minced, or 1 teaspoon ground thyme

1. In a large skillet, heat the oil and add the chicken breasts, onion, and fresh mushrooms (and garlic). Cook for about 5 minutes per side.
2. Add the wine (and canned mushrooms and thyme).
3. Cover and simmer for about 10 minutes or until the chicken is done and the juices run clear when the meat is slit with a knife.
4. Place 1/2 ounce (15 g) of cheese on top of each cooked chicken breast. Cover the pan and simmer for another 3 minutes or until the cheese is melted.
5. Serve by placing the chicken on top of a bed of mushrooms.

Yield: 4 servings

NUTRITION INFORMATION: 1,200 total calories; 300 calories per serving; 10 g carbohydrate; 42 g protein; 10 g fat

CHICKEN WITH PASTA AND SPINACH

This recipe is not only quick and easy but also includes three food groups (grain, protein, and vegetable), creating a well-balanced meal. Food variety can help keep you strong to the finish—as can the spinach itself.

1 pound (500 g) pasta, such as fettuccine

2 tablespoons oil, preferably olive or canola

1 pound (500 g) boneless, skinless chicken breasts, thinly sliced

1 to 4 cloves garlic, finely chopped, or 1/4 to 1 teaspoon garlic powder

1 10-ounce (300 ml) can chicken broth

1 pound (500 g) fresh spinach, washed, drained, and roughly chopped

salt and pepper to taste

Optional: 10 ounces (300 g) mushrooms, sliced; 1/4 cup (25 g) Parmesan cheese

1. Cook the pasta according to the package directions.
2. While the pasta is cooking, heat the oil in a large skillet and saute the sliced chicken breasts for 30 seconds.
3. Toss in the garlic (and mushrooms) and stir well. Cook for about 5 minutes.
4. Pour in the chicken broth and bring it to a simmer. Add the spinach, stirring until it wilts.
5. Drain the pasta and return it to the cooking pot. Pour in the chicken and spinach mixture and toss well. Heat for 2 minutes.
6. Season to taste with salt and pepper (and Parmesan cheese, as desired).

Yield: 5 servings

NUTRITION INFORMATION: 2,800 total calories; 560 calories per serving; 75 g carbohydrate; 40 g protein; 11 g fat

GREEN CHILI CHICKEN ENCHILADA CASSEROLE

A family favorite, this recipe is easy to make and yummy to eat. The green chilies in the enchilada sauce add a special flavor and a nice change from the traditional red enchilada sauce. This recipe is adapted from dietitian Brenda Ponichtera's best-selling book, *Quick & Healthy Recipes and Ideas.*

1 1/2 pounds (700 g) boneless, skinless chicken breasts

1 medium onion, finely diced, or 1/4 cup (30 g) dried onion

1 large can (28 oz, or 840 ml) green chili enchilada sauce

1 can (4.5 oz, or 135 g) diced green chilies

1/2 cup (115 g) sour cream, fat free or low fat

1 cup (4 oz, or 120 g) low-fat cheddar cheese, grated

12 corn tortillas (6 in., or 15 cm)

1. Put an inch (2.5 cm) of water in a medium saucepan, add the chicken breasts, cover, and bring to a boil. Simmer over low heat for 10 minutes or until juices run clear when it is pricked with a fork. Drain off the broth, and let the chicken cool briefly.

2. While the chicken cooks, dice the onion, and then microwave it in a small bowl for 2 minutes.

3. In a medium bowl, combine the onion, 1 1/2 cups (360 ml) of the enchilada sauce, sour cream, green chilies, and 1/2 cup (60 g) of the grated cheese.

4. Preheat the oven to 350 °F (180 °C), and spray a 9- × 13-inch (23 × 33 cm) baking pan with cooking spray.

5. Place 4 tortillas in the pan, tearing them to fill any empty spaces.

6. Top with half of the chicken mixture. Add another layer of 4 tortillas, and top with the remaining chicken mixture and the remaining 4 tortillas.

7. Pour the remaining enchilada sauce over the top. Bake uncovered for 30 to 40 minutes. Top with the remaining grated cheese and return to the oven for 5 minutes.

Yield: 4 large servings

NUTRITION INFORMATION: 1,800 total calories, 450 calories per serving; 55 g carbohydrate; 35 g protein; 10 g fat

CHICKEN SALAD WITH ALMONDS AND MANDARIN ORANGES

This is nice served on a bed of salad greens and accompanied by whole-grain bread.

1 pound (480 g) boneless, skinless chicken breasts

1/4 to 1/2 cup (30 to 60 g) slivered almonds

1 can (11 oz, or 310 g) mandarin oranges, drained

Optional: 1 can (8 oz, or 240 g) pineapple chunks, 1 can (6 oz, or 180 g) sliced water chestnuts, 1/2 cup (80 g) raisins or chopped dates

Lemon Dressing

1/2 to 1 cup (115 to 230 g) low-fat lemon yogurt, or a mixture of half yogurt, half low-fat mayonnaise

Asian Dressing

2 tablespoons hoisin sauce

2 tablespoons juice from the mandarin oranges

4 tablespoons low-fat mayonnaise

Optional: 1/2 teaspoon dry mustard, 1/4 teaspoon garlic powder

Alternative Dressing

1/2 cup (115 g) low-fat mayonnaise

1. Simmer the chicken in 1 cup (240 ml) of water in a covered pan for about 20 minutes or until the juices run clear when chicken is pricked with a fork. Cool; dice and place in a large bowl with the almonds and oranges (and pineapple, water chestnuts, and raisins or dates).
2. For the lemon dressing, add the lemon yogurt and mix well. For the Asian dressing, in a small bowl, mix the hoisin sauce, mandarin orange juice, and low-fat mayonnaise (and mustard and garlic).
3. If time allows, chill. Serve on a bed of salad greens.

Yield: 4 servings

NUTRITION INFORMATION: 1,100 total calories with lemon dressing; 275 calories per serving; 12 g carbohydrate; 40 g protein; 7 g fat

1,200 total calories with Asian dressing; 300 calories per serving; 17 g carbohydrate; 40 g protein, 8 g fat

Courtesy of Barbara Day, RD.

CHICKEN BLACK BEAN SOUP

Fitness enthusiast and chef Peter Herman gave me this simple yet delicious and nutritious recipe. It's a tasty way to add more fiber-rich beans to your diet. You can make it a heartier meal by adding cooked pasta.

4 boneless, skinless chicken breasts

5 cups (1.2 L) chicken broth or water

2 carrots, peeled and sliced

2 tomatoes, chopped

1/2 onion, chopped

3 to 5 cloves garlic, crushed

2 16-ounce (480 g) cans black beans, rinsed and drained

1 tablespoon fresh oregano leaves or 1 teaspoon dried oregano

Optional: 1/2 cup (120 ml) Marsala wine; 2 to 4 cups cooked pasta, shells, or bow ties; 2 ounces

(60 g) grated cheddar cheese; hot red pepper flakes

1. In a large stockpot, place the chicken breasts, broth or water, carrots, tomatoes, onion, garlic, beans, and seasonings (and wine). Cover and bring to a boil, reduce the heat, and simmer for about 20 minutes or until done.

2. Remove the chicken pieces from the broth and set them aside to cool. Keep the broth warm over low heat. (*Optional:* Add the cooked pasta.)

3. Dice the chicken into small pieces. Return it to the soup and heat it through.

4. Garnish with grated cheese and red pepper flakes, if desired.

Yield: 4 servings

NUTRITION INFORMATION: 1,200 total calories; 300 calories per serving; 33 g carbohydrate; 35 g protein; 3 g fat

Reprinted by permission from Peter Herman.

CHICKEN AND WHITE BEANS

This one-pot meal offers a tasty carbohydrate–protein combination with carbohydrate from the beans to refuel your muscles and protein from the chicken, beans, and cheese to build and repair your muscles. If you are using leftover chicken or turkey, about 1 1/2 cups diced will do the job!

> 1 1/2 pounds (720 g) boneless, skinless chicken breasts or thighs
>
> 1 can (15 oz, or 450 ml) chicken broth
>
> 1 tablespoon olive oil
>
> 1 small onion, chopped
>
> 1/4 teaspoon garlic powder or 1 clove garlic, minced
>
> 1 can (4 oz, or 120 g) chopped green chilies
>
> 1 teaspoon ground cumin
>
> 2 cans (15 oz, or 450 g) white beans, undrained
>
> 1/2 cup (120 g) grated low-fat cheese, such as Monterey Jack or white cheddar
>
> *Optional:* 1 seeded jalapeno pepper, chopped; 1 dash ground cloves; 1 dash cayenne pepper

1. Simmer the chicken in the chicken broth for about 10 minutes.
2. While the chicken is cooking, heat the olive oil in a large saucepan over medium heat. Stir in the chopped onion and cook until tender, 5 to 7 minutes.
3. Mix in the garlic, green chilies, cumin, (jalapeno, cloves, cayenne). Continue to cook and stir until tender, about 3 minutes.
4. Add the onion and chili mixture into the chicken broth. Add the beans, and bring to a boil.
5. Turn down heat and simmer uncovered for 10 minutes, stirring occasionally. It should be a little soupy. To make the broth thicker, mash about half of the beans using a potato masher.
6. Serve topped with grated cheese. If desired, garnish with cilantro, salsa, chopped tomato, scallions, and avocado or guacamole. To complete the meal, serve with fresh, warmed tortillas on the side.

Yield: 4 servings

NUTRITION INFORMATION: 1,700 total calories; 425 calories per serving; 38 g carbohydrate; 42 g protein; 12 g fat

CHICKEN, KALE, AND BLACK BEAN QUESADILLAS

What better way to use leftover rotisserie chicken (or freshly cooked chicken breast) than to make it into a quesadilla! Recipe contributor and elite triathlete Michele Tuttle, RD, considers this recipe to be superfuel for athletes. It's easy to make, yummy, and a healthy combination of nourishing carbohydrate and protein. This is adapted from one of several recipes for simple sports foods created for the Wheat Food Council, available at www.centerfornutritionandathletics.org.

2 cups (135 g) baby kale

1 tablespoon oil, preferably olive or canola

1/4 teaspoon salt

1 can (15 oz, or 450 g) black beans, rinsed and drained

1/2 cup (130 g) salsa

2 cups (480 g) chopped or shredded cooked chicken

6 flour tortillas (8 in., or 20 cm), preferably whole wheat

1 1/2 cups (6 oz, or 180 g) shredded Mexican blend cheese

1. Heat oil is a medium-sized skillet. Add kale and salt; stir until the kale is wilted.
2. Place half the beans in the skillet and mash them with a fork. Add remaining beans and salsa; heat.
3. Place a spoonful of bean mixture on half of a tortilla. Top with chicken and shredded cheese. Fold each tortilla in half over the filling.
4. Heat another skillet to medium; coat with a little oil. Add 2 quesadillas, cook until lightly browned on each side (about 2 minutes per side). Set aside on a serving plate and make the remaining 4 quesadillas.
5. Cut each quesadilla into 3 pieces for easy eating.

Yield: 6 quesadillas

NUTRITION INFORMATION: 2,400 total calories; 400 calories per quesadilla; 37 g carbohydrate, 30 g protein, 15 g fat

Courtesy of centerfornutritionandathletics.org.

SAVORY AFRICAN PEANUT STEW

This stew is creamy, savory, just plain yummy—and versatile. This is a fun recipe to cook with a few friends because there's a bit of chopping and dicing for everyone. If you are preparing the meal on your own and want to make the process easier, simply use frozen diced peppers and onions, minced garlic (from a jar) or garlic powder, and ground ginger (instead of fresh—although fresh is really worth the effort). I had to buy coriander just for this recipe, but because I frequently make the recipe, I'm happy to have that spice on my shelf.

You could make this recipe with chickpeas or tofu in place of the pork or chicken; white potato or cauliflower in place of the sweet potato; and kale, collard greens, asparagus tips, or green beans in place of the spinach. For a thin broth, use 1/2 cup (130 g) peanut butter; the 3/4 cup (175 g) makes the broth thick and creamy. *Note:* This recipe is relatively low in carbohydrate, so add extra sweet potato if you want to fully fuel your muscles.

This recipe is courtesy of busy mom, food blogger (www.jugglingwith-julia.com), and registered dietitian Julia Robarts, RD.

3 tablespoons olive oil

1 medium sweet bell pepper, diced (about 1 cup, or 150 g)

1 medium onion (yellow or Vidalia), diced (about 1 cup, or 160 g)

1 pound (480 g) chicken or pork tenderloin, cut in bite-sized pieces

1 1/2 teaspoons salt

1 teaspoon ground black pepper

1 1/2 teaspoons minced garlic, or 1/4 teaspoon garlic powder

1 tablespoon fresh ginger, diced

2 teaspoons ground coriander

1/8 teaspoon cayenne pepper, or to taste

1 can (15 oz, or 450 g) diced tomatoes, undrained

2 large sweet potatoes (about 2 lb, or 900 g), peeled and chopped

3 cups (720 ml) chicken broth

1/2 to 3/4 cup (130 to 175 g) natural peanut butter

Optional: 1 to 2 cups (65 to 135 g) baby spinach, 1 to 2 tablespoons apple cider vinegar (brightens the flavors), 1/2 cup (60 g) peanuts for topping

1. In a large soup pot, heat the olive oil over medium-high heat. Add the diced peppers and onions and saute until softened, 3 to 5 minutes. While that is cooking, sprinkle the salt and pepper over the chicken (or pork) pieces.

2. Add the chicken (or pork) to the pot and brown the meat on all sides, about 2 minutes. Drop in the garlic, ginger, coriander, and cayenne, and saute for 1 minute more.

3. Pour in the canned tomatoes; add the sweet potatoes and broth.

4. Cover and bring to a boil, and then reduce heat to a gentle boil for 15 to 18 minutes, until the sweet potatoes are softened.

5. Add the peanut butter, and whisk until smooth. Add the spinach. Cover and cook for an additional 1 to 2 minutes.

6. Remove from heat; (stir in the vinegar).

7. Taste, and adjust seasonings (salt, cayenne, pepper) as desired.

Yield: 6 servings

NUTRITION INFORMATION: 2,600 total calories; 430 calories per serving, 28 g carbohydrate, 32 g protein; 21 g fat

Courtesy of Julia Robarts, RD. www.JugglingWithJulia.com.

TURKEY CRAN-APPLE WRAP

Simple to make, yet unique and tasty, this wrap is a favorite lunch or supper from Boston-area registered dietitian and food writer Heidi McIndoo (www.appleadaynutrition.net). You can make it as a wrap, or put it on a pita, crusty whole-grain baguette, or sliced bread. It's a perfect recovery food—a nice combination of protein, carbohydrate, and good taste. On a winter day, zap it briefly in the microwave oven. Yum!

Per Sandwich

1 to 2 tablespoons cranberry sauce

1 wrap or whole-grain roll or 2 slices whole-grain bread

1 ounce (30 g) sliced cheddar cheese, preferably low fat

2 ounces (60 g) turkey breast, sliced

1/4 apple, such as Granny Smith, sliced very thin

1. Spread the cranberry sauce on the wrap, the bottom of the roll, or a slice of bread.
2. Add sliced cheese, turkey breast, and very thinly sliced apple.
3. Roll up the wrap, or add the top of the roll or the second slice of bread.
4. If desired, heat briefly in the microwave oven.

Yield: 1 sandwich

NUTRITION INFORMATION: 400 total calories; 400 calories per serving; 60 g carbohydrate; 25 g protein; 6 g fat

Courtesy of Heidi McIndoo, RD. www.appleadaynutrition.net.

TURKEY MEATBALLS WITH TANGY CRANBERRY SAUCE

These turkey meatballs are yummy as an appetizer! When served with toothpicks, they disappear in no time. If you want to incorporate them into a meal, serve them with (brown) rice and a green vegetable.

This recipe comes from the dietitians at Hy-Vee stores. They often use this recipe in cooking demonstrations to teach people how to enjoy ground turkey (or ground chicken) as an alternative to fattier hamburger.

1 pound (480 g) ground turkey

1/2 cup (60 g) seasoned bread crumbs

1 large egg

1 can (14 oz, or 420 g) whole-berry cranberry sauce

1 can (8 oz, or 240 ml) tomato sauce

1 to 2 tablespoons horseradish

1 tablespoon Worcestershire sauce

1 tablespoon lemon juice

1. Mix the ground turkey, bread crumbs, and egg in a bowl.
2. Shape into small (1 in., or 2.5 cm) balls.
3. Cook the meatballs in a 10-inch (25 cm) nonstick skillet over medium-high heat for about 10 minutes, turning once or twice. (You can also bake the meatballs in a 350 °F [180 °C] oven for about 20 minutes.)
4. Add the cranberry sauce, tomato sauce, horseradish, Worcestershire sauce, and lemon juice to the skillet, stirring carefully to avoid damaging the meatballs.
5. Heat to boiling and reduce the heat. Simmer uncovered for about 10 minutes, stirring occasionally

Yield: 30 small meatballs

NUTRITION INFORMATION: 1,500 total calories; 300 calories per serving (6 meatballs, including 1/5 of the sauce); 40 g carbohydrate; 18 g protein; 7 g fat

Courtesy of Hy-Vee. www.Hy-Ve.com

CHAPTER 22

FISH AND SEAFOOD

Fish meals tend to be more popular in restaurants than at home because many people don't know how to buy or prepare fish. The following tips will take the mystique out of fish cookery; fish is actually one of the easiest foods to prepare.

Fresh fish, when properly handled, has no fishy odor whether it is raw or cooked. The odor comes with aging and bacterial contamination. Whenever possible, ask to smell the fish you want to buy. After buying fresh fish, use it quickly, preferably within a day. Keep it in the coldest part of the refrigerator.

When buying commercially frozen fish, be sure the box is firm and square, showing no sign of thawing and refreezing. To thaw, defrost the fish in the refrigerator or microwave oven. Do not refreeze.

For each serving, allow 1 pound (480 g) of uncooked whole fish (such as trout or mackerel) or 1/3 to 1/2 pound (160 to 240 grams) uncooked fish fillets or steaks (such as salmon, swordfish, halibut, or sole). To rid your hands of any fishy smell, rub them with lemon juice or vinegar. Wash cooking utensils with 1 teaspoon of baking soda per quart of water.

Here are a few tips to help you prepare your "catch":

- If possible, cook fish in its serving dish; fish is fragile, and the less it is handled, the more attractive it is.

- Seasonings that go well with fish include lemon, dill, basil, rosemary, and parsley. Add paprika for color.

- To test for doneness, gently pull the flesh apart with a fork. It should flake easily and not be translucent.

- Use leftover fish, warm or cold, in sandwiches as a change from chicken or turkey.

Here are four ways to cook fish.

- **Broiling.** Place fish on a broiling pan that has been lightly oiled or treated with cooking spray to prevent sticking. Sprinkle with a little olive oil and seasonings (if desired), or spread with a mixture of equal parts low-fat mayonnaise and Dijon mustard. Place it 4 to 6 inches (10 to 15 cm) from the heat source. Thin fillets (such as sole and bluefish) can be cooked in 5 minutes without turning; thicker fillets (such as salmon and swordfish) may require 5 to 6 minutes per side.

- **Baking.** Set the fish in a baking dish that has been lightly oiled or treated with cooking spray, season as desired, cover, and bake at 400 °F (200 °C) for 15 to 20 minutes, depending on thickness.

- **Poaching.** Set the fish in a nonstick skillet, and cover the fillets with water, white wine, or milk. Season as desired with herbs and garlic, cover, and gently simmer on the stove top for about 10 minutes. For an Asian twist, add scallions and a little soy sauce.

- **Microwaving.** If possible, place the thickest part of the fillet toward the outside of the dish, overlapping thin portions to prevent over-cooking. Season as desired, cover with waxed paper, and microwave for the minimum amount of time to prevent the fish from becoming tough and dry. Remove from the oven before the fish is totally cooked, and allow it to stand for 5 minutes to finish cooking before serving. Whitefish fillets may need 4 minutes; salmon steaks, 6 to 7 minutes.

RECIPE FINDER

Broiled salmon with mustard-maple glaze	421
Simple salmon patties	422
Fish and spinach bake	423
Shrimp and shells	424
Tuna pasta salad	425
Shrimp marinara	426
Fish in foil, Mexican style	427

BROILED SALMON WITH MUSTARD-MAPLE GLAZE

This simple topping nicely complements salmon and could also be used with chicken. Cutting the salmon into two pieces before cooking makes it easier to serve.

1 pound (480 g) salmon

1 tablespoon mustard, preferably Dijon

1 tablespoon maple syrup

Optional: juice of 1/2 a lemon, sprinkle of garlic powder

1. Preheat the broiler. Place the salmon pieces on a broiler pan lined with foil (for easy cleanup).
2. In a small bowl, combine the mustard and maple syrup (and lemon juice and garlic powder). Spread on the salmon fillet.
3. Broil for 5 to 8 minutes (depending on the thickness of the salmon fillet) until the salmon is just cooked through and flakes easily when pierced with a fork.

Yield: 3 large servings

NUTRITION INFORMATION: 750 total calories; 250 calories per serving; 4 g carbohydrate; 32 g protein; 14 g fat

SIMPLE SALMON PATTIES

These salmon patties are made with canned salmon, an inexpensive source of health-protective omega-3 fat. Enjoy them with pasta with mushrooms and asparagus (see chapter 19) or brown rice and a green vegetable for a complete meal.

> 1 14-ounce (420 g) can pink salmon, drained and flaked (remove the skin, but keep the bones for added calcium)
>
> 1 cup (120 g) crushed whole-wheat saltine crackers or bread crumbs
>
> 1 egg, slightly beaten
>
> 1 cup (150 g) diced pepper, green or red
>
> 1/2 diced onion, preferably a sweet onion such as a Vidalia
>
> 1/4 cup (60 ml) milk, preferably low fat
>
> lemon pepper or black pepper, as desired
>
> 1 to 2 tablespoons olive or canola oil, for cooking
>
> *Optional:* 1 teaspoon Worcestershire sauce or soy sauce, dash of hot pepper sauce, 1/2 teaspoon dried dill or 2 teaspoons fresh dill

1. In a large bowl, stir together the salmon, crackers or bread crumbs, egg, bell pepper, and onion. Mix in milk (and Worcestershire sauce and hot pepper sauce, as desired). Add pepper (and dill), and mix well with your hands. Lightly press the mixture into 8 patties.

2. Heat oil in a large saute pan on medium heat. Once the oil is hot, place the patties in the pan and cook on both sides until lightly browned, 3 to 5 minutes.

Yield: 4 servings (8 patties)

NUTRITION INFORMATION: 1,200 total calories; 300 calories per serving (2 patties); 24 g carbohydrate; 27 g protein; 11 g fat (2 g omega-3)

Courtesy of Kelly Leonard, MS, RD.

FISH AND SPINACH BAKE

This recipe goes nicely with rice and a loaf of crusty whole-grain bread. If you want a fancier recipe, saute 1/2 teaspoon of minced garlic, 1/2 pound (240 g) of sliced mushrooms, and 1/4 teaspoon of oregano in a little olive oil; then add that to the spinach before placing it in the baking dish.

1 10-ounce (300 g) box frozen chopped spinach
2 ounces (60 g) shredded mozzarella cheese
1 pound (480 g) fish fillets
salt, pepper, and lemon juice, as desired

1. Preheat the oven to 400 °F (200 °C).
2. Thaw the spinach, and squeeze out excess moisture. Spread it on the bottom of a small baking dish.
3. Sprinkle with the cheese and top with the fish. Season as desired.
4. Cover with foil. Bake for 20 minutes or until the fish flakes easily.

Yield: 2 servings

NUTRITION INFORMATION: 560 total calories (made with cod); 280 calories per serving; 6 g carbohydrate; 50 g protein; 6 g fat

SHRIMP AND SHELLS

This is a quick and easy-to-prepare pregame meal. Some athletes choose it before an event because it is low in fiber and easy to digest and has a mild flavor. It's unlikely to "talk back to you." (You can jazz it up by adding a dash of red pepper!) Serve it with green vegetables (such as peas, green beans, or broccoli) that you steam while the pasta is cooking.

> 6 ounces (175 g) pasta shells (or other pasta shape)
>
> 1 tablespoon margarine or olive oil
>
> 1 8-ounce (250 g) package frozen, peeled, and deveined shrimp
>
> 1/2 teaspoon chicken bouillon granules or 1 cube (or 1/2 tsp salt)
>
> 1 tablespoon cornstarch mixed into
>
> 1 cup (240 ml) milk, preferably low fat
>
> 2 to 4 tablespoons grated Parmesan cheese
>
> *Optional:* 1 clove garlic, minced, or 1/8 teaspoon garlic powder; 2 tablespoons white wine; tomatoes and parsley for garnish

1. In a large pot, cook the pasta according to package directions.
2. While the pasta is cooking, heat a large nonstick skillet, and add the margarine, and then the shrimp and chicken bouillon (or salt and garlic). Stir-fry for 3 to 4 minutes or until the shrimp turn pink.
3. Stir the cornstarch into the milk, then pour the mixture into the cooked shrimp. Cook, stirring constantly, until thick and bubbly. Stir in the cheese (and wine, as desired).
4. Add the cooked, drained pasta; toss to combine. Garnish with more Parmesan, tomatoes, and parsley, as desired.

Yield: 2 large servings

NUTRITION INFORMATION: 1,100 total calories; 550 calories per serving; 70 g carbohydrate; 40 g protein; 12 g fat

Adapted from a recipe contributed by Helen Baker.

TUNA PASTA SALAD

This is a classic favorite, perfect for summer gatherings or brown-bag lunches that you bring to work. You can adjust the ingredients to your liking, such as add less onion, more pasta, whatever. If the salad gets dry with standing, add milk for moistness.

2 1/2 cups (300 g) uncooked pasta, such as small shells, elbows, or wagon wheels

2/3 to 1 cup (152 to 230 g) light mayonnaise

1 10-ounce (300 g) package frozen petite green peas

1 12-ounce (360 g) can of tuna

1 cup (160 g) celery, diced

1 cup (240 g) low-fat shredded cheddar cheese

1/4 to 1/2 cup (40 to 80 g) chopped onion, preferably red or Vidalia

2 tablespoons chopped sweet pickles

salt and pepper, as desired

1. Cook pasta according to directions. Drain and rinse under cold water.
2. In a large bowl, combine the mayonnaise, green peas (they will thaw during preparation), tuna, celery, grated cheese, onion, chopped pickle, and salt and pepper, as desired.
3. Add the drained pasta, mix thoroughly, chill, and serve.

Yield: 4 servings as a main dish (8 as a side dish)

NUTRITION INFORMATION: 1,800 total calories; 450 calories per main dish serving; 45 g carbohydrate; 34 g protein; 15 g fat

SHRIMP MARINARA

I adapted this recipe from sports nutritionist Eileen Stellefson Myers, MPH, RD, from Nashville. It makes a quick and easy—yet somewhat special— dinner. It's light and easy to digest and good for preevent fueling!

Eileen recommends letting the tomato sauce simmer for about 25 minutes, to thicken it. I get impatient and settle for 5 minutes. Serve with salad and whole-grain rolls.

> 1 28-ounce (840 g) can diced tomatoes that come seasoned
>   with basil, garlic, and oregano
> 1/4 teaspoon red pepper
> 3 tablespoons olive oil
> 1 pound (480 g) raw shrimp, shelled and deveined
> 12 ounces (360 g) uncooked pasta, preferably whole wheat
> *Optional:* 1 to 2 cloves minced garlic; 2 tablespoons parsley,
>   cut fine

1. Cook the pasta according to the package directions.
2. While the pasta water is coming to a boil, in a large skillet combine the olive oil, red pepper, and diced tomatoes. Heat to a low boil; then let simmer for 5 to 25 minutes while the pasta cooks.
3. Add shrimp and cook until just pink. Garnish with parsley, as desired.
4. Serve over pasta.

Yield: 4 hearty servings

NUTRITION INFORMATION: 2,400 total calories; 600 calories per serving; 82 g carbohydrate; 35 g protein; 12 g fat

Sauce only: 1,100 total calories; 275 calories per serving; 20 g carbohydrate; 25 g protein; 11 g fat

Adapted by permission from a recipe contributed by Eileen Stellefson Myers, MPH, RD.

FISH IN FOIL, MEXICAN STYLE

Fish always comes out moist and flavorful when cooked in foil. For variety, you can bake the fish Asian style (with soy sauce, sesame oil, and scallions) or Italian style (with tomatoes, onions, and oregano). The recipe also works well with boneless, skinless chicken breasts.

This recipe produces two servings. Be sure to double it if you're feeding the family.

2 18-inch (46 cm) pieces of heavy-duty foil

1 pound (480 g) whitefish fillets

1/2 cup (130 g) salsa

Optional: 1 diced green pepper and 1 diced small onion, sauteed in 1 teaspoon olive oil; 1/8 teaspoon garlic powder; salt and pepper; low-fat grated cheddar cheese

1. If desired, saute the onion and pepper in olive oil.
2. In the middle of each piece of foil, place 1/2 pound (240 g) of fish. Cover with 1/4 (65 g) cup salsa (add peppers, onions, and other ingredients or seasonings, as desired).
3. Wrap by bringing together two edges of the foil, folding them over, and then folding up the ends and crimping the edges.
4. Bake or grill the packets for 15 to 20 minutes. Lift with a spatula and open, being careful not to burn yourself with the escaping steam.

Yield: 2 servings

NUTRITION INFORMATION: 400 total calories; 200 calories per serving; 4 g carbohydrate; 42 g protein; 2 g fat

CHAPTER 23

BEEF AND PORK

Despite popular belief, lean beef and pork can be a part of a heart-healthy diet. They are excellent sources of protein, iron, and zinc—nutrients important for everyone, particularly athletes. The main health concern about red meat is its fat content and large portions. The solution is to choose lean cuts, trim the fat, eat smaller portions, and balance it into an environmentally friendlier, plant-rich weekly menu.

These are the leanest cuts of beef:

- Top round roast and steak
- Bottom round roast
- Eye of round
- Boneless rump roast
- Tip roast and steak
- Round, strip, and flank steak
- Lean stew beef

And here are the leanest cuts of pork:

- Sirloin roast and chops
- Loin chops
- Top loin roast
- Tenderloin
- Cutlets

RECIPE FINDER

Meatballs by the gallon	430
Enchilada casserole	431
Boston baked beans and rice	432
Burger that's better for you	433
Honey-glazed pork chops	434
Stir-fried pork with fruit	435

See also: skillet lasagna. southwestern rice and bean salad (chapter 19); pumpkin chili (chapter 24).

MEATBALLS BY THE GALLON

Friend and retired sports nutritionist Sue Luke of Fort Mill, South Carolina, likes to always have these meatballs in her freezer. When all else fails for dinner, spaghetti and meatballs or a meatball sub is readily available, accompanied by cut-up peppers and baby carrots or a salad.

2 pounds (1 kg) extra-lean ground beef or ground turkey

4 eggs, slightly beaten

1 1/2 cups (180 g) seasoned bread crumbs

2 medium onions, finely chopped

2 teaspoons Italian seasoning

1 teaspoon pepper

Optional: 2 to 6 cloves garlic, minced

1. Put all the ingredients in a large bowl.
2. Wash your hands well (or use sterile latex gloves); then mix the ingredients with your hands.
3. Shape into meatballs of whatever size you desire.
4. Place on a large cookie sheet sprayed with cooking spray (or lined with foil that you have oiled), and bake at 350 °F (180 °C) for 25 to 30 minutes.
5. Cool. Place in a 1-gallon (at least 3 L) freezer bag and freeze.
6. When you are ready to eat the meatballs, take out the number needed. Thaw them in the microwave or in a pot of simmering spaghetti sauce.

Yield: 28 2-inch (5 cm) meatballs

NUTRITION INFORMATION: 2,800 total calories; 200 calories per serving (2 meatballs); 10 g carbohydrate; 22 g protein; 8 g fat

Courtesy of Sue Luke, RD.

ENCHILADA CASSEROLE

Here's a family favorite that everyone enjoys. This particular recipe is made with beef, but you could just as easily make it with ground turkey, diced tofu, or kidney beans. For color and crunch, top the casserole with diced peppers.

1 pound (480 g) extra-lean ground beef

1 28-ounce (840 g) can diced tomatoes, drained, or fresh tomatoes, chopped

1 10-ounce (300 ml) can enchilada sauce

1 16-ounce (480 g) can refried beans, preferably low fat

6 ounces (180 g) corn chips, preferably baked

4 ounces (120 g) cheddar cheese, preferably reduced fat

Optional: 1 medium onion, chopped; 1 teaspoon chili powder; 1/2 teaspoon dried basil; 1 green pepper, diced

1. Brown the ground beef (and onion) in a large nonstick skillet.

2. Drain any fat; then add the diced tomatoes, enchilada sauce, and refried beans (and chili powder and basil, as desired). Heat until bubbly.

3. Preheat the oven to 350 °F (180 °C). Crumble the corn chips, and spread all but 1 cup in the bottom of a 9- × 13-inch (23 × 33 cm) baking pan.

4. Pour the beef and enchilada mixture over the chips.

5. Grate the cheese and sprinkle it over the top. Sprinkle with 1 cup corn chips (and diced green pepper, if desired).

6. Bake for 15 minutes or until the cheese is melted.

Yield: 6 servings

NUTRITION INFORMATION: 2,800 total calories; 470 calories per serving; 52 g carbohydrate; 30 g protein; 16 g fat

BOSTON BAKED BEANS AND RICE

This recipe falls into the category of quick and easy, hearty recovery food. The baked beans add a sweetness that is welcome after a hard workout, as well as carbs to refuel, and protein to repair and build muscles.

Serve with pepper strips and baby carrots to add crunch to the meal.

> 1 16-ounce (480 g) can baked beans
> 1 pound (480 g) lean ground beef
> 1/2 cup (100 g) rice, uncooked
> 1/3 cup (75 g) ketchup

1. Cook the rice according to directions on the package and drain.
2. While the rice is cooking, brown the ground beef in a skillet; drain the grease.
3. Add to the skillet the can of baked beans, cooked rice, and the ketchup. Mix until combined.

Yield: 3 generous servings

NUTRITION INFORMATION: 1,725 total calories; 575 calories per serving; 65 g carbohydrate, 45 g protein, 15 g fat

BURGER THAT'S BETTER FOR YOU

What if I told you there was a way to enjoy a delicious, juicy burger that was low in saturated fat and good for you? Well, here you are! The key is to simply replace part of the ground beef (or ground bison or turkey) with finely chopped mushrooms. Add a side of (sweet potato) oven fries and you have a family-pleasing meal. Thanks to Laura McCann, RD, for sharing this recipe from her blog www.myfamilyfork.com.

1/2 pound (225 g) mushrooms finely chopped or pulsed in a food processor

1 pound (480 g) 93 percent lean ground beef (or bison)

Optional: 1 teaspoon soy sauce, 1 teaspoon Worcestershire sauce

1. Finely chop the mushrooms or pulse them in a food processor.
2. Mix together the ground beef, diced mushrooms, (soy sauce and Worcestershire sauce).
3. Shape into 4 patties.
4. Grill or cook in a lightly oiled pan on the stove top.

Yield: 4 servings

NUTRITION INFORMATION: 725 total calories; 170 calories per patty; 2 g carbohydrate, 26 g protein, 8 g fat.

Courtesy of Laura McCann, RD: www.MyFamilyFork.com.

HONEY-GLAZED PORK CHOPS

The combination of honey, cinnamon, and applesauce makes a nice glaze for pork chops. Enjoy these with rice, using the pan juices as a gravy.

4 extra-lean pork chops or pork cutlets, well trimmed (about 5 oz, or 150 g, each, raw)

Honey Glaze

2 tablespoons honey

1/4 cup (57 g) applesauce

1/4 teaspoon cinnamon

salt and pepper, as desired

1. In a small bowl, combine the honey, applesauce, and cinnamon (and salt and pepper, as desired).
2. Heat a nonstick skillet; then brown the pork for 3 minutes on one side.
3. Turn the pork; then spoon the glaze on top. Cover and cook for 3 minutes.
4. Uncover and cook over medium-low heat for 10 minutes or until done, turning once.
5. Serve the pork with rice, spooning the glaze over both the rice and the pork.

Yield: 4 servings

NUTRITION INFORMATION: 1,000 total calories; 250 calories per serving; 10 g carbohydrate; 30 g protein; 10 g fat

STIR-FRIED PORK WITH FRUIT

This is a popular family food that appeals to children and adults alike. Pineapple is a nice addition to the mandarin oranges.

1 teaspoon oil

1 pound (480 g) boneless pork cutlets, trimmed and sliced into thin strips

1/2 cup (120 ml) water

1/4 cup (60 ml) vinegar

2 tablespoons molasses or honey

2 tablespoons soy sauce

1 11-ounce (330 g) can mandarin oranges

1 tablespoon cornstarch

1 tablespoon water

Optional: 1/2 cup (125 g) pineapple chunks; 1 green pepper cut into chunks; 1 medium apple, diced; 1/4 cup (40 g) raisins; 1/4 cup (30 g) chopped toasted nuts

1. In a large nonstick skillet, heat the oil and add the sliced pork. Stir until browned.
2. Add the water, vinegar, molasses, soy sauce, and mandarin oranges (and pineapple, green pepper, apple, and raisins, as desired).
3. Bring to a boil; cover and simmer for 5 minutes.
4. Thicken the broth by slowly adding the cornstarch and water mixture and cooking until thickened to the desired consistency.
5. Sprinkle with chopped nuts, as desired.

Yield: 4 servings

NUTRITION INFORMATION: 1,200 total calories; 300 calories per serving; 30 g carbohydrate; 25 g protein; 8 g fat

CHAPTER 24

BEANS AND TOFU

When I wrote the first edition of this *Sports Nutrition Guidebook* in 1990, beans and tofu were low on the list of popular foods. Today, as more active people are choosing a vegetarian option, beans and tofu are mainstream. I have even added bean-based desserts as a way to show the versatility of these health-promoting sports foods.

Here are recipes to enjoy on Meatless Mondays—if not every day. *Note*: Recipes that you might expect to have gluten, but do not, have "GF" (gluten-free) after the recipe name.

Beans

Beans are some of nature's greatest foods; they are rich in protein and contain little fat and no cholesterol. They help lower blood cholesterol, control blood sugar, fight cancer, reduce problems with constipation, build muscles (with their protein), fuel muscles (with their carbohydrate), and nourish muscles (with lots of B vitamins, iron, zinc, magnesium, copper, folic acid, and potassium).

Because beans are a healthy source of both protein and carbohydrate, vegetarian meals such as chili, hummus, bean and rice casseroles, and other bean meals are perfect for a sports diet. When beans are the only protein source, be sure to eat them in large quantities to consume adequate protein (see chapter 7). If you are a meat eater who wants to become more of a vegetarian, replace part or all of the meat in recipes with more beans, for example, replace ground beef in chili or lasagna with kidney beans.

For more information about preparing homemade beans and creating bean dishes, read cook books that specialize in vegetarian cookery (appendix A has suggestions) or search the Internet for "cooking with beans."

Tofu

Tofu, also known as bean curd, is made from an extract of soybeans. It is a complete protein that contains all the essential amino acids and healthy fat. Tofu has no cholesterol and is relatively low in calories and sodium. It is a popular alternative to meat and can be a source of calcium for people who limit their intake of dairy foods.

Tofu is found in most supermarkets in the refrigerated vegetable section. You can buy soft or firm tofu cakes that are packaged in water; be sure to check the "sell by" date, and buy the freshest brand. Soft or silken tofu is preferable for blending into a smooth cream; firm tofu is good to crumble or slice.

Tofu itself has very little flavor; it takes on the flavors of the foods it's prepared with. For example, tofu mixed with soy sauce takes on the soy sauce's flavor; likewise, with chili. Because of this versatility, tofu lends itself to many recipes: spaghetti, salads, chili, Chinese stir-fry, and even salad dressings. To achieve an interesting, spongy texture, freeze the tofu for at least two days. After it has thawed, squeeze out the water (as if it were a kitchen sponge), tear the tofu into chunks, and add them to spaghetti sauce, chili, soups, or other dishes.

RECIPE FINDER

Quick and easy bean ideas	439
Sweet-n-sour tofu bites	440
Buddha bowl ideas	441
Pumpkin chili	442
Turkey chili with quinoa and beans	444
Pasta and white bean soup with sun-dried tomatoes	446
Kale and cannellini bean soup	447
Chick pea, curry, and peanut butter soup	448
Tofu burritos	449
Cookie dough hummus snack GF	450
Chocolate cake batter dessert hummus GF	451

See also: skillet lasagna, southwestern rice and bean salad (chapter 19); chicken black bean soup, chicken and white beans, chicken and kale and black bean quesadillas, savory African peanut stew (chapter 21); enchilada casserole, Boston baked beans and rice (chapter 23); smoothie suggestions (chapter 25).

QUICK AND EASY BEAN IDEAS

Here are suggestions for preparing and serving beans:

- In a blender, mix black or pinto beans, salsa, and cheese. Heat in the microwave and use as a dip or on top of tortillas or potatoes.
- Blend black beans, Greek yogurt, salsa, and taco seasoning mix for a dip with chips or green pepper strips.
- Saute garlic and onions in a little oil, add canned beans (whole or mashed), and heat together. Eat with rice or rolled in a tortilla.
- Add beans to salads, spaghetti sauce, soups, and stews for a protein booster.
- In a large tortilla, wrap heated vegetarian refried beans, a dollop of cottage cheese, salsa, chopped lettuce, and tomato, as desired. Roll into a burrito.
- Combine black beans, refried beans, and salsa to taste. Spoon onto a tortilla, and top with more salsa and cheese, as desired.
- Sprinkle beans, salsa, shredded cheese, and whatever else sounds good (shredded chicken, diced tomato, ground beef) on top of baked corn chips. Heat in the oven until the cheese is melted.

SWEET-N-SOUR TOFU BITES

Adults and kids who claim that they don't like tofu end up chowing down on this dish by Julie Negrin, RD. For a snack, serve the tofu bites with toothpicks. For a meal, serve with rice and a green vegetable.

1 cake (14 to 16 oz, or 420 to 480 g) tofu (firm or extra firm)

1 tablespoon canola oil

4 tablespoons soy sauce or tamari

4 tablespoons maple syrup

4 tablespoons water

1. Drain the water from the tofu package. Wrap the tofu in a clean dish towel or cheesecloth for at least 10 minutes to absorb the excess moisture (you can put a heavy plate or pan on top to speed this process along). Carefully cut the tofu into 1-inch (2.5 cm) cubes.

2. Heat the oil in a large, wide skillet on medium heat. Add the tofu to the pan and cook it for about 10 minutes, flipping the cubes over frequently with a spatula so that each piece becomes golden and a little crispy.

3. While the tofu is cooking, whisk the soy sauce, maple syrup, and water together in a small bowl. Make sure that the mixture is well combined before adding it to the pan, or the maple syrup will separate from the tamari.

4. Pour the sauce over the tofu, and continue to cook it until most of the sauce has been absorbed by the tofu, 12 to 15 minutes. Remove the pan from the heat and transfer the tofu to a serving bowl.

Yield: 4 servings as an appetizer on toothpicks, or 2 servings as an entree with rice

NUTRITION INFORMATION: 700 total calories; 175 calories per appetizer serving; 15 g carbohydrate; 10 g protein; 8 g fat

Adapted with permission from a recipe in *Easy Meals to Cook with Kids,* by Julie Negrin, © 2010. www.mykitchennutrition.com

BUDDHA BOWL IDEAS

A Buddha bowl is a big bowl of food, piled up with a rounded "belly" on top, much like the belly of Buddha. They are popular with not only vegans and vegetarians, but also anyone looking for a wholesome meal in a bowl. Depending on what you toss into the bowl, it can be savory, sweet, spicy, warm, or cold. Depending on when you eat the bowl, it could be breakfast, lunch, or dinner. Because of the varying ingredients, we are unable to include nutrition information with this recipe.

1. To create your Buddha bowl, start with a wholesome grain as the first layer: quinoa, (brown) rice, farro.

2. Add roasted vegetables: bite-size chunks of roasted winter squash, beets, brussels sprouts, carrots, cauliflower, broccoli, sweet potato, kale.

3. Add raw greens: spinach, kale, arugula.

4. Add fruit: diced avocado, apple, pear, craisins, berries, raisins.

5. Add plant-based protein: (seasoned) chickpeas, tofu cubes, pinto beans, edamame, almonds, cashews, sunflower seeds.

6. Add animal protein (blasphemy!): shredded cheese, hard-boiled egg, shredded chicken, fish.

7. Add a (spicy) dressing, as desired, that might have Asian flavors (ginger, soy sauce, garlic).

PUMPKIN CHILI

Who would have thought that pumpkin blends nicely with chili? Not me! But thanks to recipe contributor, sports dietitian, runner, and yoga instructor Enette Larson Meyer PhD, RD, CSSD, I now know it's a yummy combination. This recipe is adapted from her book *Plant-Based Sports Nutrition: Expert Fueling Strategies for Training, Recovery, and Performance* a resource that athletes choosing a plant-based diet should add to their sports nutrition library.

This basic recipe tastes great, and it becomes more flavorful when you add some or all of the optional ingredients. For a vegan chili, use soy crumbles (textured vegetable protein), a cake of diced tofu, or a third can of beans. For a meaty chili, include one pound of browned ground turkey, beef, or pork. Add water or broth, if needed, to reach the desired consistency. As desired, top with diced avocado, sour cream, and/or grated cheese; serve with a green salad.

1 to 2 tablespoons oil, preferably olive or canola

1 medium onion, chopped

1 medium pepper, diced

2 cans (15 oz, or 450 g) black, pinto, or kidney beans

1 cup (170 g) textured vegetable protein (TVP)

1 can (28 oz, or 840 g) diced tomatoes

1 can (15 oz, or 430 g) tomato sauce

1 can (16 oz, or 450 g) pumpkin

2 tablespoons chili powder

1 to 2 tablespoons cumin

Optional: Replace TVP with 1 pound (480 g) lean ground beef, ground turkey, or ground pork.

Add 2 to 3 cups (340 to 510 g) of diced vegetables (corn, carrots, green beans, zucchini, etc.); 1 can (4 oz, or 120 g) green chilies; 1 to 2 cloves garlic, minced, or 1/4 to 1/2 teaspoon garlic powder; 1/2 teaspoon cinnamon, cayenne pepper, as desired; 1 tablespoon sugar, 1 to 2 tablespoons cocoa powder

1. In a large pot, briefly saute diced onion and peppers (and other vegetables, as desired) until soft (about 5 minutes). *Optional*: Add the ground beef, turkey, or pork; brown and drain any grease.

2. Stir in beans, diced tomatoes, tomato sauce, pumpkin, and spices. Cover and simmer for 25 to 45 minutes.

Yield: 5 servings

NUTRITION INFORMATION: 2,000 total calories; 400 calories per serving; 65 g carbohydrate, 24 g protein, 3 g fat

---

Adapted from *Plant-Based Sports Nutrition: Expert Fueling Strategies for Training, Recovery, and Performance* by Enette Larson Meyer, RD.

TURKEY CHILI WITH QUINOA AND BEANS

This turkey chili recipe, adapted from food blogger and dietitian Samina Qureshi, RD, is a simple and delicious one-pot meal that can be on the table in just 30 minutes. It differs from traditional chili in that it doesn't have a heavy tomato base, but rather a lighter broth-base. To make this a vegetarian meal, simply replace the turkey with tofu or another can of beans. For more nutrients, add diced carrots, green beans, zucchini, or other vegetables of your choice. Samina makes the chili in her Instant Pot; I do it the old-fashioned way on my stove. For more yummy recipes, check out Samina's blog, www.wholesomestart.com.

2 to 3 tablespoons oil, preferably olive, canola, or avocado

1 medium onion, diced (about 1 cup, or 160 g)

1 pound (480 g) ground turkey

1 can (15 oz, or 450 g) tomatoes, diced

1 can (15 oz, or 450 g) kidney, black, or pinto beans, drained and rinsed

1 cup (170 g) uncooked quinoa

1 1/2 cup (360 ml) chicken broth or water

1 tablespoon ketchup

1 tablespoon Dijon mustard

1/4 to 1 teaspoon ground black pepper, as desired

1 tablespoon ground cumin

1 to 2 teaspoons garlic powder, as desired

1/4 to 1 teaspoon ground cayenne pepper, as desired

Optional: 1/2 cup (120 g) cilantro, chopped; 2 cups diced vegetables (carrots, celery, zucchini, etc.)

1. In a large pot, heat the oil, add the diced onions and cook until the onions are translucent.

2. Add the ground turkey and once it has browned, add the canned tomatoes, beans, quinoa, and broth (and additional vegetables).

3. Mix in the ketchup, mustard, black pepper, cumin, garlic powder, cayenne (and cilantro).

4. Cover, bring to a boil, and then simmer for 15 minutes.

    Optional: Top with low-fat sour cream and shredded cheese and enjoy!

Yield: 5 servings

NUTRITION INFORMATION: 2,000 total calories; 400 calories per serving; 40 g carbohydrate, 30 g protein, 13 g fat

Courtesy of Samina Oureshi, RD. www.wholesomestart.com.

PASTA AND WHITE BEAN SOUP WITH SUN-DRIED TOMATOES

This soup is delicious and worth the trip to the store to get the sun-dried tomatoes. If desired, add more beans and pasta—and even diced chicken—to the soup, and you'll have a heartier meal.

1 tablespoon oil, preferably olive or canola

1 large onion, diced

1 medium carrot, diced

1/4 to 1/2 teaspoon red pepper flakes

1 12-ounce (360 g) can cannellini beans, drained

5 cups (1.2 L) chicken or vegetable broth, homemade, canned, or from bouillon

3 ounces (about 2/3 cup, or 90 g) dry bow tie or shell pasta

1/3 cup (35 g) sun-dried tomatoes, diced

salt and pepper, as desired

3 tablespoons fresh parsley

Optional: 1 clove garlic, minced, or 1/4 teaspoon garlic powder; 1 bay leaf; grated Parmesan cheese

1. In a large pot, heat the oil over medium heat. Saute the onion, carrot, and red pepper flakes (and garlic).
2. Cover and cook for 10 minutes, stirring occasionally.
3. Pour in the broth and add the beans (and bay leaf). Bring the mixture to a boil.
4. Add the pasta and sun-dried tomatoes. Reduce the heat and simmer for about 10 minutes (or until the pasta is tender).
5. Season with salt and pepper, and add the parsley.
6. Serve with grated Parmesan cheese, if desired.

Yield: 4 servings

NUTRITION INFORMATION: 900 total calories; 225 calories per serving; 38 g carbohydrate; 9 g protein; 4 g fat

Adapted from recipe contributed by Terri Smith, RD.

KALE AND CANNELLINI BEAN SOUP

Simple, yummy, and healthy—that's the kind of food that athletes like. And that's why this soup is popular with busy, sports-active people like recipe contributor and registered dietitian Angela Moore. Angela makes this recipe with finely chopped spicy sausage. You can make it with just the beans for protein, or add diced chicken or ground turkey. If you have thyme in your spice cabinet, a pinch adds a really nice flavor. Top with grated cheese, and you have a satisfying meal in a bowl.

1 to 2 tablespoons oil, preferably olive or canola

1 medium onion, chopped (about 1 cup, or 160 g)

1 to 3 cloves garlic, minced

3 to 4 cups (720 to 960 ml) chicken broth, canned, fresh, or from bouillon cubes

2 cans (15.5 oz, or 450 g) cannellini (white) beans, rinsed and drained

4 to 6 cups (270 to 400 g) kale, chopped

salt and pepper, as desired

Optional: 2 diced chicken sausages, 1/4 teaspoon thyme, 1/4 cup (30 g) grated Parmesan cheese

1. Heat oil in a large saucepan over medium-high heat. Add onion and garlic (and sausage, chicken, or ground turkey) to pan; saute 5 minutes or until onions are tender.
2. While onions cook, drain the beans and rinse well.
3. Add the broth and beans to the saucepan; bring to a boil. Partially mash beans with potato masher.
4. Stir in kale, salt, and pepper (and thyme); cook over medium heat for 6 minutes.

Optional: Sprinkle with grated Parmesan cheese.

Yield: 3 servings

NUTRITION INFORMATION: 1,000 total calories; 330 calories per serving; 50 g carbohydrate; 20 g protein, 6 g fat

Courtesy of Angela Moore, RD.

CHICKPEA, CURRY, AND PEANUT BUTTER SOUP

Unlike many soups that you need to cook for hours, you can toss this soup together with ingredients you likely have on hand and eat it in minutes. It may seem like a strange combination, but it's amazingly tasty! For a heartier soup, cook chicken with the broth, or add leftover diced chicken, TVP, or tofu. You can also add rice (or replace the chickpeas with rice).

I adapted this recipe from Cheryl Harris, RD, who offers many other gluten-free recipes on her website: www.harriswholehealth.com.

> 2 14-ounce (420 ml) cans broth, chicken or vegetable
>
> 1 14-ounce (420 g) can diced tomatoes, with juice
>
> 1/2 cup (130 g) peanut butter or another nut butter
>
> 1 tablespoon curry powder
>
> 1 10-ounce (300 g) box frozen spinach (thawed in the micro-wave) or 1 pound (480 g) chopped fresh kale or collards
>
> 1 15-ounce (450 g) can chickpeas, drained
>
> *Optional:* 1/2 teaspoon ginger (or 1 teaspoon fresh minced ginger), squeeze of lemon

1. In a large pot, combine the broth, tomatoes, peanut butter, and curry powder (and ginger). Bring to a boil, and if you are patient, simmer it for a few minutes so the flavors meld.

2. Add drained chickpeas and spinach (or greens of your choice) and simmer until the greens are cooked.

Yield: 4 servings

NUTRITION INFORMATION: 1,300 total calories; 325 calories per serving; 26 g carbohydrate; 14 g protein; 18 g fat

Courtesy of Cheryl Harris, MPH, RD, www.HarrisWholeHealth.com.

TOFU BURRITOS

This is a simple lunch, dinner, or even breakfast. I like it with a dollop of hummus.

- 2 teaspoons olive or canola oil
- 1 small onion, diced
- 1 green pepper, diced
- 1 14-ounce (420 g) cake firm tofu, crumbled
- 4 tortillas, white, whole wheat, or corn, warmed
- salt and pepper, as desired
- *Optional:* raisins, chopped walnuts, and curry powder; sesame seeds, sesame oil (instead of margarine), and soy sauce; garlic powder; hummus

1. In a skillet, heat the oil; then add the onion and green pepper. Saute until tender.
2. Add the crumbled tofu and desired seasonings; heat thoroughly.
3. Place 1/4 of the mixture in the middle of a tortilla, fold over one end, fold in one side, and roll up.

Yield: 4 small servings (or 2 large)

NUTRITION INFORMATION: 1,200 total calories; 300 calories per serving (small); 40 g carbohydrate; 15 g protein; 9 g fat

COOKIE DOUGH HUMMUS SNACK GF

Hungry athletes often want a snack that offers health value. Here it is! Sports dietitians Sarah Charton, RD, and Uriell Carlson, RD, both contributed this recipe. They report that athletes allergic to dairy and eggs, or in need of gluten-free foods will welcome this "cookie dough." Whether eaten by the spoonful, enjoyed with slices of apple or pear, or dipped into with graham cracker sticks or pretzel thins, it will satisfy a sweet tooth.

If you have the patience to do so, remove the skins from the chickpeas to make a smoother texture. The longer you blend the ingredients, the more the recipe will have the texture of real cookie dough.

> 1 15.5-ounce (450 g) can chickpeas, rinsed well (three times) and drained (about 1 1/2 cups)
>
> 1/3 to 1/2 cup (85 to 130 g) peanut or cashew butter, depending on the nut taste you want
>
> 1/3 cup (115 g) maple syrup, honey, or agave
>
> 2 teaspoons vanilla extract
>
> 1/3 cup (80 g) chocolate chips
>
> *Optional:* 1/8 to 1/4 teaspoon salt, 1/2 teaspoon cinnamon

1. Put all the ingredients in a blender or food processer and puree until smooth.
2. To adjust to the desired moistness, add a bit of milk or water.
3. Dig in with a spoon or pretzel sticks!

Yield: 10 servings

NUTRITION INFORMATION: 1,500 total calories; 150 calories per serving; 20 g carbohydrate; 4 g protein; 6 g fat

Courtesy of Sarah Charton, RD, and Uriell Carlson, RD.

CHOCOLATE CAKE BATTER DESSERT HUMMUS GF

This dessert is a treat not only for athletes on a gluten-free diet but also for anyone who hankers for a spoonful of chocolate cake batter. As a long-distance backpacker and registered dietitian, Aaron Owens Mayhew reports, "This recipe is quite addictive and dangerous to keep in the house. It's just plain delicious." You can find more recipes like this in her cookbook: *Backcountry Foodie: Ultralight Recipes for Outdoor Explorers*. Aaron dehydrates this dessert (adding the peanut butter at the time of consumption) and enjoys it as a treat on long hikes, along with a chocolate mint Honey Stinger Waffle. I enjoy it when I want comfort food.

The texture of the batter will be a little gritty unless you have the time and patience to remove the skins from the garbanzo beans (chickpeas).

1 can (15 oz, or 450 g) garbanzo beans, drained and rinsed

1/2 cup (100 g) cocoa powder

1/2 cup (100 g) sugar

1 1/2 teaspoons vanilla extract

1/2 teaspoon table salt

1/2 cup (120 ml) water (or to desired consistency)

2 tablespoons nut butter

1. Put all ingredients in a food processor or blender and puree until smooth, adding water to the desired consistency.
2. Get your spoon and dig in!

Yield: 4 servings

NUTRITION INFORMATION: 800 total calories; 200 calories per serving; 34 g carbohydrate; 6 g protein; 5 g fat

Reprinted by permission from Aaron Owens Mayhew, RD, *Backcountry Foodie: Ultralight Recipes for Outdoor Explorers.*

CHAPTER 25

BEVERAGES AND SMOOTHIES

Beverages are not only a way to quench your thirst and replace fluids lost through sweat but also a way to refuel your muscles with carbohydrate and boost recovery with protein. Some smoothies can be a quick meal that you pour into a travel coffee mug and sip on the way to work. Others are an easy way to boost your fruit intake with minimal effort.

RECIPE FINDER

Homemade sports drink	454
Maple sports drink	455
Smoothie suggestions	456
Banana-date smoothie	458
PB & J smoothie	459
Beet-cherry smoothie	460
Thick and frosty milk shake	461
Hot cocoa	462

HOMEMADE SPORTS DRINK

The nutrition profile of commercial sports drinks is 50 to 70 calories per 8 ounces (240 ml), with about 110 milligrams of sodium. Following is a simple recipe that offers this profile, but at a much lower cost than the expensive store-bought brands—and without additives, colors, or preservatives.

You can make this recipe without the lemon juice, but the flavor will be weaker. Don't be afraid to be creative; you can dilute many combinations of juices (such as cranberry and lemonade) to 50 calories per 8 ounces (240 ml) and then add a pinch of salt. More precisely, add 1/4 teaspoon salt per quart (liter) of liquid. Some people use flavorings such as sugar-free lemonade to enhance the flavor yet leave the calories in the 50 to 70 per 8-ounce range. The trick is to always test the recipe during training, not during an important event. You want to be sure it tastes good when you are hot and sweaty and settles well when you're working hard.

> 1/4 cup (50 g) sugar
>
> 1/4 teaspoon salt
>
> 1/4 cup (60 ml) hot water
>
> 1/4 cup (60 ml) orange juice (not concentrate) plus 2 table-
> spoons lemon juice
>
> 3 1/2 cups (840 ml) cold water

1. In the bottom of a pitcher, dissolve the sugar and salt in the hot water.
2. Add the juice and the remaining water; chill.
3. Quench that thirst!

Yield: 1 quart (1 L)

NUTRITION INFORMATION: 200 total calories; 50 calories per 8 ounces (240 ml); 12 g carbohydrate; 110 mg sodium

MAPLE SPORTS DRINK

This easy-to-make maple syrup recipe is delicious and settles well because it is not acidic and is low in FODMAPs (see chapter 9). When you are working out for more than an hour, enjoy this all-natural sports beverage to energize your workouts.

Note: Maple syrup is also a tasty alternative to gels. Put some in a small flask and take nips during extended exercise.

> 3 3/4 cups (900 ml) cold water
> 1/4 cup (60 ml) pure maple syrup
> 1/4 teaspoon salt

1. Mix all ingredients together in a 1-quart (1 L) bottle.
2. Shake well and enjoy!

Yield: 1 quart (1 L); four 8-ounce (240 ml) servings

NUTRITION INFORMATION: 50 calories per 8-ounce (240 ml) serving; 12 g carbohydrate; 0 g protein; 0 g fat; 110 mg sodium

SMOOTHIE SUGGESTIONS

Fruit and vegetable smoothies are popular for breakfasts and snacks. The ingredients can vary according to individual tastes. Some tried-and-true combinations are banana and strawberries in orange juice and melon and pineapple in pineapple juice. Almost any combination works. Just don't judge a smoothie by its color! If you add colored fruit with spinach, kale or other greens, you will end up with a gray smoothie the color of cement. By putting it into an opaque travel mug, you won't have to look at it and can simply enjoy its yummy taste and nutritional goodness.

For a thick, frosty shake, use fruit that has been frozen. To have fruit ready for blending into a smoothie, simply slice a surplus of ripe fresh fruit (that might otherwise spoil) into chunks; then freeze the chunks on a flat sheet. When frozen, pack them into sealable bags. (If you freeze them in the bag, you'll end up with one big chunk of frozen fruit that is hard to break apart.)

You don't need a recipe to make smoothies. Just toss into a blender some fruit and vegetables, a source of protein (yogurt, nut butter, powdered milk, protein powder, silken tofu), a liquid (juice, milk, ice cubes), and sweetener as desired. If you don't have frozen fruit handy, you can add ice cubes to the smoothie for that cool and frosty feeling. To spur your creativity, here is a template for making smoothies, with many tried-and-true combinations on the next page.

> 1/2 cup (115 g) low-fat (Greek) yogurt (plain or flavored) or milk
> 1 cup (240 ml) fruit juice
> 1/2 to 1 cup (80 to 160 g) fruit, fresh, frozen, or canned
> *Optional:* 1/4 cup (30 g) milk powder; chia seeds, ground flax, dry oatmeal, graham crackers, peanut butter, dash cinnamon or nutmeg; sweetener as desired; whatever else suits your fancy.

1. Place all ingredients in a blender.
2. Cover, and whip until smooth.

Yield: 1 serving

NUTRITION INFORMATION: 220 to 290 total calories; 50 to 60 g carbohydrate; 5 g protein; 0 to 3 g fat

Fruit or vegetable	Protein	Liquid	Extra
Frozen strawberries and banana chunks	Milk powder	Orange juice	Uncooked oats
Coconut flakes	Vanilla Greek yogurt	Ice cubes	Instant coffee powder (decaf or regular)
Peaches	Soy milk	Vanilla frozen yogurt	Nutmeg
Dates	Vanilla Greek yogurt Walnuts	Milk of your choice	Maple syrup Flax oil
Frozen banana chunks	Protein powder	Pineapple juice	Chia seeds
Canned pumpkin and 1/2 banana	Almond butter	Milk of your choice	Pumpkin pie spice Molasses
Frozen strawberries Spinach	Hemp hearts	Coconut water	Fresh mint
Frozen cherries	Chocolate milk	Tart cherry juice	Cocoa powder garnish
Frozen blueberries Frozen banana	Cannellini beans	Kefir	Honey
Pineapple Baby carrots	Greek yogurt	Orange juice	Nutmeg
Frozen raspberries	Silken tofu	Cranberry juice	Ground flax Honey
Frozen banana chunks	Peanut or sunflower butter	(Soy) milk	Graham crackers
Applesauce	Ricotta cheese	Milk of your choice	Maple syrup
Zucchini, kale Frozen banana	Walnuts	Milk of your choice	Ginger
Avocado Spinach	Almonds or almond butter	Vanilla yogurt	Flax oil
Frozen mango Pineapple chunks	Cottage cheese	Coconut water	Cardamom
Frozen cherries	Vanilla Greek yogurt	(Tart) cherry juice	Graham crackers

BANANA-DATE SMOOTHIE

Dates offer a lovely sweetness to a smoothie as well as health-protective phytochemicals. Your job is to eat a rainbow of colorful fruits and vegetables; let dates represent the brown color group. This prize-winning recipe was created by chef and aspiring dietitian Suzy McClain, who is known for her cooking demonstrations in the Las Vegas school system and online cooking channels.

1/2 cup (115 g) Greek yogurt, plain or vanilla

1/2 cup (120 ml) milk, 1 percent

1 frozen banana

2 to 3 dates

Optional: 1 teaspoon nut butter, garnish with a sprinkling of old fashioned rolled oats, 1/2 teaspoon cocoa powder, and a dash of salt

1. Put into the blender the yogurt, milk, frozen banana chunks, and dates.
2. Blend well.
3. *Optional:* Garnish with a sprinkling of dry oats, cocoa powder, and salt.

Yield: 1 serving

NUTRITION INFORMATION: 350 total calories; 57 g carbohydrate, 20 g protein, 5 g fat

Recipe contributed by Suzy McClain.

PB & J SMOOTHIE

This smoothie recipe from sports dietitian Lauren Trocchio, RD, includes cottage cheese for a boost of not only protein but also sodium (400 mg per 1/2 cup [115 g] cottage cheese). The sodium heightens the sweetness from the cherries and helps replace electrolytes lost in sweat. It's a recovery meal in a travel mug for athletes on the go, or a bedtime snack for athletes trying to gain weight.

As with all smoothies, you can be creative and toss whatever you want into the blender: a teaspoon of chia seeds, Greek yogurt or protein powder instead of the cottage cheese, more fruit, chocolate syrup, or a graham cracker or two.

Note: If you have extra cherries, enjoy them in the recipe for beet-cherry smoothie.

1/2 cup (115 g) 2 percent cottage cheese

1 cup (240 ml) milk of your choice, preferably dairy or soy

2 tablespoons peanut butter (or any nut butter)

1 banana (room temperature or frozen)

1 cup (160 g) frozen cherries

Yield: 1 large smoothie

NUTRITION INFORMATION: 600 total calories; 72 g carbohydrate; 35 g protein; 21 g fat; 700 mg sodium; 1,400 mg potassium

Courtesy of Lauren Trocchio, RD. www.NutritionUnlockedLLC.com

BEET-CHERRY SMOOTHIE

Beets are rich in nitrates, which can enhance blood flow to the muscles and improve athletic performance (see chapter 11). This smoothie is a tasty way to add beets to your sports diet and is a perfect energy booster before your workout. The cherries add a sweetness that nicely balances any bitterness from the beets. Any leftover frozen cherries can be used another time in the recipe for the PB & J smoothie.

If you don't want to cook your own beets, look for cooked and peeled beets in the refrigerated produce section at grocery stores such as Trader Joe's and Kroger.

> 1 cup (160 g) diced cooked and peeled beets
>
> 1/2 cup (80 g) frozen sweet cherries
>
> 1/2 cup (120 ml) orange juice or 2 to 3 mandarin oranges, peeled

1. Add ingredients to blender.
2. Blend until smooth and enjoy!

Yield: 1 serving

NUTRITION INFORMATION: 220 total calories; 52 g carbohydrate; 5 g protein; 0 g fat

Recipe courtesy of Laura McCann, MS, RD, and family food blogger at www.myfamilyfork.com.

THICK AND FROSTY MILK SHAKE

This thick and tasty milk shake is a healthy alternative to shakes made with ice cream. The instant pudding powder adds a thick texture, and the ice cubes make it frosty and refreshing. I like to make these for kids—an enjoyable way to boost their protein and calcium intake. (Chia seeds are an alternative thickener.)

By varying the flavor of the pudding (vanilla, lemon, chocolate), you can create numerous variations. You can also add fruit (preferably frozen chunks) for extra nutritional value. *Note:* The shake thickens upon standing; add more (or less) pudding powder, depending on how thick you like your shakes. If pieces of ice cubes remain in the shake, worry not—they'll just keep the beverage cool.

> 1 cup (240 ml) low-fat milk
> 1/4 cup (35 g) instant pudding powder
> 1/4 cup (30 g) powdered milk
> 3 ice cubes
> *Optional:* 1/2 to 1 cup (80 to 160 g) (frozen) fruit chunks

1. Place all ingredients in a blender.
2. Blend until smooth.

Yield: 1 serving

NUTRITION INFORMATION: 280 total calories; 55 g carbohydrate; 15 g protein; 0 g fat

HOT COCOA

While a chug of cold chocolate milk is a wonderful recovery food in warm weather, a steaming mugful of hot cocoa is a welcome warm-me-up after cold-weather running, hiking, or skating. Making your own hot cocoa is simple. No need to buy packets. Cocoa is plant based and rich in health-protective phytochemicals. Enjoy this guilt free!

1 cup (240 ml) milk, low fat or skim

1 tablespoon cocoa powder

1 tablespoon brown sugar or sweetener of your choice

Optional: dash salt (this makes the flavors "pop")

1. Put the cocoa, sugar, and milk in a 12-ounce (360 ml) mug. *Note:* The cocoa will not dissolve in the cold milk, so don't bother to stir it yet.

2. Heat the mixture for a minute in the microwave oven; stir until it is well blended.

3. Finish heating to the desired temperature, being careful not to boil the milk or it will curdle.

4. Enjoy!

Yield: 1 serving

NUTRITION INFORMATION: 150 total calories (made with 1 percent milk); 25 g carbohydrate; 8 g protein; 2 g fat

CHAPTER 26

SNACKS AND DESSERTS

Many athletes enjoy snacks and desserts as part of their daily food plans. Fresh fruits are ideal choices for either, yet there is a time and a place for other sweets. The trick is to choose snacks and desserts that are low in saturated fat and rich in wholesome carbohydrate. These recipes provide healthy alternatives to empty-calorie temptations.

RECIPE FINDER

Quick and easy nut butter snacks	464
Sweet and crispy almond bars	465
Super-seedy granola bars	466
Sugar and spice trail mix	468
Chia seed pudding	469
Vanilla chia seed pudding	470
Strawberry chia seed pudding	471
Apple crisp	472
Banana ice cream	473
Healthy-ish heart oatmeal raisin cookies with chocolate chips	474
Chocolate lush	475
Carrot cake	476

See also: banana bread, peanut butter and dark chocolate chip muffins (chapter 18); cookie dough dessert hummus, chocolate cake batter dessert hummus (chapter 24); smoothie suggestions, thick and frosty milk shake, (chapter 25).

QUICK AND EASY NUT BUTTER SNACKS

Peanut butter and other nut butters like almond, cashew, and sunflower seed are a staple for hungry athletes who want a satisfying, wholesome snack. Nut butters offer a lot of calories from fat, but the fat is unsaturated and can healthfully fit into your sports diet.

If you are a nut butter lover, you can spread it on bread, bananas, graham crackers, and apple slices. For a real treat, slit open a few dates (remove the pit, if needed), stick in a few dark-chocolate chips, and top with a dab of peanut butter. Now that will cure your sweet tooth!

If nut butter sandwiches are your tried-and-true, go-to sports food, here are a few suggestions to add variety beyond jelly:

- Honey
- Cinnamon or cinnamon sugar
- Raisins
- Banana slices
- Apple slices
- Chopped dates
- Applesauce, raisins, and cinnamon
- Sprouts
- Granola or sunflower seeds
- Cottage cheese
- Dill pickle slices (no kidding!)

You can also make yourself a homemade milk shake by combining 1 cup (240 ml) milk, 1 banana, 1 tablespoon peanut butter, and sweetener as desired. Check out the PB & J smoothie in chapter 25.

SWEET AND CRISPY ALMOND BARS

Whether eating them for breakfast on the run, a preexercise snack, or an afternoon treat, you'll enjoy these crispy bars. When measuring the honey, add a little more than the 1/2 cup (170 g), so the mixture sticks together better. You'll need to pack the ingredients firmly into the pan; otherwise, the bars will fall apart (but the crumbs are tasty—especially in yogurt or sprinkled on top of your morning bowl of cereal).

2 cups (160 g) uncooked oats

2 cups Rice Krispies cereal or puffed brown rice cereal

1 cup (120 g) slivered almonds

1/2 cup (heaping) (170 g) honey

1/2 cup (130 g) almond butter

Optional: 1/2 teaspoon salt

1. Lightly coat a 9- × 13-inch (23 × 33 cm) baking dish with oil or cooking spray.
2. In a large bowl, combine the oats, Rice Crispies, and slivered almonds.
3. In a medium microwavable bowl, combine the honey and almond butter. Microwave for 2 to 3 minutes, stirring occasionally.
4. Slowly pour the almond butter mixture over the cereal, stirring until all the ingredients are well coated.
5. Transfer the mixture into the prepared pan and press firmly while still warm. (Butter your fingers so the mixture does not stick to them.) Cool to room temperature.
6. Cut into 20 bars and store them in an airtight container.

Yield: 20 servings

NUTRITION INFORMATION: 3,400 total calories; 170 calories per serving; 24 g carbohydrate; 5 g protein; 6 g fat

SUPER-SEEDY GRANOLA BARS

These crunchy, seedy bars offer fiber, protein, and healthy fats. Allegra Egizi, who developed this recipe when she was a nutrition student at Simmons University, likes them because they contain several heart-healthy foods, including chia, nut butter, and sunflower seeds—and they are super easy to make. You can mix and match ingredients. That is, don't fret if you have no chia (although the chia seeds add a fun crunch) or if you want to use chopped walnuts instead of sunflower seeds.

These are best stored in the fridge for a quick and hearty snack. At room temperature, they can be very crumbly (but you can enjoy the crumbs by the spoonful or as a tasty topping for yogurt or oatmeal).

1 1/2 cup (120 g) oats, quick-cooking or old fashioned

1/2 cup (60 g) sunflower seeds, hemp hearts, or chopped nuts of your choice

3 tablespoons chia seeds

1/4 cup (40 g) dried fruit of your choice such as raisins, chopped dates, craisins

1 teaspoon ground cinnamon

1 cup (260 g) peanut butter or nut butter of your choice

1/2 cup (170 g) honey

Optional: 1 teaspoon vanilla extract, 1/2 teaspoon salt

1. Line a 9- × 9-inch (23 × 23 cm) square pan with parchment paper or plastic wrap with enough overhang for easy removal.
2. In a mixing bowl, combine oats, sunflower seeds, chia seeds, dried fruit, cinnamon, and salt.
3. In a small microwaveable bowl, combine peanut butter, honey (and vanilla extract); warm in the microwave oven (30 to 60 seconds), and then mix together until very smooth.
4. Pour the peanut butter mixture over the dry ingredients. Using a sturdy spoon, stir until evenly combined.
5. Transfer the mixture to the prepared pan. Using the back of the spoon or a spatula, firmly press the mixture evenly into the pan.
6. Cover and refrigerate for at least 1 hour or overnight.
7. Gently lift the parchment or plastic overhang to remove from pan and slice into 16 bars. Enjoy immediately or wrap individual bars and place in a freezer-safe bag to store in the fridge or freezer.

Yield: 16 bars

NUTRITION INFORMATION: 2,900 total calories; 180 calories per bar; 20 g carbohydrate; 5 g protein; 9 g fat

Courtesy of Allegra Egizi.

SUGAR AND SPICE TRAIL MIX

Shannon Weiderholt, RD, likes this recipe as a snack for calming the afternoon munchies on the trail, at home, or at work. Keep this in a resealable plastic bag in your desk drawer or gym bag, and you'll have energy to enjoy your day. It's sweet, but not too sweet.

> 3 cups (165 g) oat squares cereal
> 3 cups mini pretzels (165 g), salted or unsalted, as desired
> 2 tablespoons tub margarine, melted
> 1 tablespoon packed brown sugar
> 1/2 teaspoon cinnamon
> 1 cup (160 g) dried fruit bits or raisins

1. Preheat oven to 325 °F (160 °C).
2. Combine the oat squares and pretzels in a large resealable plastic bag or a plastic container with a lid. Set aside.
3. Melt the margarine in a small microwavable bowl.
4. Add the brown sugar and cinnamon to the margarine and mix well.
5. Pour the cinnamon and sugar mixture over the cereal and pretzels, and seal the bag or container. Shake gently until the mixture is coated. Pour onto a baking sheet and spread evenly.
6. Bake for 15 to 20 minutes, stirring once or twice.
7. Remove from the oven, allow to cool, and then mix in the dried fruit.
8. Store in an airtight container or single-serving resealable bags.

Yield: 10 servings

NUTRITION INFORMATION: 2,000 total calories; 200 calories per serving; 40 g carbohydrate; 5 g protein; 2 g fat

Adapted from American Heart Association, www.deliciousdecisions.org.

CHIA SEED PUDDING

Chia seeds are similar in size to poppy seeds, are typically black or white, and because they are not a grain, are gluten free. They offer heart-healthy omega-3 fats (but not enough to displace fish from your dinner), a little protein (one tablespoon has 3 to 4 grams of protein—the amount in half an egg), and other trace minerals such as magnesium and manganese. Chia seeds are easily digested. You eat them dry (sprinkled on cereal or toast for a fun crunch) or hydrated in a smoothie.

These recipes for chia pudding are just two examples of ways to enjoy chia. The possibilities are endless when you use different fruits, fluids, and sweeteners. If you want chia pudding with a smooth texture, put the ingredients in a blender and process on high for 1 to 2 minutes. *Note:* Chia seeds that have gone through the blender acquire a greyish look. You can blend the strawberry chia seed pudding because the ingredients hide the gray color, but you might prefer to leave this vanilla pudding as is.

VANILLA CHIA SEED PUDDING

1 cup (240 ml) milk of your choice (dairy, soy, coconut, almond) or fruit juice

1/4 cup (30 g) chia seeds

1/4 teaspoon vanilla

2 tablespoons sweeter: maple syrup, honey, agave, jam

Optional: 1/4 teaspoon cinnamon or nutmeg; 2 tablespoons cocoa; coconut flakes; diced fresh or dried fruit as desired

1. Put all the ingredients in an empty (peanut butter) jar. Shake well.
2. Refrigerate for 4 hours or overnight.

Yield: 3 servings

NUTRITIONAL INFORMATION: 500 total calories; 170 calories per serving; 21 g carbohydrate; 6 g protein, 7 g milk (if made with 2 percent milk)

Recipe courtesy of Allegra Egizi.

STRAWBERRY CHIA SEED PUDDING

1 cup (160 g) fresh or frozen whole strawberries

1 tablespoon honey (more if desired)

1 cup (230 g) kefir, plain, low-fat

1/2 cup (120 ml) milk, 1 percent, low-fat

5 tablespoons chia seeds

1. Place the strawberries, honey, and kefir in a blender or food processor and blend on high until smooth, about 2 minutes.
2. In a medium bowl, combine the milk and chia seeds. Add the strawberry mixture and stir to combine.
3. Cover and refrigerate for at least 8 hours or overnight before eating.

Yield: 2 servings

NUTRITIONAL INFORMATION: 500 total calories; 250 calories per serving; 32 g carbohydrate; 9 g protein; 11 g fat; 9 g fiber

Recipe courtesy of healthy eating blogger Elizabeth Ward MS, RD, author of www.betteristhe-newperfect.com and *Expect the Best: Your Guide to Healthy Eating Before, During, and After Pregnancy.*

APPLE CRISP

When making apple crisp, I prefer to leave the peels on the apples for added fiber and nutrients. The small amount of spices allows for a nice apple flavor to shine through the "crisp." For a crisp topping, the margarine or butter should be thoroughly worked into the flour, coating each granule.

> 6 cups sliced apples (about 4 to 5 apples), preferably half Granny Smith, half McIntosh
>
> 1/4 cup (50 g) sugar
>
> 1/2 cup (70 g) flour
>
> 1/3 to 1/2 cup (65 to 100 g) sugar, preferably half white, half packed brown sugar
>
> 1/4 teaspoon cinnamon
>
> 3 to 4 tablespoons cold margarine or butter
>
> *Optional:* 3/4 cup (90 g) chopped almonds or pecans, 1/4 teaspoon nutmeg, 1/4 teaspoon salt

1. Core, slice, and place the apples in an 8- × 8-inch (20 × 20 cm) baking pan. Coat with 1/4 cup (50 g) sugar.
2. Heat oven to 375 °F (190 °C).
3. In a medium bowl, mix the flour, sugar, and cinnamon (and nutmeg and salt). Add the margarine or butter, pinching it into the flour with your fingers until it looks like crumbly wet sand. Add nuts, as desired.
4. Distribute the topping evenly over the apples.
5. Bake for 40 minutes. If you want a crisper topping, turn the oven up to 400 °F (200 °C) for the last 5 minutes.

Yield: 6 servings

NUTRITION INFORMATION: 1,560 total calories; 260 calories per serving; 50 g carbohydrate; 1 g protein; 6 g fat

BANANA ICE CREAM

Blenderized frozen bananas taste amazingly like ice cream. The next time you are confronted with too many ripe bananas, peel them, cut them into 1/2-inch (1.3 cm) slices, lay them on a flat pan, and place them in the freezer for an hour or so. Once frozen, they are ready to be made into banana "ice cream." You can then be creative with the mix-ins. Here are examples:

- Blend in peanut butter, honey, or frozen berries.
- Sprinkle chopped walnuts, mini chocolate chips, or fresh berries on top.
- Drizzle a little chocolate sauce on top.
- Make banana "frozen yogurt" by freezing Greek yogurt in ice cube trays, and then tossing a few cubes into the blender along with the bananas.

1 large banana, sliced and frozen

Optional: mini chocolate chips, chopped walnuts, slivered almonds, fresh berries, frozen cubes of Greek yogurt

1. Put frozen banana slices in a blender or food processor. Blend until smooth, while scraping down the sides.
2. *Optional:* Add in frozen Greek yogurt cubes.
3. Transfer to a serving dish and sprinkle with toppings of your choice (chocolate chips, chopped walnuts, slivered almonds) or blend them into the ice cream.

Yield: 1 serving

NUTRITION INFORMATION: 150 total calories (using 1 large 6 oz, or 180 g, banana, no toppings); 37 g carbohydrate; 1 g protein; 0 g fat

HEALTHY-ISH HEART OATMEAL RAISIN COOKIES WITH CHOCOLATE CHIPS

A problem with most cookies is they are made with butter (saturated fat). If you swap butter for oil (unsaturated fat), the cookies lose their crispness. This recipe solves that problem! By adding one tablespoon of cornstarch per 1/2 cup (120 ml) of oil, you end up with pleasingly crisp cookies.

You can easily make this cookie gluten free by swapping the wheat flour with oat flour (or uncooked oats pulverized in the blender). You might have to form the cookies on the pan, but during baking they will become unified.

> 1 1/2 cups (120 g) (old fashioned) oats
>
> 3/4 cup (105 g) flour, preferably half white and half whole wheat
>
> 1/2 teaspoon baking soda
>
> 1/2 teaspoon baking powder
>
> 1/2 teaspoon salt
>
> 2/3 cup (80 g) sugar, preferably half brown and half white
>
> 1 tablespoon cornstarch
>
> 1/2 cup (120 ml) oil
>
> 2 eggs
>
> 1 cup (240 g) (dark) chocolate chips, preferably mini-chips
>
> *Optional:* 1/2 teaspoon cinnamon; 1/4 cup nut butter; 1 cup raisins (or other diced dried fruit); 1/2 cup sunflower seed kernels, chopped nuts, or peanuts

1. Preheat oven to 350 °F (180 °C).
2. In a medium bowl, mix together the oats, flour, baking soda, baking powder, salt, sugar, and cornstarch.
3. Make a well in the middle of the dry ingredients, and in it put the oil and eggs (and cinnamon and nut butter). Blend those three ingredients, and then stir them into the dry ingredients.
4. Mix in the chocolate chips (mini-chips blend in better than bigger chips), (sunflower seeds and raisins).
5. Place a tablespoon of dough on an ungreased baking sheet and bake for 12 to 15 minutes or until golden and just after they fall.

Yield: 30 cookies

NUTRITIONAL INFORMATION: 3,325 total calories; 110 calories per cookie; 12 g carbohydrate; 2 g protein; 6 g fat

CHOCOLATE LUSH

What I like best about this brownie pudding is that it's a low-fat yet tasty treat for those who want a chocolate fix. It forms its own sauce during baking. If you need to rationalize eating chocolate, remember that cocoa contains health-protective phytochemicals.

1 cup (140 g) flour

3/4 cup (150 g) sugar

2 tablespoons unsweetened dry cocoa

2 teaspoons baking powder

1 teaspoon salt

1/2 cup (120 ml) milk

2 tablespoons oil, preferably canola

2 teaspoons vanilla

3/4 cup (150 g) brown sugar

1/4 cup (35 g) unsweetened dry cocoa

1 3/4 cups (420 ml) hot water

Optional: 1/2 cup (60 g) chopped nuts

1. Preheat the oven to 350 °F (180 °C).
2. In a medium bowl, stir together the flour, white sugar, 2 tablespoons cocoa, baking powder, and salt; add the milk, oil, and vanilla (and nuts). Mix until smooth.
3. Pour into an 8- × 8-inch (20 × 20 cm) square pan that is nonstick, lightly oiled, or treated with cooking spray.
4. Combine the brown sugar, 1/4 cup (35 g) of cocoa, and hot water. Gently pour this mixture on top of the batter in the pan.
5. Bake for 40 minutes or until lightly browned and bubbly.

Yield: 9 servings

NUTRITION INFORMATION: 2,100 total calories; 230 calories per serving; 46 g carbohydrate; 3 g protein; 4 g fat

Courtesy of Sue Westin.

CARROT CAKE

Avid cyclist and dietitian Jenny Hegmann, RD, suggests that if you are destined to eat cake, at least have one filled with fruit, vegetables, and nuts. This carrot cake recipe fills that bill. Unlike most carrot cakes, which are extremely high in fat, Jenny's recipe offers a lower-fat option—with a heart-healthy fat at that—canola oil.

1 1/2 cups (300 g) sugar

3/4 cup (180 ml) canola oil

3 eggs

2 cups (220 g) grated carrot, lightly packed

1 cup (250 g) crushed canned pineapple with juice

2 teaspoons vanilla extract

1 teaspoon salt

1 teaspoon cinnamon

1 teaspoon baking powder

1/2 teaspoon baking soda

2 1/2 cups (350 g) flour

Optional: 1 cup (120 g) chopped walnuts, 1 cup (160 g) raisins

Frosting

4 ounces (125 g) low-fat cream cheese, at room temperature

2 1/2 cups (250 g) confectioners' sugar, sifted

1 teaspoon vanilla extract or 2 teaspoons grated orange peel

1 to 2 tablespoons milk or orange juice

1. Treat a 9- × 13-inch (23 × 33 cm) baking pan with cooking spray, or line with waxed paper. Preheat the oven to 350 °F (180 °C).

2. In a medium mixing bowl, beat together the sugar and oil and then the eggs.

3. Add the grated carrot, pineapple and its juice, and vanilla. Mix well.

4. Add the salt, cinnamon, baking powder, and baking soda (and nuts and raisins, if desired). Gently blend in the flour, being careful not to overbeat.

5. Pour the batter into the prepared pan. Bake for 35 to 40 minutes. Cool completely before frosting.

6. In a small mixing bowl, beat the cream cheese and confectioners' sugar. Add vanilla and milk (or orange juice and grated orange peel), and beat until smooth and creamy. Spread the frosting on the cake.

Yield: 24 pieces

NUTRITION INFORMATION: 4,200 total calories (plain cake); 175 calories per serving; 26 g carbohydrate; 2 g protein; 7 g fat

With frosting: 5,500 total calories; 230 calories per serving; 37 g carbohydrate; 3 g protein; 8 g fat

Courtesy of Jenny Hegmann, RD.

APPENDIX A

For More Information

This appendix provides a variety of sources, including books, websites, and newsletters, where you can find additional information about many of the topics discussed in this book. Some of the books listed are classics; some are new releases. A few titles are primarily for professionals, but most are appropriate for the public. You can look for the books in your local library or bookstore or order them online. Alternatively, many are available through the following sources of reliable nutrition materials:

NCES Health and Nutrition Education

www.ncescatalog.com

877-623-7266

Eating Disorders Resource Catalogue

www.EDCatalogue.com

800-756-7533

Human Kinetics

www.humankinetics.com

800-747-4457

The websites and newsletters listed provide quality nutrition, sports nutrition, and health information. The list reflects information gathered in December 2018. It is by no means complete; many other excellent resources and websites are available.

Because I am frequently asked how to become a sports nutritionist, I have included at the end of this appendix some information on starting down that road. Health professionals who want sports nutrition teaching materials can find handouts and slides on my website, www.nancyclarkrd.com, and find online courses at www.NutritionSportsExerciseCEUs.com.

Aging

Rosenbloom, C., and B. Murray. 2018. *Food and fitness after 50: Eat well, move well, be well.* Chicago, IL: Academy of Nutrition and Dietetics.

American College of Sports Medicine position statement: Exercise and physical activity for older adults. 2009. *Medicine and Science in Sports and Exercise* 41 (7): 1510-1520. doi: 10.1249/MSS.0b013e3181a0c95c.

Alcohol

Fletcher, A. 2013. *Inside rehab: The surprising truth about addiction treatment and how to get help that works.* New York: Viking.

Adult Children of Alcoholics

Woititz, J. 2002. *The complete adult children of alcoholics sourcebook: Adult children at home, at work and in love.* Deerfield Beach, FL: Health Communications.

The following websites offer resources for people who want to stop their problem drinking and resources for their loved ones.

www.smartrecovery.org

www.aa.org (Alcoholics Anonymous)

www.moderation.org

Amenorrhea

Muir, T. 2019 *Overcoming amenorrhea: Get your period back. Get your life back.* Amazon Digital Services LLC.

Rinaldi N., S. Buckler, L. Sanfilippo Waddell. 2016. *No Period. Now What?: A guide to regaining your cycles and improving your fertility.* Antica Press LLC.

Backpacking and Hiking

Mayhew, A.O. 2018. *Ultralight recipes for outdoor explorers.* Millcreek, WA: Backcountry Foodie LLC.

www.backcountryfoodie.com.

Body Fat (see also Weight Management, Obesogens)

International Society of Sports Nutrition position stand: Diets and body composition. 2017. *Journal of the International Society of Sports Nutrition* 14:16. doi.org/10.1186/s12970-017-0174-y.

This website has a body fat calculator.
www.calculator.net/body-fat-calculator.html

Body Image (see also Eating Disorders)

Creekmore, H. 2017. *Compared to who? A proven path to improve your body image.* Abilene, TX: Leafwood Publishers.

Scritchfield, R. 2016. *Body kindness: Transform your health from the inside out—and never say diet again.* New York, NY: Workman Publishing.

www.EDCatalogue.com offers a large assortment of books about body image, and the following websites promote positive self-esteem in women of all ages:

www.bodypositive.com

https://now.org/now-foundation/love-your-body

www.about-face.org

Caffeine

International Society of Sports Nutrition position stand: Caffeine and performance. 2010. *Journal of the International Society of Sports Nutrition* 7: 5. doi.org/10.1186/1550-2783-7-5.

Calories (see also Dietary Analysis and Nutrition Assessment; Feed Trackers)

www.calorieking.com

www.MyFitnessPal.com

www.webmd.com/diet/healthtool-food-calorie-counter

Cancer (see also Healthy Eating; Herbs, Medicinal; Supplements)

LaMantia, J., and N. Berinstein, MD. 2012. *The essential cancer treatment nutrition guide and cookbook.* Toronto: Robert Rose.

The American Cancer Society's site has answers to all your questions about prevention and treatment.

www.cancer.org/healthy/eat-healthy-get-active/acs-guidelines-nutrition-physical-activity-cancer-prevention.html

The American Institute for Cancer Research offers dietary information about eating for a healthier life.

www.aicr.org

The World Cancer Research Fund offers the latest evidence on food, nutrition, physical activity, and the prevention of cancer.

www.dietandcancerreport.org

Celiac Disease

Case, S. 2016. *Gluten-free diet: The definitive resource guide.* Saskatchewan, Canada: Case Nutrition Consulting, Inc.

Shelley Case, RD, offers this website for people with celiac disease.

http://shelleycase.com

The Celiac Disease Awareness Campaign sponsored by National Institutes of Health offers resources for professionals and clients.

www.celiac.nih.gov

Visit these websites of the Celiac Disease Foundation, the Gluten Intolerance Group, and the National Institute of Diabetes and Digestive and Kidney Diseases (NIDDK) for more information and resources about celiac disease.

https://celiac.org

https://gluten.org

www.niddk.nih.gov

Childhood Obesity

Satter, E. 2005. *Your child's weight: Helping without harming.* Madison, WI: Kelcy Press.

We Can! is a national education program that offers parents and families tips and fun activities to encourage healthy eating, increase physical activity, and reduce sedentary or screen time.

www.nhlbi.nih.gov/health/educational/wecan

Growth charts for assessing children's weight are available at the Centers for Disease Control and Prevention website.

www.cdc.gov/growthcharts

Children and Nutrition

Satter, E. 2008. *Secrets of feeding a healthy family.* Madison, WI: Kelcy Press.

These sites promote healthy eating and physical activity among kids and parents.

www.kidnetic.org

www.superkidsnutrition.com

Clothing

The following site offers running shorts and other exercise apparel with pockets for holding sports foods.

www.raceready.com

Complementary and Alternative Medicine (see also Herbs, Medicinal)

The websites of the National Center for Complementary and Integrative Health and the National Institutes of Health Office of Dietary Supplements provide abundant information about alternative medicine, herbs, and dietary supplements.

https://nccih.nih.gov

https://ods.od.nih.gov

Cookbooks and Recipes (see also Vegetarian Nutrition)

American Heart Association. 2017. *New American Heart Association cookbook.* New York, NY: Harmony Books.

Flanagan, S. 2018. *Run fast. Cook fast. Eat slow.* Emmaus, PA: Rodale.

Flanagan S. 2016. *Run fast. Eat slow: Nourishing recipes for athletes.* Emmaus, PA: Rodale.

Thomas, B., and A. Lim. 2011. *The feed zone cookbook: Fast and flavorful food for athletes.* Boulder, CO: Velopress.

Visit these sites for recipes and additional cooking information.

www.cookinglight.com

www.cooksillustrated.com

www.eatingwell.com

Creatine

International Society of Sports Nutrition position stand: Safety and efficacy of creatine supplementation in exercise, sport, and medicine. 2017. *Journal of the International Society of Sports Medicine* 14: 18. doi: 10.1186/s12970-017-0173-z.

Diabetes

American Diabetes Association. 2018. *Managing type 2 diabetes for dummies*. Hoboken, NJ: John Wiley and Sons.

Colberg, S. 2020. *The Athelete's Guide to Diabetes*. Champaign, IL: Human Kinetics.

Geil, P., and T. Ross. 2015. *What do I eat now? A step-by-step guide to eating right with type 2 diabetes*. Alexandria, VA: American Diabetes Association.

Founded by a registered dietitian with diabetes, this site offers practical information.

http://diabeteseveryday.com

The National Diabetes Education Program, part of the NIDDK, offers information on how to improve diabetes care.

www.ndep.nih.gov

The American Diabetes Association offers information and resources for diabetes care.

www.diabetes.org

Dietary Analysis and Nutrition Assessment (see also Calories)

These are sites you can use to track your calorie and nutrient intake.

www.eaTracker.ca

www.MyFitnessPal.com

www.MyFoodRecord.com

https://ndb.nal.usda.gov/ndb (designed for nutrition professionals)

Dietitian (how to find one locally)

The Academy of Nutrition and Dietetics' referral network can help you find a registered dietitian (RD) in your area.

www.eatright.org

This is the referral network of the Academy of Nutrition and Dietetics' Sports, Cardiovascular and Wellness Nutrition practice group.

www.scandpg.org

You can also find an RD by calling the nutrition department at your local hospital or sports medicine clinic. Select a name followed by *RD* or *RDN*.

Eating Disorders (see also Body Image)

Costin, C. 2017. *8 keys to recovery from an eating disorder.* New York, NY: W.W. Norton and Company.

Gaudiani, J. 2018. *Sick enough: A guide to the medical complications of eating disorders.* New York, NY: Routledge Press

Hicks, S. *Emily's guide to eating disorders: A workbook for children ages 5 to 11.* Denver, CO: Outskirts Press. (This is a guide for children whose mothers are going into treatment.)

Siegel, M., J. Brisman, and M. Weinshel. 2009. *Surviving an eating disorder: Perspectives and strategies for family and friends.* New York, NY: HarperCollins Publishers.

Schaefer, J. 2014. *Life without Ed: How one woman declared independence from her eating disorder.* New York, NY: McGraw-Hill Education.

Schauster, H. 2018. *Nourish: How to heal your relationship with food, body, and self.* Somerville, MA: Hummingbird Press.

Steil, R. 2016 *Running in silence: My drive for perfection and the eating disorder that fed it.* Virginia Beach, VA: Koehler Books.

Tribole, E., and E. Resch. 2017. *The intuitive eating workbook: Ten principles for nourishing a healthy relationship with food.* Oakland, CA: New Harbinger Publications.

The Academy of Nutrition and Dietetics (AND) and SCAN, the sports nutrition dietary practice group of AND, offer a referral service for sports nutritionists skilled in handling eating disorders.

www.eatright.org

www.scandpg.org

This website offers information about eating disorders and body image and provides a hotline, screening tool, referral network, and educational materials.

www.nationaleatingdisorders.org

This website offers information about eating disorders and a bookstore with more than 200 titles on eating disorders.

www.EDCatalogue.com

This site is for the National Association for Males With Eating Disorders, Inc.
https://namedinc.org

Ergogenic Aids

IOC Consensus Statement: Dietary supplements and the high performance athlete. 2018. *International Journal of Sport Nutrition and Exercise Metabolism* (28) 2: 104-125. doi: 10.1123/ijsnem.2018-0020.

Exercise and Exercise Physiology (see also Weight Management)

Textbooks (see also Sports Nutrition Textbooks)

McArdle, W., F. Katch, and V. Katch. 2014. *Exercise physiology: Nutrition, energy, and human performance.* Philadelphia, PA: Lippincott Williams & Wilkins.

Powers, S., and E. Howley. 2017. *Exercise physiology: Theory and application to fitness and performance.* New York, NY: McGraw-Hill Education.

The American College of Sports Medicine is the largest group of sports medicine and sports science professionals in the world.

www.acsm.org

The Gatorade Sports Science Exchange offers many articles about exercise physiology and the science of fueling for performance.

www.gssiweb.org

2018 Physical Activity Guidelines Advisory Committee scientific report. https://health.gov/paguidelines/second-edition/report.

Female Athlete Triad and RED-S

IOC consensus statement: Beyond the female athlete triad—Relative energy deficiency in sport (RED-S). 2014. *British Journal of Sports Medicine* (7): 491-7. doi: 10.1136/bjsports-2014-093502.

IOC consensus statement on relative energy deficiency in sport (RED-S): 2018 update. 2018. *International Journal of Sport Nutrition and Exercise Metabolism* 28 (4): 316-331. doi: 10.1123/ijsnem.2018-0136.

FODMAP Information for People With Intestinal Distress

Kate Scarlata, RD, and Patsy Catsos, RD, have written books and educational materials about using the FODMAP diet to treat people with irritable bowel syndrome (IBS).

www.KateScarlata.com

www.VeryWellFit.com

Catsos, P. 2017. *The IBS elimination diet and cookbook: A plan for eating well and feeling great.* New York, NY: Harmony Books.

Scarlata, K. 2017. *The low FODMAP diet step by step: A personalized plan to relieve the symptoms of IBS and other digestive disorders—with more than 130 deliciously satisfying recipes.* New York, NY: De Capo Press.

Food Information

The International Food Information Council offers information about all aspects of food and food safety.

https://foodinsight.org

Food Labels

Sponsored by the U.S. Department of Agriculture, this site offers a guide to understanding food labels.

www.fda.gov/Food/LabelingNutrition/ucm20026097.htm

Food Trackers (also called calorie counters)

These are just a few of the websites (with apps) my clients commonly use to track their food intake:

www.MyFitnessPal.com

www.livestrong.com

www.LoseIt.com

www.sparkpeople.com

Heart Disease

American Heart Association scientific statement: Recommended dietary pattern to achieve adherence to the American Heart Association/American College of Cardiology (AHA/ACC) Guidelines. 2016. *Circulation* 134: e505-e529. doi.org/10.1161/CIR.0000000000000462.

Presidential advisory from the American Heart Association on dietary fats and cardiovascular disease. 2017. *Circulation* 136: e1-e23. doi.org/10.1161/CIR.0000000000000510.

Healthy Eating

Duyff, R. 2017. *The American Dietetic Association's complete food and nutrition guide.* Hoboken, NJ: John Wiley and Sons.

Read healthy living topics at the American Heart Association's website:

www.heart.org

The Food and Nutrition Information Center at the U.S. Department of Agriculture features nutrition information for infants, children, teens, adults, and seniors.

www.nal.usda.gov/fnic

The Office of Disease Prevention and Health Promotion provides information on how to eat for health.

https://health.gov

Many registered dietitians (RDs) are food bloggers. If you search the Internet for "food bloggers," choose authors with RD or RDN after their names. Here are popular blogs:

Amidor, RD, T. https://tobyamidornutrition.com/my-blog

Helm, RD, J. www.nutritionunplugged.com

Weiss, RD, L. www.LizsHealthyTable.com

Herbs, Medicinal (see also Complementary and Alternative Medicine)

The Memorial Sloan Kettering Cancer Center offers information about herbs, botanicals, supplements, and more.

https://www.mskcc.org/cancer-care/diagnosis-treatment/symptom-management/integrative-medicine/herbs

The Herb Research Foundation offers science-based information on the health benefits and safety of herbs.

www.herbs.org

Hoaxes

This site offers a guide to health fraud and quackery and enhances your ability to make intelligent decisions regarding sports supplements and herbs.

www.quackwatch.org

Locally Grown Food

This site can help you find farm stands and farmers' markets in your area.

www.localharvest.org

Medical Information

These sites offer the latest medical and nutrition information.

www.webmd.com

www.mayoclinic.org

Mediterranean Diet (and other cultural food traditions)

Oldways offers information about the Mediterranean diet and other cultural food traditions.

https://oldwayspt.org

Menopause

Northrup, C. 2012. *The wisdom of menopause.* New York, NY: Bantam Books.

The North American Menopause Society's site is devoted to promoting women's health through menopause and beyond.

www.menopause.org

Muscle Dysmorphia (see also Body Image)

Pope Jr., H.G., K.A. Phillips, and R. Olivardia. 2002. *The Adonis complex: How to identify, treat and prevent body obsession in men and boys.* New York, NY: Touchstone.

Newsletters

Tufts University Health & Nutrition Letter

P.O. Box 8547, Big Sandy, TX 757555-8517

800-274-7581, on the Web: www.nutritionletter.tufts.edu

University of California, Berkeley Wellness Letter

P.O. Box 433235, Palm Coast, FL 32143

800-829-9170, on the Web: www.berkeleywellness.com

Obesogens (see also Body Fat, Weight Management)

The following websites provide more information about obesogens, which I briefly introduced in chapter 1.

http://en.wikipedia.org/wiki/Obesogen

www.niehs.nih.gov/health/topics/conditions/obesity/obesogens/index.cfm

Obesity pathogenesis: An Endocrine Society scientific statement. 2017. *Endocrine Reviews* 38 (4): 2670296. doi.org/10.1210/er.2017-00111.

Osteoporosis

Nelson, M., and S. Wernick. 2006. *Strong women, strong bones: Everything you need to know to prevent, treat, and beat osteoporosis.* New York, NY: Penguin Group.

The National Osteoporosis Foundation offers a variety of information and resources.

www.nof.org

Performance-Enhancing Drugs (lists of banned substances)

World Anti-Doping Agency (WADA) prohibited drug list: www.usada.org/substances/prohibited-list

National Collegiate Athletic Association (NCAA) banned drug list: www.ncaa.org/2018-19-ncaa-banned-drugs-list

U.S. Food and Drug Administration tainted supplement list: www.accessdata.fda.gov/scripts/sda/sdNavigation.cfm?sd=tainted_supplements_cder

Personal Trainers

Professional organizations that certify personal trainers include the American College of Sports Medicine, American Council on Exercise, IDEA Health and Fitness Association, and National Strength and Conditioning Association.

Use these websites to find a personal trainer:

www.acsm.org/get-stay-certified/find-a-pro

www.acefitness.org/education-and-resources/lifestyle/find-ace-pro

www.ideafit.com/find-personal-trainer

Pesticides

The websites for the USDA Pesticide Data Program, the Environmental Protection Agency (EPA), and the Environmental Working Group provide information about pesticides.

www.ams.usda.gov/AMSv1.0/pdp

www.EPA.gov/pesticides

www.ewg.org

Pregnancy

Erick, M. 2004. *Managing morning sickness: A survival guide for pregnant women.* Boulder, CO: Bull Publishing Company.

Luke, B., and T. Eberlein. 2017. *When you are expecting twins, triplets or quads.* New York, NY: HarperCollins Publishers.

Ward, E. 2017. *Expect the best: Your guide to healthy eating before, during, and after pregnancy.* Chicago, IL: Academy of Nutrition and Dietetics.

www.eatrightpro.org/practice/position-and-practice-papers/position-papers/nutrition-and-lifestyle-for-a-healthy-pregnancy-outcome.

Protein

Jager R., C. Kerksick, B. Campbell, et al. 2017. International Society of Sports Nutrition position stand: Protein and exercise. 2017. *Journal of the International Society of Sports Nutrition* 14: 20. https://jissn.biomedcentral.com/articles/10.1186/s12970-017-0177-8.

Probiotics

"One size fits all" does not work for probiotics. Various strains and dosages are recommended for various goals. The Clinical Guide to Probiotic Products can help you determine which probiotic might be suited for a specific health issue.

www.usprobioticguide.com (U.S. products)

www.probioticchart.ca/PBCAdultHealth.html (Canadian products)

Relative Energy Deficiency in Sport (RED-S) (see Female Athlete Triad)

Sleep

Athletes who travel across time zones will benefit from this information from the American Sleep Association.

www.SleepAssociation.org

Sports Nutrition (see also Supplements)

Position of the Academy of Nutrition and Dietetics, American College of Sports Medicine and the Dietitians of Canada: Nutrition and athletic performance: 2016. *Journal of the Academy of Nutrition and Dietetics* 116 (3): 501-528. doi.org/10.1016/j.jand.2015.12.006.

ACSM, and D. Benardot. 2018. *ACSM's nutrition for exercise science.* Philadelphia, PA: Wolters Kluwer.

Castle, J. 2015. *Eat like a champion: Performance nutrition for your young athlete.* New York, NY: American Management Association.

Kleiner, S., and M. Greenwood. 2019. *The new power eating: More muscle, more energy, less fat.* Champaign, IL: Human Kinetics.

Larson-Meyer, D.E. 2019. *Plant-based sports nutrition: Expert fueling strategies for training, recovery, and performance.* Champaign, IL: Human Kinetics.

Karpinski, C. 2017. *Sports nutrition: A handbook for professionals,* 6th ed. Chicago, IL: Academy of Nutrition and Dietetics.

Sports Nutrition Textbooks (see also Exercise Physiology)

Nancy Clark's Sports Nutrition Guidebook is a popular textbook for high school and college students (for non-nutrition majors or as a supplemental text for nutrition majors). For information about the instructor's guide, visit www.humankinetics.com.

Jeukendrup, A., and M. Gleeson. 2019. *Sports nutrition,* 3rd ed. Champaign, IL: Human Kinetics.

Spano, M., L. Kruskall, and T. Thomas. 2017. *Nutrition for sport, exercise and health.* Champaign, IL: Human Kinetics.

The Australian Institute of Sport website offers sports nutrition information, including advice about sports supplements.

www.ausport.gov.au/ais/nutrition

This is the professional website of the Academy of Nutrition and Dietetics' Sports, Cardiovascular and Wellness Nutrition (SCAN) practice group.

www.scandpg.org

The websites for the Gatorade Sports Science Institute and for PowerBar offer resource for both professionals and the public.

www.gssiweb.com

www.powerbar.com

The National Library of Medicine offers access to the latest research in medical and scientific journals.

www.pubmed.gov

Stress Management and Relaxation

The World Wide Online Meditation Center, designed for both novices and experienced meditators, includes various types of "meditation rooms," complete with audio for stress reduction, healing, and centering.

www.meditationcenter.com

Supplements (see also Herbs, Medicinal; Sports Nutrition)

Maughan, R., and L. Burke. 2018. IOC consensus statement: Dietary supplements and the high-performance athlete. *British Journal of Sports Medicine* 52 (7):439-455. doi: 10.1136/bjsports-2018-099027. Free full text available.

Position of the Academy of Nutrition and Dietetics: Micronutrient supplementation. 2018. *Journal of the Academy of Nutrition and Dietetics.* www.eatrightpro.org/practice/position-and-practice-papers/position-papers/nutrient-supplementation.

Here's an A to Z list of herbs and other supplements, including background information, dosages, safety, interactions, and references.

https://medlineplus.gov

The National Agricultural Library's Food and Nutrition Information Center offers information on the safe use of dietary supplements as well as links to sites and sources with credible information.

www.nal.usda.gov/fnic/dietary-supplements

This site contains published, peer-reviewed scientific literature on dietary supplements, including vitamins, minerals, and herbs. The site is a joint effort between the NIH's Office of Dietary Supplements and the National Library of Medicine.

https://ods.od.nih.gov/Research/PubMed_Dietary_Supplement_Subset.aspx

The website for the National Collegiate Athletic Association provides information about supplements that have been banned for use by college athletes. It also provides information on sports nutrition for student athletes.

www.ncaa.org

The National Institute on Drug Abuse offers information on the science of drug abuse and addiction.

www.drugabuse.gov

ConsumerLab provides the results of dietary supplement testing for quality and purity.

www.consumerlab.com

Supplement Safety Information

Athletes should confirm any supplements they take are safe and not contaminated with illegal drugs. The World Anti-Doping Agency prohibited list is https://www.wada-ama.org/en/content/what-is-prohibited

Reputable supplement companies include Klean Athlete, Thorne Douglas, Labs Garden of Life, and Nordic Naturals. Website and an app that can confirm approved supplements are NSF International Certified for Sport and Informed-Choice™: http://www.nsfsport.com/

Vegetarian Nutrition

Larson-Meyer, D.E. 2019. *Plant-based sports nutrition: Expert fueling strategies for training, recovery, and performance.* Champaign, IL: Human Kinetics.

Position of the Academy of Nutrition and Dietetics: Vegetarian diets. 2016. *Journal of the Academy of Nutrition and Dietetics.* www.eatrightpro.org/practice/position-and-practice-papers/position-papers/vegetarian-diets.

This website offers practical information from the Vegetarian Nutrition Dietetic Practice Group of the Academy of Nutrition and Dietetics.

http://vegetariannutrition.net

The Vegetarian Resource Group is a nonprofit organization dedicated to educating the public on the interrelated issues of nutrition, ecology, ethics, and world hunger.

www.vrg.org

This website claims to offer the world's largest collection of vegetarian recipes, blogs, articles, and vegan information.

www.vegweb.com

Vitamin Supplements

Position of the Academy of Nutrition and Dietetics: Micronutrient supplementation. 2018. *Journal of the Academy of Nutrition and Dietetics* 118 (11): 2162-2173.

Weight Management (see also Exercise and Exercise Physiology, Obesogens)

Tribole, E., and E. Resch. 2012. *Intuitive eating: A revolutionary program that works.* New York, NY: St. Martin's Press.

Position of the Academy of Nutrition and Dietetics: Interventions for the treatment of overweight and obesity in adults. 2016. *Journal of the Academy of Nutrition and Dietetics.*

www.eatrightpro.org/practice/position-and-practice-papers/position-papers/interventions-treatment-overweight-obesity-in-adults.

International Society of Sports Nutrition position stand: Diets and body composition. 2017.

Journal of the International Society of Sports Nutrition 14: 16. doi. org/10.1186/s12970-017-0174-y.

National Athletic Trainers' Association position statement: Safe weight loss and maintenance practices in sport and exercise. 2011. *Journal of Athletic Training.* http://natajournals.org/doi/pdf/10.4085/1062-6050-46.3.322.

How to Become a Sports Nutritionist

Every week I receive e-mails from people who have read my books or articles and want to know where they can go to school to learn more about nutrition and exercise. Some even want to become sports nutritionists. Here's what I tell them.

More and more institutions are offering sports nutrition majors, particularly if they have departments in both nutrition and exercise science. You can often combine the two programs to create a major that suits your needs.

• For a list of sports nutrition degree programs, visit www.scandpg. org, the website of Sports, Cardiovascular and Wellness Nutrition (SCAN), a dietetic practice group of the Academy of Nutrition and Dietetics (AND).

• For a list of academic programs in nutrition accredited and approved by AND, visit www.eatright.org. For a list of academic programs in exercise science, visit www.acsm.org, the website of the American College of Sports Medicine.

• If you just want to further your personal knowledge, you can take one or two classes in nutrition or exercise science without committing to four years of advanced education. I recommend the full program, however, for people who want to develop a career in sports nutrition.

• If you want to be a nutrition counselor, you should become a registered dietitian (RD). This means that you are recognized by the Academy of Nutrition and Dietetics, the largest organization of nutrition professionals in the United States. Career doors will open up to you. Some people take short certificate courses, but these cannot match the education you receive in four years of undergraduate schooling, plus an internship and a master's degree in nutrition. Getting proper education and credentials is an important professional responsibility.

• By becoming a registered dietitian, you will also be eligible to join SCAN, the sports nutrition interest group of the Academy of Nutrition and Dietetics. SCAN members are the leading sports nutritionists. Once you have experience, you can sit for an exam and become a board-certified specialist in sports dietetics (CSSD). See www.scandpg.org for more information.

Although your career goals may be to work with athletes and other active, healthy people, I strongly recommend that students and new graduates work first in clinical settings, such as hospitals, to learn more about how to handle heart disease, diabetes, cancer, and many of the ailments of aging that you will encounter in your work with athletes and fitness exercisers. This knowledge will help you keep people well and enhance your work experience. One or two years of clinical work is a good investment in your career.

Get involved as a volunteer with a high school sports team, in youth soccer, at the YMCA, or in any area that interests you. Work on nutrition and fitness programs sponsored by the dietetic association or council on physical fitness in your area. Practice what you preach. Write articles for the local newspaper or the newsletter of your local bicycle or running club. Try to develop networks that will help you meet other local sports nutritionists and sports medicine professionals. Networking might open doors that eventually lead to paid work.

Sports nutrition is now an integral part of many programs dealing with sports and athletes, so job opportunities are available. Some places to look for (or create) jobs include health clubs, training centers, spas, YMCAs, corporate wellness programs, sports medicine practices, high schools, college and university athletic departments, and professional and semiprofessional sports teams. Be creative!

You might have to knock on several doors before finding a welcoming venue. Or you make your own job using their personal contacts. For example, some registered dietitians who are mothers of teenage athletes have started sports nutrition classes targeted to parents, coaches, and students. Some RDs who love tennis, ballet, or gymnastics have become known as the sports nutritionist for their sports. Many who work out at health clubs have started to work with the members of their clubs. You can create your dream job, and with lots of hard work and time, you'll achieve your goals. Have fun!

With best wishes,
Nancy

APPENDIX B

Selected References

Academy of Nutrition and Dietetics. 2016. Position of the Academy of Nutrition and Dietetics: Interventions for the treatment of overweight and obesity in adults. *J Acad Nutr Diet* 116: 129-147.

Ackland T.R., T.G. Lohman, J. Sundgot-Borgen, et al. 2012. Current status of body composition assessment in sport: Review and position statement on behalf of the ad hoc research working group on body composition, health and performance, under the auspices of the I.O.C. Medical Commission. *Sports Med* 42 (3): 227-249.

Ackermark, C., I. Jacobs, M. Rasmussan, and J. Karlsson. 1996. Diet and muscle glycogen concentration in relation to physical performance in Swedish elite ice hockey players. *Int J Sports Nutr and Exerc Metab* 6 (3): 272-284.

Affenito, S. 2007. Breakfast: A missed opportunity. *J Amer Diet Assoc* 107 (4): 565-569.

Ainslie, P., I. Campbell, K. Frayn, et al. 2002. Energy balance, metabolism, hydration, and performance during strenuous hill walking: The effect of age. *J Appl Physiol* 93 (2): 714-723.

American College of Sports Medicine (ACSM). 2007. ACSM position stand on exercise and fluid replacement. *Med Sci Sports Exerc* 39 (2): 377-390.

American College of Sports Medicine (ACSM), Academy of Nutrition and Dietetics, and Dietitians of Canada. 2016. Joint position statement: Nutrition and athletic performance. *Med Sci Sports Exerc* 48 (3): 543-568.

American Psychiatric Association. 2013. *Diagnostic and statistical manual of mental disorders*, 5th ed. Washington, DC: Author.

Appel, L., F. Sacks, V. Carey, et al. 2005. Effects of protein, monounsaturated fat, and carbohydrate intake on blood pressure and serum lipids: Results of the OmniHeart randomized trial. *JAMA* 294: 2455-64.

Antoni, R., T. Robertson, M. Denise, et al. 2018. A pilot feasibility study exploring the effects of moderate time-restricted feeding intervention on energy intake, adiposity and metabolic physiology in free-living human subjects. *J Nutr Sci* 7e 22.

Aragon, A., B. Schoenfeld, R. Wildman, et al. 2017. International Society of Sports Nutrition position stand: Diets and body composition. *J Int Soc Sports Nutr* 14 (1): 16.

Archer, E. 2018. In defense of sugar. *Prog Cardiovas Dis* 61 (3-4): 386-387. doi. org/10.1016/j.pcad.2018.07.013.

Armstrong, L. 2002. Caffeine, body fluid-electrolyte balance, and exercise performance. *Int J Sports Nutr and Exerc Metab* 12: 189-206.

Armstrong, L., A. Pumerantz, M. Roti, et al. 2005. Fluid, electrolyte, and renal indices of hydration during 11 days of controlled caffeine consumption. *Int J Sport Nutr Exerc Metab* 15: 252-265.

Artioli, G., B. Gualano, A. Smith, J. Stout, and A. Lancha Jr. 2010. Role of beta-alanine supplementation on muscle carnosine and exercise performance *Med Sci Sports Exerc* 42 (6): 1162-1173.

Bailey, W., D. Jacobsen, and J. Donnelly. 2002. Changes in total daily energy expenditure as a result of 16 months of aerobic training: The Midwest Exercise Trial. *Am J Clin Nutr* 75 (Suppl. no. 2): 363.

Barnes, J., J. Wagganer, J. Loenneke, R. Williams Jr, Y. Arja, G. Kirby, and T. Pujol. 2012. Validity of bioelectrical impedance analysis instruments for the measurement of body composition in collegiate gymnasts. *Med Sci Sports Exerc* 44 (5S): S592.

Barr, S., K.C. Janelle, and J.C. Prior. 1995. Energy intakes are higher during the luteal phase of ovulatory menstrual cycles. *Am J Clin Nutr* 61: 39-43.

Beals, K., and M. Manore. 2000. Behavioral, psychological, and physical characteristics of female athletes with subclinical eating disorders. *Int J Sports Nutr and Exerc Metab* 10 (2): 128-143.

Beals, K., and M. Manore. 2002. Disorders of the female athlete triad among collegiate athletes. *Int J Sports Nutr and Exerc Metab* 12: 281-293.

Beelen, M., L. Burke, M. Gibala, and L. van Loon. 2010. Nutritional strategies to promote postexercise recovery. *Int J Sports Nutr Exerc Metab* 20 (6): 515-532.

Bergstrom, J., L. Hermansen, E. Hultman, and B. Saltin. 1967. Diet, muscle glycogen, and physical performance. *Acta Physiol Scand* 71: 140-150.

Blackburn, G. 2001. The public health implications of the Dietary Approaches to Stop Hypertension Trial. *Am J Clin Nutr* 74: 1-2.

Bo, K, R. Artal, R. Barakat, et al. 2018. Exercise and pregnancy in recreational and elite athletes: 2016/2017 evidence summary from the IOC expert group meeting, Lausanne. Part 5. Recommendations for health professionals and active women. *Br J Sports Med* 52: 1080-1085.

Borjian, A., C. Ferrari, A. Anouf, and L. Touyz. 2010. Pop-cola acids and tooth erosion: An *in vitro, in vivo*, electron-microscopic, and clinical report. *Int J Dent* 2010: 957842. doi: 10.1155/2010/957842.

Bouchard, C. 1990. Heredity and the path to overweight and obesity. *Med Sci Sports Exerc* 23 (3): 285-291.

Braakhuis, A. 2012. Effect of vitamin C supplements on physical performance. *Curr Sports Med Reports* 11 (4): 180-184.

Bradbury, K., A. Balkwill, E. Spencer, et al. 2014. Organic food consumption and the incidence of cancer in a large prospective study of women in the United Kingdom. *Br J Cancer* 110 (9): 2321-2326.

Bartlett, J., J. Hawley, and J. Morton. 2015 Carbohydrate availability and exercise training adaptation: Too much of a good thing? *Eur J Sport Sci* 15 (1): 3-12.

Bratland-Sanda, S., J. Sundgot-Borgen. 2013. Eating disorders in athletes: Overview of prevalence, risk factors and recommendations for prevention and treatment. *Eur J Sports Sci* 13 (5): 499-508.

Bray, G., S.J. Nielsen, and B. Popkin. 2004. Consumption of high-fructose corn syrup in beverages may play a role in the epidemic of obesity. *Am J Clin Nutr* 79: 537-543.

Breyere, O., C. Cooper, J. Pelletier, et al. 2016. A consensus statement on the European Society for Clinical and Economic Aspects of Osteoporosis and Osteoarthritis (ESCEO) algorithm for the management of knee osteoarthritis-From evidence-based medicine to the real-life setting. *Semin Arthritis Rheum* 45 (4 Suppl): S3-11.

Brik, M., I. Fernandez-Buhigas, and A. Martin-Arias. 2019. Does exercise during pregnancy impact on maternal weight gain and fetal cardiac function? A randomized controlled study. *Ultrasound Obstet Gynecol* 53(5): 583-589. doi: 10.1002/uog.20147.

Brown L., A. Midgley, R. Vince, L.A. Madden, and L.R. McNaughton. 2013. High versus low glycemic index 3-h recovery diets following glycogen-depleting exercise has no effect on subsequent 5-km cycling time trial performance. *J Sci Med Sport* 16 (5): 450-454.

Bryant S., K. McLaughlin, K. Morgaine, and B. Drummond. 2011. Elite athletes and oral health. *Int J Sports Med* 32 (9): 720-724.

Buijsse, B., E. Feskens, F. Kok, and D. Kromhout. 2006. Cocoa intake, blood pressure, and cardiovascular mortality: The Zutphen Elderly Study. *Arch Intern Med* 166 (4): 411-417.

Burdon, C., I. Spronk. H. Cheng, and H.T. O'Connor. 2017. Effect of glycemic index of a pre-exercise meal on endurance exercise performance: A systematic review and meta-analysis. *Sports Med* 47 (6): 1087-1101.

Burke, L. 2010. Fueling strategies to optimize performance: Training high or training low? *Scand J Med Sci Sports* 20 (Suppl. no. 2): 48-58.

Burke, L., G. Collier, and M. Hargreaves. 1998. Glycemic index: A new tool in sports nutrition? *Int J Sport Nutr* 8: 401-415.

Burke, L., and J. Hawley. 2018. Swifter higher, stronger: What's on the menu? *Science* 362: 781-787.

Burke, L., J. Hawley, S. Wong and A. Jeukendrup. 2011. Carbohydrates for training and competition. *J Sports Sci* 29 (Suppl. no. 1): S17-S27.

Burke, L., M. Ross, L. Garvican-Lewis, et al. 2017. Low carbohydrate, high fat diet impairs exercise economy and negates the performance benefit from intensified training in elite race walkers. *J Physiol.* 595 (9): 2785-2807.

Burke L., L. van Loon, and J. Hawley. 2017. Postexercise muscle glycogen resynthesis in humans. *J Appl Physiol* 122: 1055-1067.

Campbell, C., D. Prince, E. Applegate, and G. Casazza. 2007. Effect of carbohydrate supplementation type on endurance cycling performance in competitive athletes. *Med Sci Sports Exerc* 39 (Suppl. no. 5): Abstract 1760.

Carrera, O., R. Adan, E. Gutierrez, U. Danner, H. Hoek, et al. 2012. Hyperactivity in anorexia nervosa: Warming up not just burning-off calories. *PLoS ONE* 7 (7): e41851. doi:10.1371/journal.pone.0041851.

Case, S. 2016. *Gluten-free diet: The definitive resource guide.* Regina, Saskatchewan: Case Nutrition Consulting.

Casa, D., L. Armstrong, S. Montain, et al. 2000. National Athletic Trainers' Association position statement: Fluid replacement for athletes. *J Athletic Training* 35 (2): 212-224.

Casa, D., J. DeMartini, and M. Bergeron. 2015. National Athletic Trainers' Association position statement: Exertional heat illness. *J Athl Train* 50 (9): 986-1000.

Centers for Disease Control and Prevention. *National diabetes statistics report, 2017.* Atlanta, GA: Centers for Disease Control and Prevention, U.S. Department of Health and Human Services.

Center for Science in the Public Interest (CSPI). 2006a. Are you deficient? *Nutrition Action Healthletter* 33 (9): 3-7.

Center for Science in the Public Interest (CSPI). 2006b. Pour better or pour worse: How beverages stack up. *Nutrition Action Healthletter* 33 (5): 3-7.

Center for Science in the Public Interest (CSPI). 2012. Going organic: What's the payoff? https://cspinet.org/tip/going-organic-whats-payoff.

Chapman, C., C. Benedict, S. Brooks, and H. Schioth. 2012. Lifestyle determinants of the drive to eat: A meta-analysis. *Am J Clin Nutr* 96 (3): 492-497.

Chowdhury, R., S. Warnakula, S. Kunutsor, F. Crowe, et al. 2014. Association of dietary, circulating, and supplement fatty acids with coronary risk: A systematic review and meta-analysis. *Annals Intern Med* 160 (6): 398-406.

Clancy, R.L., M. Gleeson, A. Cox, et al. 2006. Reversal in fatigued athletes of a defect in interferon gamma secretion after administration of *Lactobacillus acidophilus*. *Br J Sports Med* 40 (4): 351-354.

Clayton, D., A. Barutcu, C. Machin, et al. 2015. Effect of breakfast omission on energy intake and evening exercise performance. *Med Sci Sports Exerc* 47 (12): 2645-2652.

ConsumerLab.com. 2007. Product review: Joint supplements. www.consumerlab.com/results/gluco.asp.

Consumer Reports. 2018. Arsenic, lead found in popular protein supplements. www.consumerreports.org/dietary-supplements/heavy-metals-in-protein-supplements.

Cook, N.R., J. Cutler, E. Obarzanek, et al. 2007. Long-term effects of dietary sodium reduction on cardiovascular disease outcomes: Observational follow-up of the trials of hypertension prevention (TOHP). *Br Med J* 334 (7599): 885.

Costill, D., R. Bowers, G. Branam, and K. Sparks. 1971. Muscle glycogen utilization during prolonged exercise on successive days. *J Appl Physiol* 31 (6): 834-838.

Costill, D.L., D.S. King, R. Thomas, and M. Hargreaves. 1985. Effects of reduced training on muscular power in swimmers. *Phys Sportsmed* 13 (2): 94-101.

Costill, D.L., W. Sherman, W. Fink, C. Maresh, M. Witten, and J. Miller. 1981. The role of dietary carbohydrate in muscle glycogen resynthesis after strenuous exercise. *Am J Clin Nutr* 34: 1831-1836.

Costill, D.L., R. Thomas, R.A. Robergs, et al. 1991. Adaptations to swimming training: Influence of training volume. *Med Sci Sports Exerc* 23 (3): 371-377.

Cribb, P., and A. Hayes. 2006. Effects of supplement timing and resistance exercise on skeletal muscle hypertrophy. *Med Sci Sports Exerc* 38 (1): 1918-1925.

Cribb, P., A. Williams, and A. Hayes. 2007. A creatine-protein-carbohydrate supplement enhances responses to resistance training. *Med Sci Sports Exerc* 39 (11): 1960-1968.

Davis, S., C. Castelo-Branco, P. Chedrual, M. Lumsden, R. Nappi, D. Shah, P. Villaseca, and Writing Group of the Society from World Menopause Day 2012. 2012. Understanding weight gain at menopause. *Climacteric* 15 (5): 419-429.

Davison, G., M. Gleeson, and S. Phillips. 2007. Antioxidant supplementation and immunoendocrine responses to prolonged exercise. *Med Sci Sports Exerc* 39 (4): 645-652.

DellaValle, D., and J. Haas. 2011. Impact of iron depletion without anemia on performance in trained endurance athletes at the beginning of a training season: A study of female collegiate rowers. *Int J Sports Nutr Exerc Metab* 21 (6): 501-506.

de Oliveira Otto, M., R. Lemaitre, X. Song, I. King, D. Siscovick, and D. Mozaffarian. 2018. Serial measures of circulating biomarkers of dairy fat and total and cause-specific mortality in older adults: The Cardiovascular Health Study. *Am J Clin Nutr* 108 (3): 476-484.

de Oliveira Otto, M., D. Mozaffarian, D. Kromhout, A. Bertoni, C. Sibley, D. Jacobs Jr, and J. Nettleton. 2012. Dietary intake of saturated fat by food source and incident cardiovascular disease: The multi-ethnic study of atherosclerosis. *Am J Clin Nutr* 96 (2): 397-404.

de Souza R., A. Mente, A. Maroleanu, et al. 2015. Intake of saturated and trans unsaturated fatty acids and risk of all cause mortality, cardiovascular disease, and type 2 diabetes: Systematic review and meta-analysis of observational studies. *BMJ* 11:351:h3978. doi: 10.1136/bmj.h3978.

Demura, S., S. Yamaji, F. Goshi, and Y. Nagasawa. 2002. The influence of transient change of total body water on relative body fats based on three bioelectrical impedance analyses methods. Comparison between before and after exercise with sweat loss, and after drinking. *J Sports Med Phys Fitness* 42 (1): 38-44.

Denny, K., K. Loth, M. Eisenberg, and D. Neumark-Sztainer. 2013. Intuitive eating in young adults: Who is doing it, and how is it related to disordered eating behaviors? *Appetite* 60 (11): 13-19.

Deutz, R., D. Benardot, D. Martin, and M. Cody. 2000. Relationship between energy deficits and body composition in elite female gymnasts and runners. *Med Sci Sports Exerc* 32 (3): 659-668.

DiNioloantonio, J., and J. O'Keefe. 2018. In critique of "In Defense of Sugar": The nuance of whole foods. *Prog Cardiovas Dis* 61 (3-4): 384-385. doi.org/10.1016/j.pcad.2018.07.006.

Doering, T., D. Jenkins, P. Reaburn, et al. 2016. Lower integrated muscle protein synthesis in masters compared with younger athletes. *Med Sci Sports Exerc* 48 (8): 1613-1618.

Doherty, M., and P. Smith. 2005. Effects of caffeine ingestion on the rating of perceived exertion during and after exercise: A meta-analysis. *Scand J Med Sci Sports* 15 (2): 69-78.

Dolan, E., B. Gualano, E. Rawson. 2018. Beyond muscle: The effects of creatine supplementation on brain creatine, cognitive processing, and traumatic brain injury. *Eur J Sports Sci* Aug 7: 1-14. doi: 10.1080/17461391.2018.1500644.

Dolan, E., and C. Sale. 2019. Protein and bone health across the lifespan. *Proc Nutr Sci* 78 (1): 45-55.

Dominguez, J., L. Goodman, S. Sen Gupta, et al. 2007. Treatment of anorexia nervosa is associated with increases in bone mineral density, and recovery is a biphasic process involving both nutrition and return of menses. *Am J Clin Nutr* 86 (1): 92-99.

Drewnowski, A., and F. Bellisle. 2007. Liquid calories, sugar, and body weight. *Am J Clin Nutr* 85: 651-661.

Dueck, C., K. Matt, M. Manore, and J. Skinner. 1996. Treatment of athletic amenorrhea with a diet and training intervention program. *Int J Sport Nutr and Exerc Metab* 6 (1): 24-40.

Environmental Working Group. 2018. Shopper's guide to pesticides in produce. www.ewg.org/foodnews/dirty-dozen.php.

Environmental Protection Agency. n.d. www.epa.gov/ghgemissions/inventory-us-greenhouse-gas-emissions-and-sinks. Accessed November 4, 2018.

Erskine, R., G. Fletcher, B. Hanson, and J. Folland. 2012. Whey protein does not enhance the adaptations to elbow flexor resistance training. *Med Sci Sports Exerc* 44 (9): 1791-1800.

Expert Panel on Detection, Evaluation, and Treatment of High Blood Cholesterol in Adults. 2001. Executive summary of the third report of the National Cholesterol Education Program Expert Panel on detection, evaluation, and treatment of high cholesterol in adults. *JAMA* 285: 2486-2497.

Fallaize, R., L. Wilson, J. Gray, L.M. Morgan, and B. Griffin. 2013. Variation in the effects of three different breakfast meals on subjective satiety and subsequent intake of energy at lunch and evening meal. *Eur J Nutr,* 52 (4): 1353-1359.

Fairchild, T., S. Fletcher, P. Steele, C. Goodman, B. Dawson, and P. Fournier. 2002. Rapid carbohydrate loading after a short bout of near maximal-intensity exercise. *Med Sci Sports Exerc* 34 (6): 980-986.

Ferreira, S.E., M.T. de Mello, S. Pompeia, and M.L. de Souza-Formigoni. 2006. Effects of energy drink ingestion on alcohol intoxication. *Alcohol Clin Exp Res* 30 (4): 598-605.

Fiolet, T., B. Srour, L. Sellem, et al. 2018. Consumption of ultra-processed foods and cancer risk: Results from NutriNet-Santé prospective cohort. *BMJ* 14:360:k322. doi: 10.1136/bmj.k322.

Flakoll, P., T. Judy, K. Flinn, C. Carr, and S. Flinn. 2004. Postexercise protein supplementation improves health and muscle soreness during basic military training in marine recruits. *J Appl Physiol* 96 (3): 951-956.

Floegel, A., T. Pischon, M. Bergmann, B. Teucher, R. Kaaks, and H. Boeing. 2012. Coffee consumption and risk of chronic disease in the European Prospective Investigation into Cancer and Nutrition (EPIC)—German study. *Am J Clin Nutr* 95 (4): 901-908.

Flores-Mateo, G., D. Rojas-Rueda, J. Basora, E. Ros, and J. Salas-Salvado. 2013. Nut intake and adiposity: Meta-analysis of clinical trials. *Am J Clin Nutr* 97 (6): 1346-1355.

Food and Nutrition Board, Institute of Medicine. 1998/2000. *Dietary reference intakes.* Lanover, MD: National Academy Press.

Forman, J., J. Silverstein, Committee on Nutrition, and Council on Environmental Health. 2012. Organic foods: Health and environmental advantages and disadvantages. *Pediatrics* 130 (5): e1406-1415.

Forouhi, N., R. Krauss, G. Taubes, and W. Willet. 2018. Dietary fat and cardiometabolic health: Evidence, controversies, and consensus for guidance *BMJ* 361:k2139.

Franz, M.J. 2003. Glycemic index: Not the most effective nutrition therapy intervention. *Diabetes Care* 26: 2466-2468.

Fredericson, M., and K. Kent. 2005. Normalization of bone density in a previously amenorrheic runner with osteoporosis. *Med Sci Sports Exerc* 37 (9): 1481-1486.

Friedmann D., G. Vick, and V. Mishra. 2017. Cellulite: A review with a focus on subcision. *Clin Cosmet Investig Dermatol* 10: 17-23.

Fuglestad, P., R. Jeffery, and N. Sherwood. 2012. Lifestyle patterns associated with diet, physical activity, body mass index and amount of recent weight loss in a sample of successful weight losers. *Int J Behav Nutr Phys Act* 26 (9): 79. doi: 10.1186/1479-5868-9-79.

Fuller N., I. Caterson, A. Sainsbury, et al. 2015. Effect of a high-egg diet on cardiovascular risk factors in people with type 2 diabetes: The Diabetes and Egg (DIABEGG) Study—a 3-month randomized controlled trial. *Am J Clin Nutr* 101 (4): 705-13.

Garner, D. 1998. The effects of starvation on behavior: Implications for dieting and eating disorders. *HWJ* 12 (5): 68-72.

Gardner, C., J. Trepanowski, L. Del Gobbo, et al. 2018. Effect of low-fat vs low-carbohydrate diet on 12-month weight loss in overweight adults and the association with genotype pattern or insulin secretion: The DIETFITS randomized clinical trial. *JAMA* 319 (7): 667-679.

Getchell, B., and W. Anderson. 1982. *Being fit: A personal guide.* New York: Wiley.

Gilhooly, C., S.K. Das, J.K. Golden, et al. 2007. Food cravings and energy regulation: The characteristics of craved foods and their relationship with eating behaviors and weight change during 6 months of dietary energy restriction. *Int J Obes* 31 (12): 1849-1858.

Gold, E., K. Leung, S. Crawford, et al. 2013. Phytoestrogen and fiber intakes in relation to incident vasomotor symptoms: Results from the study of women's health across the nation. *Menopause*, 20 (3): 305-314.

Gordon, C., K. Ackerman, S. Berga, et al. 2017. Functional hypothalamic amenorrhea: An Endocrine Society clinical practice guideline. *J Clin Endocrinol Metab* 102 (5): 1-27.

Green, H., M. Ball-Burnett, S. Jones, and B. Farrance. 2007. Mechanical and metabolic responses with exercise and dietary carbohydrate manipulation. *Med Sci Sports Exerc* 39 (1): 139-148.

Greene, R., S. Godek, A. Burkholder, and C. Peduzzi. 2007. Sweat sodium and total sodium losses in NFL players with exercise associated muscle cramps during training camp vs matched non-crampers. *Med Sci Sports Exerc* 39: 5 (Suppl) Abstract 574.

Gwacham, N., and D. Wagner. 2012. Acute effects of a caffeine-taurine energy drink on repeated sprint performance of American college football players. *Int J Sports Nutr Exerc Metab* 22 (2): 109-116.

Haakstad, L., and K. Bo. 2011. Effect of regular exercise on prevention of excessive weight gain in pregnancy: A randomised controlled trial. *Eur J Contracept Reprod Health Care* 16 (2): 116-25.

Hansen, A., C. Fischer, P. Plomgaard, J. Andersen, B. Saltin, and B. Pedersen. 2005. Skeletal muscle adaptation: Training twice every second day vs training once daily. *J Appl Physiol* 98: 93-99.

Helms, E., C. Zinn, D. Rowlands, and S. Brown. 2014. A systematic review of dietary protein during caloric restriction in resistance trained lean athletes: A case for higher intakes. *Intl J Sports Nutr Exerc Metab* 24 (2): 127-138.

Hemila H., and E. Chalker. 2013. Vitamin C for preventing and treating the common cold. *Cochrane Database Sust Rev* 31: (1) CD000980. doi: 10.1002/14651858. CD000980.pub4.

Heneghan, C., J. Howick, B. O'Neill, P. Gill, D. Lasserson, D. Cohen, R. Davis, A. Ward, A. Smith, and G. Jones. 2012. The evidence underpinning sports performance products: A systematic assessment. *BMJ Open* 2: e001702. doi:10.1136/bmjopen-2012-001702.

Heydari, M., J. Freund, and S. Boutcher. 2012. The effect of high-intensity intermittent exercise on body composition of overweight young males. *J Obes*: 480467. doi: 10.1155/2012/480467.

Hickner, R., C. Horswill, J. Welker, J. Scott, J. Roemmich, and D. Costill. 1991. Test development for the study of physical performance in wrestlers following weight loss. *Int J Sports Med* 12 (6): 557-562.

Hills, A., N. Byrne, R. Lindstrom, J. Hill. 2013. "Small changes" to diet and physical activity behaviors for weight management. *Obes Facts* 6 (3): 228-238.

Hill, J.O., W. McArdle, J. Snook, and J. Wilmore. 1992. *Commonly asked questions regarding nutrition and exercise: What does the scientific literature suggest?* Vol. 9 of *Sports Science Exchange*. Chicago: Gatorade Sports Science Institute.

Hoffman M., and K. Stuempfle. 2015. Muscle cramping during a 161-km ultramarathon: Comparison of characteristics of those with and without cramping. *Sports Med Open* 1 (1): 24.

Hollcamp, W. 2012. Obesogens: An environmental link to obesity. *Environ Health Perspect* 120 (2): a62-168. www.medscape.com/viewarticle/758210.

Holway, F., and L. Spriet. 2011. Sport-specific nutrition: Practical strategies for team sports. *J Sports Sci* 29 (Suppl. no. 1): S115-S125.

Hottenrott, K., E. Hass, M. Kraus, G. Neumann, M. Steiner, and B. Knechtie. 2012. A scientific nutrition strategy improves time trial performance by ~6% when compared with a self-chosen nutrition strategy in trained cyclists: A randomized cross-over study. *Appl Physiol Nutr Metab* 37 (4): 637-645.

Houmard, J.A., D.L. Costill, J.B. Mitchell, S.H. Park, R.C. Hickner, and J.N. Roemmich. 1990. Reduced training maintains performance in distance runners. *Int J Sports Med* 11 (1): 46-52.

Huang, H.Y., B. Caballero, S. Chang, et al. 2006. The efficacy and safety of multivitamin and mineral supplement use to prevent cancer and chronic disease in adults: A systematic review for a National Institutes of Health state-of-the-science conference. *Ann Intern Med* 145 (5): 372-385.

Howe, S., T. Hand, and M. Manore. 2014. Exercise-trained men and women: Role of exercise and diet on appetite and energy intake. *Nutrients* 6 (11): 4935-4960.

Institute of Medicine. 1994. *Fluid replacement and heat stress*. Washington, DC: National Academy Press.

Institute of Medicine. 2009. *Weight gain during pregnancy: Reexamining the guidelines*. Washington, DC: National Academies Press.

International Olympic Committee. 2011. IOC consensus on sports nutrition 2010. *J Sports Sci* 29 (Suppl. no. 1): S3-4.

Jakubowicz D., O. Froy, J. Wainstein, and M. Boaz. 2012. Meal timing and composition influence ghrelin levels, appetite scores and weight loss maintenance in overweight and obese adults. *Steroids* 77 (4): 323-331.

Janssen, G., C. Graef, and W. Saris. 1989. Food intake and body composition in novice athletes during a training period to run a marathon. *Int J Sports Med* 10: S17-21.

Jentjens, R.L., K. Underwood, J. Achten, K. Currell, C.H. Mann, and A.E. Jeukendrup. 2006. Exogenous carbohydrate oxidation rates are elevated after combined ingestion of glucose and fructose during exercise in the heat. *J Appl Physiol* 100 (3): 807-816.

Jiang, R., J.E. Manson, M.J. Stampfer, S. Liu, W.C. Willett, and F.B. Hu. 2002. Nut and peanut butter consumption and risk of type 2 diabetes in women. *JAMA* 288 (20): 2554-2560.

Johannesson, E., M. Simren, H. Strid, A. Bajor, and R. Sadik. 2011. Physical activity improves symptoms in irritable bowel syndrome: A randomized controlled trial. *Am J Gastroenterol* 106 (5): 915-922.

Johnson, C., A. Davenport, M. Hansen, and D. Bacharach. 2010. Pre-competition hydration status of high school athletes participating in different sports. *Med Sci Sports Exerc* 42 (5): S128 (Abstract 1149).

Johnson, S., H. Park, C. Gross, et al. 2018. Complementary medicine, refusal of conventional cancer therapy, and survival among patients with curable cancers. *JAMA Oncol* Published online July 19, 2018. doi:10.1001/jamaoncol.2018.2487.

Joy. E., A. Kussman, and A. Nattiv. 2016. Update on eating disorders in athletes: A comprehensive narrative review with a focus on clinical assessment and management. *Br J Sports Med* 50: 154-162.

Joy, J., R. Vogel, K. Shane Broughton, U. Kudla, N. Kerr, J. Davison, R. Wildman, and N. DiMarco. 2018. Daytime and nighttime casein supplements similarly increase muscle size and strength in response to resistance training earlier in the day: A preliminary investigation. *J Int Soc Sports Nutr* 15: 24. doi: 10.1186/s12970-018-0228-9.

Jones A., S. Bailey, and A. Vanhatalo. 2013. Dietary nitrate and O_2 consumption during exercise. *Med Sports Sci* 59: 29-35.

Joy E., A. Kussman, and A. Nattiv. 2016. 2016 update on eating disorders in athletes: A comprehensive narrative review with a focus on clinical assessment and management. *Br J Sports Med* 50: 154-162.

Jeukendrup, A. 2017. Training the gut for athletes. *Sports Med* 47 (Suppl 1): S101-S110.

Kahleova H., J. Lloren, A. Mashchak, et al. 2017. Meal frequency and timing are associated with changes in body mass index in Adventist Health Study 2. *J Nutr* 147 (9): 1722-1728.

Kahwati L., R. Weber, H. Pan, et al. 2018. Vitamin D, calcium, or combined supplementation for the primary prevention of fractures in community-dwelling adults: Evidence report and systematic review for the US Preventive Services Task Force. *JAMA* 319 (15): 1600-1612.

Kapoor, E., M. Collazo-Clavell, and S. Faubion. 2017. Weight gain in women at midlife: A concise review of the pathophysiology and strategies for management. *Mayo Clin Proc.* 92 (10): 1552-1558.

Karp, J., J. Johnston, S. Tecklenburg, T. Mickleborough, A. Fly, and J. Stager. 2006. Chocolate milk as a post-exercise recovery aid. *Int J Sports Nutr Exerc Metab* 16: 78-91.

Karppanen, H., and E. Mervaala. 2006. Sodium intake and hypertension. *Prog Cardiovasc Dis* 49 (2): 59-75.

Karsch-Volk M., B. Barrett, and K. Linde. 2015. Echinacea for preventing and treating the common cold. *JAMA* 313 (6): 618-619.

Keay, N., G. Francis, and K. Hind. 2018. Low energy availability assessed by a sport-specific questionnaire and clinical interview indicative of bone health, endocrine profile and cycling performance in competitive male cyclists. *BMJ Open Sport Exerc Med* 4 (1): e000424. doi: 10.1136/bmjsem-2018-000424.

Kerr, K., et al. 2008. Effects of pre-exercise nutrient timing on glucose responses and intermittent exercise performance. *Med Sci Sports Exerc* 40 (Suppl. no. 5): S77.

Keys, A., J. Brozek, A. Henschel, et al. 1950. *The biology of human starvation*. Vols. I and II. Minneapolis: University of Minnesota Press.

Kirk, E.P., J. Donnelly, and D. Jacobsen. 2002. Time course and gender effects in aerobic capacity and body composition for overweight individuals: Midwest Exercise Trial (MET). *Med Sci Sports Exerc* 34 (Suppl. no. 5): 120.

Knowler, W.C., E. Barrett-Conner, S.E. Fowler, et al. 2002. Reduction in the incidence of type II diabetes with lifestyle intervention or metformin. *N Eng J Med* 346: 393-403.

Kris-Etherton, P., G. Zhao, A.E. Binkoski, S.M. Coval, and T.D. Etherton. 2001. The effects of nuts on coronary heart disease. *Nutr Rev* 59 (4): 103-111.

Lambert C. 2018. Exercise training alters the glycemic response to carbohydrates and is an important consideration when evaluating dietary carbohydrate intake. *J Intl Soc Sport Med* 15: 53.

Lavie, C. 2018. Sugar wars – commentary from the editor. *Prog Cardiovasc Dis* 61 (3-4): 382-383. doi.10.1016/j.pcad.2018.07.007.

Leibel, R.L., M. Rosenbaum, and J. Hirsch. 1995. Changes in energy expenditure resulting from altered body weight. *N Engl J Med* 332: 621-628.

Leone, J., E. Sedory, and K. Gray. 2005. Recognition and treatment of muscle dysmorphia and related body image disorders. *J Athl Train* 40 (4): 352-359.

Levine, J., N. Eberhardt, and M. Jensen. 1999. Role of non-exercise activity thermogenesis in resistance to fat gain in humans. *Science* 282 (5399): 212-214.

Liu, X., G.C. Machado, J.P. Eyles, et al. 2018. Dietary supplements for treating osteoarthritis: A systematic review and meta-analysis. *Br J Sports Med.* 52: 167-175.

Lovelady, C. 2011. Balancing exercise and food intake with lactation to promote postpartum weight loss. *Proc Nutr Soc* 70 (2): 181-184.

Lowndes, J., D. Kawiecki, S. Pardo, V. Nguyen, K. Melanson, Z. Yu, and J. Rippe. 2012. The effects of four hypocaloric diets containing different levels of sucrose or high fructose corn syrup on weight loss and related parameters. *Nutr J* 11 (1): 55.

Lutter, J., and S. Cushman. 1982. Running while pregnant. *J Melpomene Institute* 1 (1): 2-4.

Macpherson, H., A. Pipingas, and M. Pase. 2013. Multivitamin-multimineral supplementation and mortality: A meta-analysis of randomized controlled trials. *Am J Clin Nutr,* 97 (2): 237-238.

Manson, J., E. Lee, W. Christen, et al. 2019. Marine n-3 Fatty Acids and Prevention of Cardiovascular Disease and Cancer. *New Eng J Med.* 380 (1): 23-32.

Marczinski, C.A., and M.T. Fillmore. 2006. Clubgoers and their trendy cocktails: Implications of mixing caffeine into alcohol on information processing and subjective reports of intoxication. *Exp Clin Psychopharmacol* 14 (4): 450-458.

Martin, W., L. Armstrong, and N. Rodriquez. 2005. Dietary protein intake and renal function. *Nutr Metab* (Lond) 20 (2): 25.

Mason, W.L., G. McConell, and M. Hargreaves. 1993. Carbohydrate ingestion during exercise: Liquid vs. solid feedings. *Med Sci Sports Exerc* 25 (8): 966-969.

Mathews, N., 2018. Prohibited contaminants in dietary supplements. *Sports Health* 10 (1): 19-30.

Maughan, R., L. Burke, J. Dvorak, et al. 2018. IOC Consensus Statement: Dietary supplements and the high-performance athlete. *Br J Sports Med* 52 (7): 439-455.

Maughan, R., P. Watson, P. Cordery, Walsh N., Oliver S., Dolci A., Rodriguez-Sanchez N., and Galloway S. 2016. A randomized trial to assess the potential of different beverages to affect hydration status: Development of a beverage hydration index. *Am J Clin Nutr* 103: 717-723.

McDermott, B.P., S. Anderson, L. Armstrong, D. Casa, S. Cheuvront, L. Cooper, W. Kenney, F. O'Connor, and W. Roberts. 2017 National Athletic Trainers' Association position statement: Fluid replacement for the physically active. *J Athl Train* 52 (9): 877-895.

McManus, K., L. Antinoro, and F. Sacks.2001. A randomized controlled trial of a moderate fat, low-energy diet compared with a low-fat, low energy diet for weight loss in overweight adults. *Int J Obes Relat Metab Disord* 25: 1503-1511.

McSwiney, F., B. Wardrop, P. Hyde, et al. 2018. Keto-adaptation enhances exercise performance and body composition responses to training in endurance athletes. *Metabolism* 81: 25-34.

Messina, M. 2010. Soybean isoflavone exposure does not have feminizing effects on men: A critical examination of the clinical evidence. *Fertil Steril* 93 (7): 2095-2104.

Miller, K., E. Lee, E. Lawson, et al. 2006. Determinants of skeletal loss and recovery in anorexia nervosa. *J Endocrinol Metab* 91 (8): 2931-2937.

Mountjoy, M., J. Sundgot-Borgen, L. Burke, et al. (2014) The IOC consensus statement: Beyond the female athlete triad—relative energy deficiency in sport (RED-S). *Br J Sports Med* 48: 491-497.

Moore, L., A. Midgley, S. Thurlow, G. Thomas, and L. McNaughton. 2010. Effect of the glycaemic index of a pre-exercise meal on metabolism and cycling time trial performance. *J Sci Med Sport* 13 (1): 182-188.

Moore D.R., Robinson M.J., Fry J.L., Tang J.E., Glover E.I., Wilkinson S.B., Prior T., Tarnopolsky M.A., and Phillips SM. 2009. Ingested protein dose response of muscle and albumin protein synthesis after resistance exercise in young men. *Am J Clin Nutr* 89 (1): 161-168.

Morgan, J., F. Reid, and J. Lacey. 1999. The SCOFF questionnaire: Assessment of a new screening tool for eating disorders. *BMJ* 319 (7223): 1467-1468.

Morton J., C. Robertson, L. Sutton, et al. 2010. Making the weight: A case study from professional boxing. *Intl J Sport Nutr Exerc Metab* 20: 80-85.

Mosca, L., C. Banka, E. Benjamin, et al. 2007. Evidence-based guidelines for cardiovascular disease prevention in women: 2007 update. *Circulation* 115 (7): 1481-1501.

Mujika, I. 2010. Intense training: The key to optimal performance. *Scand J Med Sci Sports* 20 (Suppl. no. 2): 24-31.

Mursu, J., K. Robien, L. Harnack, K. Park, and D. Jacobs. 2011. Dietary supplements and mortality rate in older women: The Iowa Women's Health Study. *Arch Intern Med* 171 (18): 1625-1633.

Napoli, N., J. Thompson, R. Civitelli, and R. Armamento-Villareal. 2007. Effects of dietary calcium compared with calcium supplements on estrogen metabolism and bone mineral density. *Am J Clin Nutr* 85: 1428-1433.

National Eating Disorders Association. 2005. No weigh! A declaration of independence from a weight-obsessed world. www.nationaleatingdisorders.org.

National Institutes of Health. 2007. National Institutes of Health state-of-the-science conference statement: Multi-vitamin and mineral supplements and chronic disease prevention. *Am J Clin Nutr* 85 (1): 257S-264S.

Nattiv, A. 2000. Stress fractures and bone health in track and field athletes. *J Sci Med Sport* 3 (3): 268-279.

Neumark-Sztainer, D., M. Wall, J. Guo, M. Story, J. Haines, and M. Eisenhberg. 2006. Obesity, disordered eating, and eating disorders in a longitudinal study of adolescents: How do dieters fare five years later? *J Amer Diet Assoc* 106: 559-568.

Nieman, D., D. Henson, S. McAnulty, et al. 2004. Vitamin E and immunity after the Kona Triathlon World Championship. *Med Sci Sports Exerc* 36 (8): 1328-1335.

Noakes, T. 2003. *Lore of running*, 4th ed. Champaign, IL: Human Kinetics.

Novak, C., C. Escande, P. Burghardt, M. Zhang. M. Barbosa, E. Chini, S. Britton, L. Koch, H. Akil, and J. Levine. 2010. Spontaneous activity, economy of activity, and resistance to diet-induced obesity in rats bred for high intrinsic aerobic capacity. *Horm Behav* 58 (3): 355-367.

O'Dea, J., and P. Rawstorne. 2001. Male adolescents identify their weight gain practices, reasons for desired weight gain, and sources of weight gain information. *J Amer Diet Assoc* 101 (1): 105-107.

Ode, J., J. Pivarnik, M. Reeves, and J. Knous. 2007. Body mass index as a predictor of percent fat in college athletes and nonathletes. *Med Sci Sports Exerc* 39 (3): 403-409.

Office of Disease Prevention and Health Promotion (ODPHP). 2018 Physical Activity Guidelines Advisory Committee scientific report. https://health.gov/paguidelines/second-edition/report.

Olivardia, R. 2002. Body image obsession in men. *HWJ* 16 (4): 59-63.

Ortega, F., D. Lee, P. Katzmarzyk, J. Ruiz, X. Sui, T. Church, and S. Blair. 2012. The intriguing metabolically healthy but obese phenotype: Cardiovascular prognosis and role of fitness. *Eur Heart J.* 34 (5): 389-397. doi: 10.1093/eurheartj/ehs174.

Otterstetter, R., J. Viar, J. Naylor, S. Krone, and K. Tessmer. 2012. Effects of acute exercise on the accuracy of air-displacement plethysmography in young adults. *Med Sci Sports Exerc* 44 (5S): S591.

Owens, D., R. Allison, G. Close. 2018. Vitamin D and the athlete: Current perspectives and new challenges. *Sports Med* 48 (Suppl 1): S3-S16.

Paoli, A., K. Grimaldi, D. D'Agostino, L. Cenci, T. Moro, A. Bianco, and A. Palma. 2012. Ketogenic diet does not affect strength performance in elite artistic gymnasts. J Int Soc Sports Nutr 9 (1): 34. doi: 10.1186/1550-2783-9-34.

Pasman, W., M. van Baak, A. Jeukendrup, and A. de Haan. 1995. The effects of different dosages of caffeine on endurance performance time. Int J Sports Med 16: 225-230.

Peterson, J., W. Repovich, M. Eash, D. Notrica, and C. Hill. 2007. Accuracy of consumer grade bioelectrical impedance analysis devices compared to air displacement plethysmography. Med Sci Sports Exerc 39 (5) (Suppl): Abstract 2105.

Petyaev I., and Y. Bashmakov. 2012. Could cheese be the missing piece in the French paradox? Med Hypotheses (12) 00385-4: S0306-9877. doi: 10.1016/j.mehy.2012.08.018. 79 (6): 746-749.

Phillips S., S. Chevalier, H. Leidy. 2016 Protein "requirement" beyond the RDA: Implications for optimizing health. Appl Phys Nutr Metab 41 (5): 565-572.

Phillips, P., B. Rolls, J. Ledingham, et al. 1984. Reduced thirst after water deprivation in healthy elderly men. N Engl J Med 311: 753-759.

Phillips, S., and van Loon, L. 2011. Dietary protein for athletes: From requirements to optimum adaptation. J Sports Sci 29 (Suppl 1): S29-S38.

Piercy, K., R. Troiano, R. Ballard, et al. 2018. The physical activity guidelines for Americans. JAMA 320 (19): 2020-2028.

Pritchard H., M. Barnes, R. Steward, J. Keogh, and M. McGuigan. 2018. Short-term training cessation as a method of tapering to improve maximal strength. J Strength Cond Res 32 (2): 458-465.

Pyne D., N. West, A. Cox, and A. Cripps. 2015. Probiotics supplementation for athletes—clinical and physiological effects. Eur J Sport Sci 15 (1): 63-72.

Reed, S., F. Levin, and S. Evans. 2008. Changes in mood, cognitive performance and appetite in the late luteal and follicular phases of the menstrual cycle in women with and without PMDD (premenstrual dysphoric disorder). Horm Behav 54 (1): 185-193.

Ristow, M., K. Zarse, A. Oberbach, et al. 2009. Antioxidants prevent health-promoting effects of physical exercise in humans. Proc. Nat. Acad. Sci USA 106 (21): 8664-8670.

Rock, C. 2007. Primary dietary prevention: Is the fiber story over? Recent Results Cancer Res 174: 171-177.

Roffe, C., S. Sills, P. Crome, and P. Jones. 2002. Randomised, cross-over, placebo controlled trial of magnesium citrate in the treatment of chronic persistent leg cramps. Med Sci Monit 8 (5): CR326-330.

Rollo, I., and C. Williams. 2011. Effect of mouth-rinsing carbohydrate solutions on endurance performance. Sports Med 41 (6): 339-361.

Rosenkilde, M., P. Auerbach, M. Reichkendler, T. Plough, B. Stallknecht, and A. Sjolin. 2012. Body fat loss and compensatory mechanisms in response to different doses of aerobic exercise: A randomized controlled trial in overweight sedentary males. Am J Physiol Regul Integr Comp Physiol 303 (6): R571-579.

Roti, M.W., D.J. Casa, A.C. Pumerantz, et al. 2006. Thermoregulatory responses to exercise in the heat: Chronic caffeine intake has no effect. Aviat Space Environ Med 77 (2): 124-129.

Saarni, S., A. Rissanen, S. Sarna, M. Koskenvuo, and J. Kaprio. 2006. Weight cycling of athletes and subsequent gain in middle age. Int J Obes 30 (11): 1639-1644.

Sacks, F., A. Lichtenstein, J. Wu, et al. 2017. Dietary fats and cardiovascular disease: Advisory from the American Heart Association. *Circulation* 136: e1-e23.

Satter, E. 2008. *Secrets of feeding a healthy family.* Madison, WI: Kelcy Press.

Schabort, E., A. Bosch, S. Welton, and T. Noakes. 1999. The effect of a preexercise meal on time to fatigue during prolonged cycling exercise. *Med Sci Sports Exerc* 31 (3): 464-471.

Schwartz, M., R. Seeley, L. Zeltser, A. Drewnowski, et al. 2017. Obesity pathogenesis: An Endocrine Society scientific statement. *Endocr Rev* 38: 267-296.

Schreiber, K. and H.A. Hausenblas. 2015. *The truth about exercise addiction: Understanding the dark side of thinspiration.* Lanham, MD: Rowman and Littlefield.

Schwellnus, M.P., J. Nicol, R. Laubscher, and T.D. Noakes. 2004. Serum electrolyte concentrations and hydration status are not associated with exercise associated muscle cramping (EAMC) in distance runners. *Br J Sports Med* 38 (4): 488-492.

Sellmeyer, D., M. Schloetter, and A. Sebastian. 2002. Potassium citrate prevents increased urine calcium secretion and bone resorption induced by a high sodium chloride diet. *J Clin Endocrinol Metab* 87 (5): 2008-2012.

Sesso H., R. Pfaffenbarger, and I. Lee. 2000. Physical activity and coronary heart disease in men: The Harvard Alumni Health Study. *Circulation* 102 (9): 975-980.

Shang, G., M. Collins, and M. Schwellnus. 2011. Factors associated with self-reported history of exercise-associated muscle cramps in Ironman triathletes: A case-control study. *Clin J Sports Med* 21 (3): 204-210.

Shaw G., A. Lee-Barthel, M. Ross, et al. 2017. Vitamin C-enriched gelatin supplementation before intermittent activity augments collagen synthesis. *Amer J Clin Nutr* 105 (1): 136-143.

Sherman, W., G. Brodowicz, D. Wright, W. Allen, J. Simonsen, and A. Dernbach. 1989. Effects of 4 h preexercise carbohydrate feedings on cycling performance. *Med Sci Sports Exerc* 21 (5): 598-604.

Sherman, W., D. Costill, W. Fink, and J. Miller. 1981. Effect of exercise-diet manipulation on muscle glycogen and its subsequent utilization during performance. *Int J Sports Med* 2: 114-118.

Shirriffs, S., P. Watson, and R. Maughan. 2007. Milk as an effective post-exercise rehydration drink. *Br J Nutr* 98: 173-180.

Shlisky, J., T. Hartman, P. Kris-Etherton, C. Rogers, N. Sharkey, and S. Nickols-Richardson. 2012. Partial sleep deprivation and energy balance: An emerging issue for consideration by dietetics practitioners. *J Acad Nutr Diet* 112: 1785-1797.

Sievert, K., S. Hussain, M. Page, et al. 2019. Effect of breakfast on weight and energy intake: systematic review and meta-analysis of randomised controlled trials. *BMJ* 2019 364: 142 http://dx.doi.org/10.1136/bmj.l42.

Sims, E. 1976. Experimental obesity, dietary induced thermogenesis, and their clinical implications. *J Clin Endocrinol Metab* 5: 377-395.

Sims, E., and E. Danforth. 1987. Expenditure and storage of energy in man. *J Clin Invest* 79: 1-7.

Sims, S.T., L. van Vliet, J. Cotter, and N. Rehrer. 2007. Sodium loading aids fluid balance and reduces physiological strain of trained men exercising in the heat. *Med Sci Sports Exerc* 39 (1): 123-130.

Siris, E.S., P.D. Miller, E. Barrett-Connor, et al. 2001. Identification and fracture outcomes of undiagnosed low bone mineral density in postmenopausal women: Results of the National Osteoporosis Risk Assessment. *JAMA* 286 (22): 2815-2822.

Slater, G., A. Rice, K. Sharpe, D. Jenkins, and A. Hahn. 2007. The influence of nutrient intake after weigh-in on lightweight rowing performance. *Med Sci Sports Exerc* 39 (1): 184-191.

Smith, D. 2012. Review: Omega-3 polyunsaturated fatty acid supplements do not reduce major cardiovascular events in adults. *Ann Intern Med* 157 (12): JC6-5.

Smith-Spangler, C., M. Brandea, G. Hunter, J. Bavinnger, et al. 2012. Are organic foods safer or healthier than conventional alternatives? A systematic review. *Ann Intern Med* 157 (5): 348-366.

St-Onge, M., L. Ard, M. Baskin, et al. 2017. Meal timing and frequency: Implications for cardiovascular disease prevention: A scientific statement from the American Heart Association. *Circulation* 135 (9): e96-e121.

Stanhope, K., M. Goran, A. Bosy-Westphal, et al. 2018. Pathways and mechanisms linking dietary components to cardiometabolic disease: Thinking beyond calories. *Obes Rev* 19 (9): 1205-1235.

Staten, M. 1991. The effect of exercise on food intake in men and women. *Am J Clin Nutr* 53: 27-31.

Stearns, R., H. Emmanuel, J. Volek, and D. Casa. 2012. Effects of ingesting protein in combination with carbohydrate during exercise on endurance performance: A systematic review with meta-analysis. *J Strength Cond Res* 24 (8): 2192-2202.

Stellingwerff, T., R. Maughan, and L. Burke. 2011. Nutrition for power sports: Middle-distance running, track cycling, rowing, canoeing/kayaking, and swimming. *J Sports Sci* 29 (S1): S79-89.

Sternfeld, B., H. Wang, C. Quesenberry, et al. 2004. Physical activity and changes in weight and waist circumference in midlife women: Findings from the study of women's health across the nation. *Am J Epidemiol* 160 (9): 912-922.

Stevenson, E., C. Williams, H. Biscoe. 2005. The metabolic responses to high carbohydrate meals with different glycemic indices consumed during recovery from prolonged strenuous exercise. *Int J Sports Nutr Exerc Metab* 15 (3): 291-307.

Sundgot-Borgen, J., and I. Garthe. 2011. Elite athletes in aesthetic and Olympic weight-class sports and the challenge of body weight and body compositions. *J Sports Sci* 29 (Suppl. no. 1): S101-114.

Sundgot-Borgen, J., N. Meyer, T. Lohman, et al. 2013. How to minimise the health risks to athletes who compete in weight-sensitive sports review and position statement on behalf of the Ad Hoc Research Working Group on Body Composition, Health and Performance, under the auspices of the IOC Medical Commission. *Br. J. Sports Med.* 47: 1012-1022.

Syrotuik D., and G. Bell. 2004. Acute creatine monohydrate supplementation: A descriptive physiological profile of responders vs. nonresponders. *J Strength Cond Res* 18 (3): 610-617.

Taheri, S., L. Lin, D. Austin, T. Young, and E. Mignot. 2004. Short sleep duration is associated with reduced leptin, elevated ghrelin, and increased body mass index. *PLoS Med* 1 (3): E62.

Taubert, D., R. Roesen, C. Lehmann, N. Jung, and E. Schömig. 2007. Effects of low habitual cocoa intake on blood pressure and bioactive nitric oxide: A randomized controlled trial. *JAMA* 298: 49-60.

Teneforde, A., M. Barrack, A. Nattiv, and M. Frederison. 2016. Parallels with the female athlete triad in male athletes. *Sports Med* 46 (2): 171-182.

Terjung, R.L., P. Clarkson, R. Eichner, et al. 2000. American College of Sports Medicine roundtable. The physiological and health effects of oral creatine supplements. *Med Sci Sports Exerc* 32 (3): 706-717.

Teixeira, F., C. Matias, C. Monteiro, et al. 2019. Leucine metabolites do not enhance training-induced performance or muscle thickness. *Med Sci Sports Exerc* 51 (1): 56-64.

Tibana, R., and Sousa, N. 2018. Are extreme conditioning programmes effective and safe? A narrative review of high-intensity functional training methods research paradigms and findings. *BMJ Open Sport Exerc Med* 4 (1): e000435. doi:10.1136/bmjsem-2018-000435.

Tipton, K., T. Elliot, M. Cree, S. Wolf, A. Sanford, and R. Wolfe. 2004. Ingestion of casein and whey proteins result in muscle anabolism after resistance exercise. *Med Sci Sports Exerc* 36 (12): 2073-2081.

Tremblay, A., J. Despres, C. Leblanc, et al. 1990. Effect of intensity of physical activity on body fatness and fat distribution. *Am J Clin Nutr* 51: 153-157.

USDA Pesticide Data Program Annual Summary, Calendar Year 2016. www.ams.usda.gov/sites/default/files/media/2016PDPAnnualSummary.

Van Loon, L. 2013. Is there a need for protein ingestion during exercise? *Sports Science Exchange* 26 (109): 1-6.

Van Loon, L.J., R. Koopman, J.H. Stegen, A.J. Wagenmakers, H.A. Keizer, and W.H. Saris. 2003. Intramyocellular lipids form an important substrate source during moderate intensity exercise in endurance-trained males in a fasted state. *J Physiol* 553 (Pt. 2): 611-625.

van Vliet, S., N.A. Burd, and L.J. van Loon. 2015. The skeletal muscle anabolic response to plant- versus animal-based protein consumption. *J Nutr* 145 (9): 1981-1991.

van Vliet, S., E. Shy, S. Abou Sawan, J. Beals, D. West, S. Skinner, A. Ulanov, et al. 2017. Consumption of whole egg promotes greater stimulation of postexercise muscle protein synthesis than consumption of isonitrogenous amounts of egg whites in young men. *Am J Clin Nutr* 106 (6): 1401-1412.

Vega-Lopez, S., L.M. Ausman, J.L. Griffith, and A.H. Lichtenstein. 2007. Inter-individual reproducibility of glycemic index values for commercial white bread. *Diabetes Care* 30: 1412-1417.

Vertanian, L., M. Schwartz, and K. Brownell. 2007. Effects of soft drink consumption on nutrition and health: A systematic review and meta-analysis. *Am J Public Health* 97: 667-675.

Voight, B., G. Peloso, M. Orho-Melander, et al. 2012. Plasma HDL cholesterol and risk of myocardial infarction: A mendelian randomisation study. *Lancet* 380 (9841): 572-580.

Wagner, M., R. Keathley, and M. Bass. 2007. Developing a social norm intervention promotion campaign for student-athletes enrolled in a Division I-AA university. *Med Sci Sports Exerc* 39 (Suppl. no. 5): Abstract 1366.

Wallis, G., D. Rowlands, C. Shaw, R. Jentjens, and A. Jeukendrup. 2005. Oxidation of combined ingestion of maltodextrins and fructose during exercise. *Med Sci Sports Exerc* 37: 426-432.

Weaver, C. 2002. Adolescence: The period of dramatic bone growth. *Endocrine* 17: 43-48.

Wesnes, K., C. Pincock, and A. Scholey. 2012. Breakfast is associated with enhanced cognitive function in schoolchildren. An internet based study. *Appetite* 59 (3): 646-649.

Westerterp, K., G. Meijer, E. Janssen, W. Saris, and F. Ten Hoor. 1992. Long term effects of physical activity on energy balance and body composition. *Br J Med* 68 (1): 21-30.

White, R. and M. Hall. 2017. Nutritional and greenhouse gas impacts of removing animals from US agriculture. *Proc Natl Acad Sci USA* 114 (48): E10301–E10308. doi: 10.1073/pnas.1707322114.

Williams, P. 2007. Maintaining vigorous activity attenuates 7-year weight gain in 8340 runners. *Med Sci Sports Exerc* 39 (5): 801-809.

Wilmore, J., K. Wambsgans, M. Brenner, et al. 1992. Is there energy conservation in amenorrheic compared with eumenorrheic distance runners? *J Appl Physiol* 72 (1): 15-22.

Wilson, J.R., J. Lowery, J. Joy, S. Walters, J. Baier, et al. 2013. B-hydroxy-B-methylbutyrate free acid reduces markers of exercise-induced muscle damage and improves recovery in resistance-trained men. *Br J Nutr* 3: 1-7.

Wing, R., S. Belle, G. Eid, G. Dakin, W. Inabnet, et al. 2008. Physical activity levels of patients undergoing bariatric surgery in the Longitudinal Assessment of Bariatric Surgery study. *Surg Obes Relat Dis* 4 (6): 721-728.

Wing, R., and S. Phelan. 2005. Long-term weight loss maintenance. *Am J Clin Nutr* 82 (Suppl. no. 1): 222-225.

Winter, C., and S. Davis. 2006. Scientific status summary: Organic foods. *J Food Science* 71 (9): R117.

Wood A., S. Kaptoge, A. Butterworth, et al. 2018. Risk thresholds for alcohol consumption: Combined analysis of individual-participant data for 599,912 current drinkers in 83 prospective studies. *The Lancet* 391: 1513-1523.

World Cancer Research Fund and the American Institute for Cancer Research Expert Panel. 2007. Food, nutrition, physical activity and the prevention of cancer: A global perspective. www.dietandcancerreport.org.

Wyatt, H.R., G.K. Grunwald, C.L. Mosca, M.L. Klem, R.R. Wing, and J.O. Hill. 2002. Long-term weight loss and breakfast in subjects in the National Weight Control Registry. *Obes Res* 10 (2): 78-82.

Yang, Y., L. Breen, N. Burd, A. Hector, T. Churchward-Venne, A. Josse, M. Tarnopolsky, and S. Phillips. 2012. Resistance exercise enhances myofibrillar protein synthesis with graded intakes of whey protein in older men. *Br J Nutr* 108 (10): 1780-1788.

Yoshioka, M., E. Doucet, S. St-Pierre, et al. 2001. Impact of high-intensity exercise on energy expenditure, lipid oxidation and body fatness. *Int J Obes Relat Metab Disord* 25 (3): 332-339.

Zelasko, C. 1995. Exercise for weight loss: What are the facts? *J Am Diet Assoc* 95 (12): 1414-1417.

INDEX

Note: The italicized *f* and *t* following page numbers refer to figures and tables, respectively.

A

alcohol 177-180, 302, 313
altitude 263-264
amenorrhea
    athletes with 256, 352-353
    bones and 53, 54-55, 154, 239
    causes 239-241
    help for 241-243
amino acids 140-141, 148, 151-153
anemia, iron-deficiency 128, 154-157, 155*t*
anorexia 148, 336-337
antioxidants 49, 215-216, 221, 224, 269
appetite, exercise and 331
artificial sweeteners 174, 186

B

back-to-back events 205-207
beans 24, 437. *See also* recipes, beans and tofu
beef 25*t*, 26, 41-43, 91, 429. *See also* recipes, beef and pork
beetroot juice 233
beta-alanine 233-234
beta-hydroxy beta-methylbutyrate (HMB) 231-232
beverages 73-77, 75*t*, 172-176, 197*t*-198*t*. *See also* recipes, beverages and smoothies; sports drinks
binge eating disorder 339, 340-341
bioelectrical impedance analysis 291
BMI (body mass index) 288
Bod Pod measurements 290
body dysmorphic disorder 282-284
body fat
    body image and 280-282
    carbohydrates and 116-117

    exercise and 277-280
    functions of 275-276
    measurement of 271, 288-292, 292*t*
    minimum 276, 332
    percentages 276-277, 276*t*
    target 292-293
    in weight loss 324, 330
body image 280-282
body mass index (BMI) 288
bone health 19-20, 53-56, 154, 236, 239
bonking 131-132
branched-chain amino acids 141, 148
breads 97, 120, 359-360, 362-363. *See also* recipes, breakfast
breakfast 61-77. *See also* recipes, breakfast
    breakfast-to-go 63-65, 66*t*, 71-72
    coffee at 73-77, 75*t*
    foods for 67-73, 68*t*, 70*f*, 359-365
    importance 61-63
bulimia 338, 349-352
B vitamins 26, 153, 225*t*

C

caffeine. *See also* coffee
    alcohol and 175
    effects of 74, 75, 166, 185
    performance and 197, 199, 233, 234
    sources of 76, 104, 168, 174-175, 197*t*-198*t*
    women and 76-77
calcium
    amenorrhea and 242-243
    boosting intake 22, 55
    lost in sweat 164*t*

calcium *(continued)*
  muscle cramps and 209
  for older athletes 269
  requirements 19-21, 21*t*, 23, 53, 224*t*
  sources of 16, 20, 23, 69, 93*t*
  supplements 20, 53-54
  in vegan diets 23, 153
calories 316
  in beverages 173, 176*t*, 178
  boosting 299-392
  protein and 142, 153
  weight loss and 316-320, 319*t*
  in winter 261-263, 262*t*
cancer 48-51, 50*t*, 56, 148
carbohydrates 111-137
  in alcohol 177-178
  body fat and 116-117
  calculating calories of 136
  carbohydrate loading 126-137, 135*t*-136*t*, 130*t*
  constipation and 127-129
  in extended exercise 126-132, 135*t*-136*t*, 130*t*, 201-205, 202*t*, 259
  food sources of 135*t*-136*t*, 134-137
  for gastric bypass athletes 270-271
  glycemic index of 117-119, 119*t*, 120
  glycogen and 121-125, 121*t*, 122*t*, 123*t*, 124*f*
  immune system and 235
  for injured athletes 266
  in intense exercise 122-124, 122*t*, 123*t*, 167-168, 201-205, 202*t*
  in ketogenic diet 125-126, 327
  liver glycogen 132
  mouth swishing 202*t*, 204
  in muscle building 297-298, 306
  preexercise guidelines 192-193, 192*t*, 195*t*
  in recovery from daily training 132-134, 133*f*
  replenishment of 124, 124*f*, 210-211
  sugar highs and lows 120-121
  during training 111, 125, 189
  types of 112-113, 116

  weight management and 6-7, 329
  in winter 261-263, 262*t*
carotenoids 49
casein 148
celiac disease 128, 185-186. *See also* gluten free diets
cellulite 279-280
cereals 67-71, 68*t*, 70*f*
cheese 23, 46, 151
chicken 95, 403. *See also* recipes, chicken and turkey
children 152, 248-250
chocolate 28, 108-109, 212, 212*t*
chondroitin 236
coconut oil 39-40
coffee 73-77, 75*t*, 156, 197*t*-198*t*. *See also* caffeine
collagen 236
colors of fruits 10, 16, 16*t*
commercial sports foods 236-237
constipation
  in carbohydrate loading 127-129, 131
  in celiac disease 128
  diet and 6, 12, 56, 67, 127, 266, 437
coolers, traveling with 93-94
cortisol, in recovery 210
creatine 231, 307

D
dairy products 16-23
  amenorrhea and 242
  benefits of 19-20
  calcium in 16-17, 18*t*, 23, 55
  fat content in 20-21
  at gas stations 93*t*
  milk 148, 204, 210, 212, 212*t*
  protein from 25*t*, 147-148, 147*t*
  in vegetarian diets 151
DASH diet 47-48
daylong events 205-207
dehydration 164-166, 169, 178, 185, 254
desserts 91-92. *See also* recipes, snacks and desserts

diabetes, adult-onset 7, 51-52, 115

diarrhea
from caffeine 185
carbohydrate loading and 129, 131
in celiac disease 128
combating 234, 236
dehydration from 169
in endurance exercise 187
fruits and fiber and 127, 129
from preexercise foods 183
probiotics and 236

dietary reference intakes (DRIs) 224-225

diets. *See also* sports diets
cancer and 48-51
DASH diet 47-48
gluten-free 104-105, 128, 364, 373
high-protein, low-carbohydrate 329-330
ketogenic 125-126, 189, 327
low-carbohydrate 327
low-FODMAP 104, 186-187
low glycemic-index 327
Paleo 327
vegan 17, 18*t*, 153, 226, 232
vegetarian 140-142, 150-154, 152*t*, 156

digestion 190*f*
of carbohydrates 112-113, 116-117, 186
during exercise 185, 203
of FODMAPS 186-187
of milk 21-22, 55, 148, 186, 226
of preexercise meals 63, 190-192, 190*f*, 233, 306
probiotics and 55
of protein 140, 148, 150, 159

dinners 85-97
meatless 89
planning and shopping for 86-88, 88*t*, 89
at restaurants 90-92
size of 85-86, 88*t*
team 97

DRIs (dietary reference intakes) 224-225

E

eating disorders 335-356. *See also* amenorrhea
anorexia 148, 336-337
balancing food and exercise in 345-347
binge eating disorder 339
bulimia 338, 349-352
exercise addicts 347-349
food obsessions 340-342
how to help 353-355, 356
hunger and 342-345
normal eating versus 351
personality traits in 336, 350*t*
preventing 335, 355
Relative Energy Deficiency in Sports 239-240, 256

eating slowly 321-322

echinacea 235

electrolytes
in recovery 213-215, 214*t*, 215*t*
requirements 163-165, 163*f*, 164*t*

endurance exercise
fueling guidelines for 126-132, 135*t*-136*t*, 130*t*
gastrointestinal distress in 187
glycemic index and 118
hyponatremia in 170-171, 170*t*
iron in 156
protein in 142, 143*t*
supplements for 233-234
ultra-endurance athletes 257-259

energy bars 102-105, 103*t*

energy drinks 174-175, 198*t*

ergogenic aids 233-234

exercise addicts 347-349

F

fast foods 94-97, 94*t*, 96*t*

fasting, intermittent 327-328

fats, dietary
as fuel 27, 129, 188-189
healthy choices 27-28, 94*t*
for injured athletes 267
in ketogenic diets 125-126
for older athletes 269

fats, dietary *(continued)*
   saturated 19, 20-21, 27, 39-40, 41, 149
   storage of 121-122, 330
female athletes 239-252
   in aesthetic sports 256
   amenorrhea in 53, 54-56, 154
   body fat in 276*t*
   caffeine and 76
   calcium and 21*t*, 53-54
   GI problems in 184
   iron and zinc for 154-157, 155*t*
   menopause 250-252
   nutrition for families of 247-248
   protein for 143*t*
   RED-S in 239-240, 256
female athlete triad 239-240, 256
ferritin 156-157
fiber 56-58
   benefits from 49-50, 56, 58, 315
   in foods 59*t*, 67-69, 68*t*, 104
   GI complaints and 185
   for older athletes 269
   types of 56-58
fish 25*t*, 26, 28, 40-41, 419-420. *See also* recipes, fish and seafood
fish oils 42, 267
fluid intake 161-180. *See also* dehydration
   after exercise 169, 211-212
   at altitude 263-264
   best choices for 172-177, 175*t*
   in carbohydrate loading 131
   coffee in 77
   commercial sports fluids 236-237
   electrolytes in 163-165, 163*f*, 164*t*
   in endurance events 258-259
   in exercise 166-169, 188, 201-202, 202*t*, 204
   hyponatremia 170-171, 170*t*
   muscle cramps and 164, 208
   for older athletes 269-270
   performance and 165-166
   in sports 254, 255
   sweating and 161-163, 164
   in weight loss 333-334
   in winter 260
FODMAPs 104, 186-187
folate/folic acid
   in foods 11*t*, 68*t*, 69, 120
   pregnancy and 8, 244-247, 246*f*
   recommended amount 225*t*
food content tables
   caffeine 197*t*-198*t*
   carbohydrates 135*t*-136*t*
   fiber 59*t*
   iron and zinc 155*t*
   potassium 214*t*
   protein 144*t*-145*t*
   sodium 45*t*, 215*t*
   vitamin D 228*t*
   vitamins and minerals 222*t*
food plans 4-6, 32-34, 33*t*
free radicals 48-49, 221
fruits
   cancer and 48
   dried 14-15
   increasing intake of 30, 57, 93, 93*t*
   pesticides residues on 29-31
   recommendations 12-14, 13*t*, 15*t*, 16*t*
   sugars in 112-113

G

gas station nutrition 92-94, 93*t*
gastric bypass athletes 270-272
gastrointestinal problems
   celiac disease and 128, 185-186
   dietary changes and 127
   FODMAPs and 186-187
   foods in 184-186
   gluten and 186
   preexercise meals and 193
   sodium bicarbonate in 234
   tips on 188
   training the gut 187
gelatin 236
GI (glycemic index) 117-119, 119*t*, 120
glucosamine 236
glucose 112-113
glutamine 235

gluten free diets 104-105, 128
    recipes specifically for 364-365,
      373, 450, 451
glycemic index (GI) 117-119, 119*t*, 120
glycemic load 119*t*
glycogen
    depletion 131-133, 133*f*
    stored in liver 132
    stored in muscles 113, 121-125,
      121*t*, 122*t*, 123*t*, 124*f*
    in training 126
grains 6-9, 25*t*, 93*t*, 120
greenhouse gas emissions 17, 30
green tea 175-176

H
heart health 36-43
    DASH diet 47-48
    dietary choices and 7, 37-43, 37*t*
    lifestyle choices 36-37, 37*t*
    potassium and 47-48
    salt intake and 44-46, 45*t*
    supplements and 43
herbs 267
high blood pressure 43-48, 45*t*
high-fructose corn syrup (HFCS) 112
high-protein, low-carbohydrate diets
    329-330
HIV/AIDS 148, 235
HMB (beta-hydroxy beta-methylbutyr-
    ate) 231-232
hormones 19, 54, 185, 232-233
hot flashes 252
Hotshot 209
hunger 342-345, 344*t*
hypertension. *See* high blood pressure
hypoglycemia 120-121
hyponatremia 170-171, 170*t*

I
ice cube craving 154
ice hockey 122
immunity boosters 234-236
indoor athletes 226-228
inflammation
    anti-inflammatory compounds 28,
      151, 267-269, 363

    diet to reduce 234
    gluten and 128
    from hard workouts 159
injured athletes 264-267
insoluble fiber 56
insulin 120, 210
intermittent fasting 327-328
iron
    altitude and 264
    blood levels of 156-157
    coffee and 74
    requirements for 154-157, 155*t*
    sources of 26, 68*t*, 69, 155*t*, 156,
      229
    in vegan diets 153
irritable bowel syndrome 186

K
kale 11, 11*t*
ketogenic diet 125-126, 189, 259, 327

L
lactose 112, 186, 226
lead 148
leucine 140-141, 231-232
locally grown foods 30
low-carbohydrate diets 327
low glycemic-index diet 327
lunches 79-85. *See also* snacks
    for dieters 81
    second lunches 79, 86, 99
    super salads 81-85, 84*t*
    timing of 79-80
    while traveling 80-81, 92-97, 94*t*,
      96*t*

M
magnesium 164*t*, 170*t*, 209
male athletes
    exercise and appetite in 331
    iron and zinc for 154
    protein for 143*t*
    RED-S in 256
maltodextrins 113
meatless meals 89
menopause 250-252
mercury, in fish 41

microbiome 4

milk. *See* dairy products

mindfulness, in eating 315

minerals
  food sources of 221-223, 222*t*
  functions of 220
  for injured athletes 267
  recommended intake of 224-225
  in supplements 221-222, 223-224

monosaccharides 112

monounsaturated fats 27, 39

mouth swishing 202*t*, 204

muscle cramps 164, 207-210

muscle dysmorphia 282*f*, 283

muscles
  creatine and 231, 307
  glycogen storage in 121-125, 121*t*,
    122*t*, 123*t*, 124*f*
  in injured athletes 266
  protein and 140
  supplements for 230-233, 307
  timing for 306-307

mushrooms, UV-treated 228

N

nitrates, dietary 233-234

nonexercise activity thermogenesis
  (NEAT) 296-297

Nutrition Facts labels 70*f*, 134-137

nuts 25*t*, 26, 28, 38, 81, 84*t*

O

oatmeal 8, 37, 361, 372-373

obesity 51-52, 248-250, 313, 332

older athletes
  GI problems in 184
  nutrition for 226, 267-270
  protein for 142, 143*t*, 158
  thirst mechanism in 152

olive oil 19, 27-28, 39-40, 48

omega-3 fatty acids 28, 38, 40, 42,
  267

orange juice 172

organic foods 29-31

osteoporosis 53, 76-77, 128, 239

overtraining 134, 216-217

P

PAD (peripheral artery disease) 233-234

Paleo diet 148, 327

pasta 89, 375-376. *See also* recipes,
  dinner starches

peanut butter 38-39, 81

peripheral artery disease (PAD) 233-
  234

pesticide residues 29-31

phytochemicals 16, 108

polyunsaturated fats 27, 39

pork 429. *See also* recipes, beef and
  pork

potassium
  in foods 12, 13*t*, 14, 15*t*, 83
  increasing intake of 47-48
  lost in sweat 164*t*, 170*t*
  in milk 20, 212*t*
  muscle cramps and 209
  in recovery 213-214, 214*t*

preexercise fuel
  for burning fat 188-189
  caffeine 197, 199
  carbohydrates 195*t*
  functions of 183
  intestinal distress factors in 183-187
  for multiple events 189-192
  sugar crashes 196-197
  training the gut 187
  before a workout 188, 192-196,
    192*t*, 197*t*-198*t*

pregnancy
  caffeine in 76
  fish in 41
  nutrition and 244-247, 244*t*, 246*f*
  supplements for 226
  weight gain in 147, 243, 246*f*

premenstrual snack attack 107

preseason training 254

probiotics 235-236

protein 139-160
  amenorrhea and 241-242
  amino acids in 140-141
  bone health and 54
  convenient sources of 93*t*, 103,
    105, 146, 150, 168

estimating intake 144-146, 144*t*-145*t*, 146*t*

excessive amounts of 148-149

in foods 9, 24-27, 25*t*, 144*t*-145*t*, 150

for injured athletes 266-267

in ketogenic diets 126

muscle building and 140-141, 297

for older athletes 268-269

postexercise 140, 141

powders, shakes, and bars 147-148, 147*t*

in power sports 255

in recovery 210-211

requirements for 23-24, 141-143, 143*t*, 158*t*

sample diet 145, 146*t*

timing of 128-129, 139-141, 143, 145, 157-159, 158*t*

in vegetarian diets 150-153, 152*t*

in weight loss 316

R

rebound hypoglycemia 196-197

recipes, beans and tofu 437-451

Buddha bowl ideas 441

chick pea, curry, and peanut butter soup 448

chocolate cake batter dessert hummus GF 451

cookie dough hummus snack GF 450

kale and cannellini bean soup 447

pasta and white bean soup with sun-dried tomatoes 446

pumpkin chili 442-443

quick and easy bean ideas 439

sweet-n-sour tofu bites 440

tofu burritos 449

turkey chili with quinoa and beans 444-445

recipes, beef and pork 429-435

burger that's better for you 433

Boston baked beans and rice 432

enchilada casserole 431

honey-glazed pork chops 434

meatballs by the gallon 430

stir-fried pork with fruit 435

recipes, beverages and smoothies 453-462

banana-date smoothie 458

beet-cherry smoothie 460

homemade sports drink 454

hot cocoa 462

maple sports drink 455

PB & J smoothie 459

smoothie suggestions 456, 457*t*

thick and frosty milk shake 461

recipes, breakfast

athlete's omelet 368

banana bread 362

bread baking tips 359-360

breakfast fruit salad 369

carrot raisin muffins 366

date nut bread 363

fluffy oatmeal pancakes 372

high-protein oatmeal pancakes GF 373

honey nut granola 370

marmalade yogurt 369

molasses muffins with flax and dates 367

oatmeal suggestions 361

peanut butter and dark chocolate chip muffins GF 364-365

protein-packed scrambled eggs 371

recipes, chicken and turkey 403-417

chicken, kale, and black bean quesadillas 413

chicken and white beans 412

chicken black bean soup 411

chicken salad with almonds and mandarin oranges 410

chicken with pasta and spinach 408

green chili chicken enchilada casserole 409

oven-fried chicken 406

quick and easy chicken ideas 405

sauteed chicken with mushrooms and onions 407

savory African peanut stew 414-415

turkey cran-apple wrap 416

turkey meatballs with tangy cranberry sauce 417

recipes, dinner starches 375-392
  angel hair Alfredo 380
  avocado potato salad 390
  cauliflower macaroni and cheese 384
  extra-creamy potatoes and cheese 388-389
  gourmet vegetarian lasagna 382-383
  oven french fries 387
  pasta cooking tips 375-376
  pasta with mushrooms and aspara-gus 385
  potato cooking tips 377-378
  quick and easy pasta toppings 379
  quick and easy potato toppings 386
  quick and easy rice or quinoa ideas 391
  rice cooking tips 376-377
  skillet lasagna 381
  Southwestern rice and bean salad 392
recipes, fish and seafood 419-427
  broiled salmon with mustard-maple glaze 421
  fish and spinach bake 423
  fish in foil, Mexican style 427
  shrimp and shells 424
  shrimp marinara 426
  simple salmon patties 422
  tuna pasta salad 425
recipes, snacks and desserts 463-477
  apple crisp 472
  banana ice cream 473
  carrot cake 476-477
  chia seed pudding 469
  chocolate lush 475
  healthy heart oatmeal raisin cookies with chocolate chips 474
  quick and easy nut butter snacks 464
  strawberry chia pudding 471
  sugar and spice trail mix 468
  super-seedy granola bars 466-467
  sweet and crispy almond bars 465
  vanilla chia pudding 470

recipes, vegetable and salads 393-402
  baked beets 401
  grilled vegetables 398
  honey-glazed sweet potatoes 402
  microwaved vegetables 397
  roasted vegetables 396
  spinach salad with Asian dressing 400
  spinach salad with sweet and spicy dressing 399
  steamed vegetables 394
  stir-fried vegetables 395
recovery 210-217
  carbohydrate plus protein in 210-211, 212-213
  from daily training 132-134, 133*f*
  electrolytes in 213-215, 214*t*, 215*t*
  fluids in 211-212
  foods in 212-213, 215-216
  overtraining 216-217
registered dietitians (RDs) 228, 311-312
Relative Energy Deficiency in Sports (RED-S) 239-240, 256
resistance training 140, 143*t*, 159, 230-233
restaurant meals 90-92, 93, 93*t*
rest days 258, 272
resting metabolic rate (RMR) 317-317, 317*t*
riboflavin 20, 153, 225*t*

S
salads 81-85, 84*t*, 96*t*. *See also* reci-pes, vegetable and salads
salt 44-45. *See also* sodium
selenium 49
self-esteem 284-286
sit-ups 279
skinfold calipers 290-291
sleep 251, 325
"sloshing" 162, 167, 171
smoothie recipes 456-460. *See also* recipes, beverages and smoothies
snacks 99-109. *See also* recipes, snacks and desserts
  energy bars 102-105, 103*t*
  fast snacks 100-102

healthy choices 92-93, 93t, 99
snack attacks 106-109
sodium
  bone health and 54
  dehydration and 164-165, 166-167
  in foods 45-46, 45t, 168, 212t, 215t
  hypertension 44
  hyponatremia 170-171, 170t
  lost in sweat 164t, 170t
  muscle cramps and 164, 208
  recommended intake of 44-45
  in recovery 213-215, 215t
  in sports drinks 168, 212t
sodium bicarbonate 234
soft drinks 172-173
soluble fiber 57-58
sorbitol 186
soy foods 151-153, 252
sports diets
  for altitude 263-264
  examples 33-34
  for extreme-sports athletes 257-259
  for gastric bypass athletes 270-272
  for injured athletes 264-267
  for older athletes 267-270
  for power sports 255
  for sports that emphasize leanness 255-257
  for team sports 253-254
  for winter athletes 260-263, 262t
sports drinks
  energy drinks 174-175, 198t
  evaluating 168-169, 174-175, 175t, 176t
  recipes for 454-455
  timing of 167, 171, 212, 212t
sports gels 236-237
stomach. See also gastrointestinal problems
  coffee and 74-75, 197
  ketogenic diet and 126
  preexercise fuel and 183-186, 192-193, 196, 331
  "sloshing" 162, 167, 171
  in winter exercise 261
stress fractures 54, 128, 154, 239-240, 242, 345

sugars
  benefits of 28, 32-33, 114-115
  diabetes and 52
  during exercise 202-203
  highs and lows from 120-121, 196-197
  sources of 69-70, 70f, 172-173, 186
  types of 112-113
sugar sensitivity 120
supplements
  calcium 20
  chondroitin and glucosamine 236
  debate on 223-224, 226, 228-229
  endurance enhancers 233-234
  fish oil 42
  glutamine 235
  hormones 232-233, 252
  iron 157
  leucine 231-232
  muscle builders 230-233
  performance-enhancing 229-230
  protein 147-148, 147t
  regulation of 223, 230
  vitamin D 227
  weight-gain 305
sweating 161-164, 164t, 167, 260

T
tapering 127-128
team sports 97, 253-254
teenage athletes 142, 143t, 156
thermogenesis 261
thirst mechanism 161-163, 167, 260
timing of nutrients 157-159. See also preexercise fuel; recovery
  of carbohydrates 195t
  for endurance events 257-259
  for extensive exercise 201-205, 202t
  at midworkout 204-205
  for multiple events 189-192, 205-207
  of protein 139-140, 143, 145, 157-159, 158t
  in recovery 211
  in team sports 255
  in weight loss 319-320, 321, 331

tofu 26, 151, 437-438. *See also* recipes, beans and tofu
tournaments 205-207
travel food 92-97, 93*t*, 94*t*, 96*t*

U
ultradistance athletes 257-259
urine 164, 188, 208, 271

V
vegan diets 17, 18*t*, 153, 226, 232
vegetable oils 39
vegetables 9-12. *See also* recipes, vegetables and salads
    cancer and 48
    intake of 10-12, 11*t*, 23-24, 57
    nutrients in 9, 13*t*, 15*t*, 23, 25*t*
    pesticide residues on 29-31
    in restaurants 91, 93, 93*t*
    sugars in 112-113
vegetarian diets 140-142, 150-154, 152*t*, 156
vitamin A 13*t*, 14, 15*t*, 225*t*
vitamin B₆ 225*t*
vitamin B₁₂ 153, 225*t*
vitamin C
    benefits from 49, 223, 235, 236
    in foods 10-12, 13*t*, 15*t*, 82
    recommended amount 221, 225*t*
vitamin D 16, 20, 23, 227, 228*t*
vitamin E 49, 50*t*, 225*t*, 235
vitamin K 225*t*
vitamins
    functions of 220-221
    for injured athletes 267
    for older athletes 269
    recommended intake of 224-225
    in recovery 215-216
    sources of 168, 222-223, 222*t*
    supplement debate 221-224

W
water 173-174. *See also* fluid intake
weight gain 295-310
    creatine in 307
    diet balancing in 307-309, 308*t*
    from dieting 313-314
    extra calories in 299-305, 303*t*, 304*t*
    factors in 296-297, 309-310
    protein in 297-299
    timing 306-307
    weightlifting by teenagers 295
weight loss 311-332
    for athletes with weight limits 332-334, 334*t*
    avoiding weight gain 313-314
    behaviors in 314-316, 321-326, 325
    calories in 252, 316-320, 319*t*
    "dieting" in 312-313, 326-328
    eating plans in 324-325
    facts and fallacies on 329-332
    food records in 321
weight management. *See also* weight gain; weight loss
    at altitude 264
    body dysmorphic disorder 282-284
    breakfast and 71
    fats and carbohydrates in 6-7
    for gastric bypass athletes 271
    gender differences in 276*t*, 279-280, 287
    health and 38, 287, 313
    for injured athletes 264-267
    in menopause 250-252
    numbers game in 252, 286-287
    off-season 254
    sleep and 251
    in sports that emphasize leanness 255-257
whey protein 147-148
winter athletes 260-263, 262*t*
women. *See* female athletes

Y
yogurt 23, 55, 151

Z
zinc
    in food 24, 26, 41, 155*t*
    recommended intake 157, 225*t*
    in vegan diets 153

ABOUT THE AUTHOR

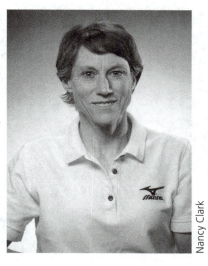

Nancy Clark

Nancy Clark, MS, RD, CSSD, is an internationally respected and trusted sports nutritionist specializing in nutrition for performance, wellness, and weight management, including helping athletes with eating disorders. At her private practice in the Boston area (Newton, Massachusetts), she counsels active people of all ages and athletic abilities—from high school athletes to Olympians—by giving one-on-one, personalized advice.

In the 40 years in which she has specialized in sports dietetics, Clark has helped thousands of casual and competitive athletes. Her more renowned clients have included members of the Boston Red Sox, Bruins, and Celtics, as well as athletes from many colleges in the area, including Boston College, Tufts University, and Brandeis University.

Clark enjoys speaking to teams, clubs, and health professionals, as well as writing as a way to teach people how to eat to win. Her best-selling book, *Nancy Clark's Sports Nutrition Guidebook,* has sold over 650,000 copies and is now in its sixth edition. Her other books include food guides for soccer players, new runners, marathoners, and cyclists. She also writes a monthly nutrition column called "The Athlete's Kitchen," which appears regularly in over 100 sports publications and websites. Her nutrition advice and photo have even graced the back of the Wheaties box!

Clark received her undergraduate degree in nutrition from Simmons University in Boston and was honored with the Simmons Distinguished Alumna Award in 2007. Her dietetic internship was at Massachusetts General Hospital. She received her graduate degree in nutrition, with a focus on exercise physiology, from Boston University. She is a fellow of both the Academy of Nutrition and Dietetics and the American College of Sports Medicine (ACSM), and she has been a member of ACSM's board of trustees. In 2015, she received the Nutrition Science Media Award from the American Society for Nutrition.

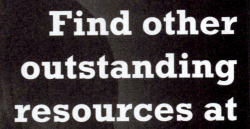